THE OFFICIAL PARENT'S SOURCEBOOK
on

CHILDHOOD ACUTE LYMPHOBLASTIC LEUKEMIA

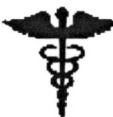

JAMES N. PARKER, M.D.
AND PHILIP M. PARKER, PH.D., EDITORS

ICON Health Publications
ICON Group International, Inc.
4370 La Jolla Village Drive, 4th Floor
San Diego, CA 92122 USA

Copyright ©2002 by ICON Group International, Inc.

Copyright ©2002 by ICON Group International, Inc. All rights reserved. This book is protected by copyright. No part of it may be reproduced, stored in a retrieval system, or transmitted in any form or by any means, electronic, mechanical, photocopying, recording or otherwise, without written permission from the publisher.

Printed in the United States of America.

Last digit indicates print number: 10 9 8 7 6 4 5 3 2 1

Publisher, Health Care: Tiffany LaRochelle
Editor(s): James Parker, M.D., Philip Parker, Ph.D.

Publisher's note: The ideas, procedures, and suggestions contained in this book are not intended as a substitute for consultation with your child's physician. All matters regarding your child's health require medical supervision. As new medical or scientific information becomes available from academic and clinical research, recommended treatments and drug therapies may undergo changes. The authors, editors, and publisher have attempted to make the information in this book up to date and accurate in accord with accepted standards at the time of publication. The authors, editors, and publisher are not responsible for errors or omissions or for consequences from application of the book, and make no warranty, expressed or implied, in regard to the contents of this book. Any practice described in this book should be applied by the reader in accordance with professional standards of care used in regard to the unique circumstances that may apply in each situation, in close consultation with a qualified physician. The reader is advised to always check product information (package inserts) for changes and new information regarding dose and contraindications before administering any drug or pharmacological product. Caution is especially urged when using new or infrequently ordered drugs, herbal remedies, vitamins and supplements, alternative therapies, complementary therapies and medicines, and integrative medical treatments.

Cataloging-in-Publication Data

Parker, James N., 1961-
Parker, Philip M., 1960-

    The Official Parent's Sourcebook on Childhood Acute Lymphoblastic Leukemia: A Revised and Updated Directory for the Internet Age/James N. Parker and Philip M. Parker, editors
        p.   cm.
    Includes bibliographical references, glossary and index.
    ISBN: 0-597-83345-1
    1. Childhood Acute Lymphoblastic Leukemia-Popular works.   I. Title.

Disclaimer

This publication is not intended to be used for the diagnosis or treatment of a health problem or as a substitute for consultation with licensed medical professionals. It is sold with the understanding that the publisher, editors, and authors are not engaging in the rendering of medical, psychological, financial, legal, or other professional services.

References to any entity, product, service, or source of information that may be contained in this publication should not be considered an endorsement, either direct or implied, by the publisher, editors, or authors. ICON Group International, Inc., the editors, or the authors are not responsible for the content of any Web pages nor publications referenced in this publication.

Copyright Notice

If a physician wishes to copy limited passages from this sourcebook for parent use, this right is automatically granted without written permission from ICON Group International, Inc. (ICON Group). However, all of ICON Group publications are copyrighted. With exception to the above, copying our publications in whole or in part, for whatever reason, is a violation of copyright laws and can lead to penalties and fines. Should you want to copy tables, graphs or other materials, please contact us to request permission (e-mail: iconedit@san.rr.com). ICON Group often grants permission for very limited reproduction of our publications for internal use, press releases, and academic research. Such reproduction requires confirmed permission from ICON Group International Inc. **The disclaimer above must accompany all reproductions, in whole or in part, of this sourcebook.**

Dedication

To the healthcare professionals dedicating their time and efforts to the study of childhood acute lymphoblastic leukemia.

Acknowledgements

The collective knowledge generated from academic and applied research summarized in various references has been critical in the creation of this sourcebook which is best viewed as a comprehensive compilation and collection of information prepared by various official agencies which directly or indirectly are dedicated to childhood acute lymphoblastic leukemia. All of the *Official Parent's Sourcebooks* draw from various agencies and institutions associated with the United States Department of Health and Human Services, and in particular, the Office of the Secretary of Health and Human Services (OS), the Administration for Children and Families (ACF), the Administration on Aging (AOA), the Agency for Healthcare Research and Quality (AHRQ), the Agency for Toxic Substances and Disease Registry (ATSDR), the Centers for Disease Control and Prevention (CDC), the Food and Drug Administration (FDA), the Healthcare Financing Administration (HCFA), the Health Resources and Services Administration (HRSA), the Indian Health Service (IHS), the institutions of the National Institutes of Health (NIH), the Program Support Center (PSC), and the Substance Abuse and Mental Health Services Administration (SAMHSA). In addition to these sources, information gathered from the National Library of Medicine, the United States Patent Office, the European Union, and their related organizations has been invaluable in the creation of this sourcebook. Some of the work represented was financially supported by the Research and Development Committee at INSEAD. This support is gratefully acknowledged. Finally, special thanks are owed to Tiffany LaRochelle for her excellent editorial support.

About the Editors

James N. Parker, M.D.

Dr. James N. Parker received his Bachelor of Science degree in Psychobiology from the University of California, Riverside and his M.D. from the University of California, San Diego. In addition to authoring numerous research publications, he has lectured at various academic institutions. Dr. Parker is the medical editor for the *Official Parent's Sourcebook* series published by ICON Health Publications.

Philip M. Parker, Ph.D.

Philip M. Parker is the Eli Lilly Chair Professor of Innovation, Business and Society at INSEAD (Fontainebleau, France and Singapore). Dr. Parker has also been Professor at the University of California, San Diego and has taught courses at Harvard University, the Hong Kong University of Science and Technology, the Massachusetts Institute of Technology, Stanford University, and UCLA. Dr. Parker is the associate editor for the *Official Parent's Sourcebook* series published by ICON Health Publications.

About ICON Health Publications

In addition to childhood acute lymphoblastic leukemia, *Official Parent's Sourcebooks* are available for the following related topics:

- The Official Patient's Sourcebook on Childhood Acute Myeloid Leukemia - Other Myeloid Malignancies
- The Official Patient's Sourcebook on Childhood Hodgkin's Disease
- The Official Patient's Sourcebook on Childhood Liver Cancer
- The Official Patient's Sourcebook on Childhood Non-hodgkin's Lymphoma
- The Official Patient's Sourcebook on Childhood Rhabdomyosarcoma
- The Official Patient's Sourcebook on Childhood Soft Tissue Sarcoma
- The Official Patient's Sourcebook on Neuroblastoma
- The Official Patient's Sourcebook on Retinoblastoma
- The Official Patient's Sourcebook on Unusual Childhood Cancers
- The Official Patient's Sourcebook on Wilm's Tumor and Other Childhood Kidney Tumors

To discover more about ICON Health Publications, simply check with your preferred online booksellers, including Barnes & Noble.com and Amazon.com which currently carry all of our titles. Or, feel free to contact us directly for bulk purchases or institutional discounts:

ICON Group International, Inc.
4370 La Jolla Village Drive, Fourth Floor
San Diego, CA 92122 USA
Fax: 858-546-4341
Web site: **www.icongrouponline.com/health**

Table of Contents

INTRODUCTION...1
   Overview..1
   Organization...3
   Scope...3
   Moving Forward...4

PART I: THE ESSENTIALS...7

CHAPTER 1. THE ESSENTIALS ON CHILDHOOD ACUTE LYMPHOBLASTIC LEUKEMIA: GUIDELINES...9
   Overview..9
   What Is Childhood Acute Lymphoblastic Leukemia?.........................11
   Stage Information...13
   Treatment Option Overview..13
   Treatment by Stage..15
   To Learn More..16
   About PDQ...17
   More Guideline Sources..19
   Vocabulary Builder..25

CHAPTER 2. SEEKING GUIDANCE..29
   Overview..29
   Cancer Support Groups...31
   The Cancer Information Service..33
   Finding Cancer Resources in Your Community..................................35
   Finding Doctors Who Specialize in Cancer Care...............................39
   Selecting Your Child's Doctor..41
   Working with Your Child's Doctor..42
   Getting a Second Opinion...43
   Finding a Cancer Treatment Facility..44
   Questions and Answers about Children's Cancer Centers..............45
   Additional Cancer Support Information..48
   Vocabulary Builder..48

CHAPTER 3. CLINICAL TRIALS AND CHILDHOOD ACUTE LYMPHOBLASTIC LEUKEMIA...51
   Overview..51
   Recent Trials on Childhood Acute Lymphoblastic Leukemia...........54
   Benefits and Risks..73
   Clinical Trials and Insurance Coverage..75
   Increasing the Likelihood of Insurance Coverage for Trials............78
   If Your Insurance Claim Is Denied after the Trial Has Begun.........80
   Government Initiatives to Expand Insurance Coverage for Trials...83
   Keeping Current on Clinical Trials...84

General References 85
Vocabulary Builder 86

PART II: ADDITIONAL RESOURCES AND ADVANCED MATERIAL 89

CHAPTER 4. STUDIES ON CHILDHOOD ACUTE LYMPHOBLASTIC LEUKEMIA 91
Overview 91
The Combined Health Information Database 91
Federally-Funded Research on Childhood Acute Lymphoblastic Leukemia 93
E-Journals: PubMed Central 103
The National Library of Medicine: PubMed 105
Vocabulary Builder 125

CHAPTER 5. BOOKS ON CHILDHOOD ACUTE LYMPHOBLASTIC LEUKEMIA 131
Overview 131
The National Library of Medicine Book Index 131
Chapters on Childhood Acute Lymphoblastic Leukemia 134
General Home References 135
Vocabulary Builder 137

CHAPTER 6. MULTIMEDIA ON CHILDHOOD ACUTE LYMPHOBLASTIC LEUKEMIA 139
Overview 139
Bibliography: Multimedia on Childhood Acute Lymphoblastic Leukemia 140
Vocabulary Builder 142

CHAPTER 7. PHYSICIAN GUIDELINES AND DATABASES 143
Overview 143
NIH Guidelines 143
What Is Childhood Acute Lymphoblastic Leukemia? 144
Risk Factors 145
Prognosis 146
Cellular Classification 148
Clinical and Laboratory Features at Diagnosis 149
Molecular and Biological Characteristics of Leukemia Cells at Diagnosis 152
Chromosome Number 155
Recurring Chromosomal Translocations 156
Treatment Option Overview 162
Treatment Options for Untreated Childhood ALL 165
Treatment Options for Childhood ALL in Remission 172
Role of Bone Marrow Transplant for Philadelphia Chromosome-Positive ALL 178
Treatment Options Under Clinical Evaluation 178
Recurrent Childhood Acute Lymphoblastic Leukemia 180

    NIH Databases 184
    Other Commercial Databases 188
    The Genome Project and Childhood Acute Lymphoblastic Leukemia 189
    Specialized References 193
    Vocabulary Builder 195

CHAPTER 8. DISSERTATIONS ON CHILDHOOD ACUTE LYMPHOBLASTIC LEUKEMIA 199
    Overview 199
    Dissertations on Childhood Acute Lymphoblastic Leukemia 199
    Keeping Current 200

PART III. APPENDICES 201

APPENDIX A. RESEARCHING YOUR CHILD'S MEDICATIONS 203
    Overview 203
    Your Child's Medications: The Basics 204
    Learning More about Your Child's Medications 205
    Commercial Databases 207
    Drug Development and Approval 208
    Understanding the Approval Process for New Cancer Drugs 209
    The Role of the Federal Drug Administration (FDA) 210
    Getting Drugs to Patients Who Need Them 213
    Contraindications and Interactions (Hidden Dangers) 215
    A Final Warning 216
    General References 217
    Vocabulary Builder 218

APPENDIX B. RESEARCHING ALTERNATIVE MEDICINE 219
    Overview 219
    What Is CAM? 220
    What Are the Domains of Alternative Medicine? 221
    Finding CAM References on Childhood Acute Lymphoblastic Leukemia 226
    Additional Web Resources 237
    General References 238

APPENDIX C. FINDING MEDICAL LIBRARIES 241
    Overview 241
    Preparation 241
    Finding a Local Medical Library 242
    Medical Libraries Open to the Public 242

APPENDIX D. YOUR CHILD'S RIGHTS AND INSURANCE 249
    Overview 249
    Your Child's Rights as a Patient 249
    Parent Responsibilities 253
    Choosing an Insurance Plan 254
    Medicaid 256

Financial Assistance for Cancer Care 257
NORD's Medication Assistance Programs 259
Additional Resources 260
Vocabulary Builder 260
APPENDIX E. TALKING WITH YOUR CHILD ABOUT CANCER 263
Overview 263
Why Should I Tell My Child? 264
Parent's Questions 264
What Should My Child Be Told? 265
Questions Children May Ask 267
Talking to Your Child with Late-Stage Cancer 268
Vocabulary Builder 269

ONLINE GLOSSARIES 271
Online Dictionary Directories 277

CHILDHOOD ACUTE LYMPHOBLASTIC LEUKEMIA GLOSSARY 279
General Dictionaries and Glossaries 292

INDEX 294

INTRODUCTION

Overview

Dr. C. Everett Koop, former U.S. Surgeon General, once said, "The best prescription is knowledge."[1] The Agency for Healthcare Research and Quality (AHRQ) of the National Institutes of Health (NIH) echoes this view and recommends that all parents incorporate education into the treatment process. According to the AHRQ:

> Finding out more about your [child's] condition is a good place to start. By contacting groups that support your [child's] condition, visiting your local library, and searching on the Internet, you can find good information to help guide your decisions for your [child's] treatment. Some information may be hard to find — especially if you don't know where to look.[2]

As the AHRQ mentions, finding the right information is not an obvious task. Though many physicians and public officials had thought that the emergence of the Internet would do much to assist parents in obtaining reliable information, in March 2001 the National Institutes of Health issued the following warning:

> The number of Web sites offering health-related resources grows every day. Many sites provide valuable information, while others may have information that is unreliable or misleading.[3]

---

[1] Quotation from http://www.drkoop.com.
[2] The Agency for Healthcare Research and Quality (AHRQ): http://www.ahcpr.gov/consumer/diaginfo.htm.
[3] Adapted from the NIH, National Cancer Institute (NCI): http://cancertrials.nci.nih.gov/beyond/evaluating.html.

Since the late 1990s, physicians have seen a general increase in parent Internet usage rates. Parents frequently enter their children's doctor's offices with printed Web pages of home remedies in the guise of latest medical research. This scenario is so common that doctors often spend more time dispelling misleading information than guiding children through sound therapies. *The Official Parent's Sourcebook on Childhood Acute Lymphoblastic Leukemia* has been created for parents who have decided to make education and research an integral part of the treatment process. The pages that follow will tell you where and how to look for information covering virtually all topics related to childhood acute lymphoblastic leukemia, from the essentials to the most advanced areas of research.

The title of this book includes the word "official." This reflects the fact that the sourcebook draws from public, academic, government, and peer-reviewed research. Selected readings from various agencies are reproduced to give you some of the latest official information available to date on childhood acute lymphoblastic leukemia.

Given parents' increasing sophistication in using the Internet, abundant references to reliable Internet-based resources are provided throughout this sourcebook. Where possible, guidance is provided on how to obtain free-of-charge, primary research results as well as more detailed information via the Internet. E-book and electronic versions of this sourcebook are fully interactive with each of the Internet sites mentioned (clicking on a hyperlink automatically opens your browser to the site indicated). Hard copy users of this sourcebook can type cited Web addresses directly into their browsers to obtain access to the corresponding sites. Since we are working with ICON Health Publications, hard copy *Sourcebooks* are frequently updated and printed on demand to ensure that the information provided is current.

In addition to extensive references accessible via the Internet, every chapter presents a "Vocabulary Builder." Many health guides offer glossaries of technical or uncommon terms in an appendix. In editing this sourcebook, we have decided to place a smaller glossary within each chapter that covers terms used in that chapter. Given the technical nature of some chapters, you may need to revisit many sections. Building one's vocabulary of medical terms in such a gradual manner has been shown to improve the learning process.

We must emphasize that no sourcebook on childhood acute lymphoblastic leukemia should affirm that a specific diagnostic procedure or treatment discussed in a research study, patent, or doctoral dissertation is "correct" or your child's best option. This sourcebook is no exception. Each child is unique. Deciding on appropriate options is always up to parents in consultation with their children's physicians and healthcare providers.

Organization

This sourcebook is organized into three parts. Part I explores basic techniques to researching childhood acute lymphoblastic leukemia (e.g. finding guidelines on diagnosis, treatments, and prognosis), followed by a number of topics, including information on how to get in touch with organizations, associations, or other parent networks dedicated to childhood acute lymphoblastic leukemia. It also gives you sources of information that can help you find a doctor in your local area specializing in treating childhood acute lymphoblastic leukemia. Collectively, the material presented in Part I is a complete primer on basic research topics for childhood acute lymphoblastic leukemia.

Part II moves on to advanced research dedicated to childhood acute lymphoblastic leukemia. Part II is intended for those willing to invest many hours of hard work and study. It is here that we direct you to the latest scientific and applied research on childhood acute lymphoblastic leukemia. When possible, contact names, links via the Internet, and summaries are provided. It is in Part II where the vocabulary process becomes important as authors publishing advanced research frequently use highly specialized language. In general, every attempt is made to recommend "free-to-use" options.

Part III provides appendices of useful background reading covering childhood acute lymphoblastic leukemia or related disorders. The appendices are dedicated to more pragmatic issues facing parents. Accessing materials via medical libraries may be the only option for some parents, so a guide is provided for finding local medical libraries which are open to the public. Part III, therefore, focuses on advice that goes beyond the biological and scientific issues facing children with childhood acute lymphoblastic leukemia and their families.

Scope

While this sourcebook covers childhood acute lymphoblastic leukemia, doctors, research publications, and specialists may refer to your child's condition using a variety of terms. Therefore, you should understand that childhood acute lymphoblastic leukemia is often considered a synonym or a condition closely related to the following:

- Acute Childhood Leukemia
- Acute Lymphocytic Leukemia
- Cancer Acute Childhood Leukemia
- Lymphoid Leukemia
- Tumor Adrenal

In addition to synonyms and related conditions, physicians may refer to childhood acute lymphoblastic leukemia using certain coding systems. The International Classification of Diseases, 9th Revision, Clinical Modification (ICD-9-CM) is the most commonly used system of classification for the world's illnesses. Your physician may use this coding system as an administrative or tracking tool. The following classification is commonly used for childhood acute lymphoblastic leukemia:[4]

- 204.0 acute lymphoblastic leukemia
- 204.0 lymphoid leukemia

For the purposes of this sourcebook, we have attempted to be as inclusive as possible, looking for official information for all of the synonyms relevant to childhood acute lymphoblastic leukemia. You may find it useful to refer to synonyms when accessing databases or interacting with healthcare professionals and medical librarians.

Moving Forward

Since the 1980s, the world has seen a proliferation of healthcare guides covering most illnesses. Some are written by parents, patients, or their family members. These generally take a layperson's approach to understanding and coping with an illness or disorder. They can be uplifting, encouraging, and highly supportive. Other guides are authored by physicians or other healthcare providers who have a more clinical outlook. Each of these two styles of guide has its purpose and can be quite useful.

---

[4] This list is based on the official version of the World Health Organization's 9th Revision, International Classification of Diseases (ICD-9). According to the National Technical Information Service, "ICD-9CM extensions, interpretations, modifications, addenda, or errata other than those approved by the U.S. Public Health Service and the Health Care Financing Administration are not to be considered official and should not be utilized. Continuous maintenance of the ICD-9-CM is the responsibility of the federal government."

As editors, we have chosen a third route. We have chosen to expose you to as many sources of official and peer-reviewed information as practical, for the purpose of educating you about basic and advanced knowledge as recognized by medical science today. You can think of this sourcebook as your personal Internet age reference librarian.

Why "Internet age"? When their child has been diagnosed with childhood acute lymphoblastic leukemia, parents will often log on to the Internet, type words into a search engine, and receive several Web site listings which are mostly irrelevant or redundant. Parents are left to wonder where the relevant information is, and how to obtain it. Since only the smallest fraction of information dealing with childhood acute lymphoblastic leukemia is even indexed in search engines, a non-systematic approach often leads to frustration and disappointment. With this sourcebook, we hope to direct you to the information you need that you would not likely find using popular Web directories. Beyond Web listings, in many cases we will reproduce brief summaries or abstracts of available reference materials. These abstracts often contain distilled information on topics of discussion.

While we focus on the more scientific aspects of childhood acute lymphoblastic leukemia, there is, of course, the emotional side to consider. Later in the sourcebook, we provide a chapter dedicated to helping you find parent groups and associations that can provide additional support beyond research produced by medical science. We hope that the choices we have made give you and your child the most options in moving forward. In this way, we wish you the best in your efforts to incorporate this educational approach into your child's treatment plan.

The Editors

PART I: THE ESSENTIALS

ABOUT PART I

Part I has been edited to give you access to what we feel are "the essentials" on childhood acute lymphoblastic leukemia. The essentials typically include a definition or description of the condition, a discussion of who it affects, the signs or symptoms, tests or diagnostic procedures, and treatments for the disease. Your child's doctor or healthcare provider may have already explained the essentials of childhood acute lymphoblastic leukemia to you or even given you a pamphlet or brochure describing the condition. Now you are searching for more in-depth information. As editors, we have decided, nevertheless, to include a discussion on where to find essential information that can complement what the doctor has already told you. In this section we recommend a process, not a particular Web site or reference book. The process ensures that, as you search the Web, you gain background information in such a way as to maximize your understanding.

CHAPTER 1. THE ESSENTIALS ON CHILDHOOD ACUTE LYMPHOBLASTIC LEUKEMIA: GUIDELINES

Overview

Official agencies, as well as federally funded institutions supported by national grants, frequently publish a variety of guidelines on childhood acute lymphoblastic leukemia. These are typically called "Fact Sheets" or "Guidelines." They can take the form of a brochure, information kit, pamphlet, or flyer. Often they are only a few pages in length. The great advantage of guidelines over other sources is that they are often written with the parent in mind. Since new guidelines on childhood acute lymphoblastic leukemia can appear at any moment and be published by a number of sources, the best approach to finding guidelines is to systematically scan the Internet-based services that post them.

The National Institutes of Health (NIH)[5]

The National Institutes of Health (NIH) is the first place to search for relatively current guidelines and fact sheets on childhood acute lymphoblastic leukemia. Originally founded in 1887, the NIH is one of the world's foremost medical research centers and the federal focal point for medical research in the United States. At any given time, the NIH supports some 35,000 research grants at universities, medical schools, and other research and training institutions, both nationally and internationally. The rosters of those who have conducted research or who have received NIH support over the years include the world's most illustrious scientists and

---

[5] Adapted from the NIH: **http://www.nih.gov/about/NIHoverview.html**.

physicians. Among them are 97 scientists who have won the Nobel Prize for achievement in medicine.

There is no guarantee that any one Institute will have a guideline on a specific medical condition, though the National Institutes of Health collectively publish over 600 guidelines for both common and rare disorders. The best way to access NIH guidelines is via the Internet. Although the NIH is organized into many different Institutes and Offices, the following is a list of key Web sites where you are most likely to find NIH clinical guidelines and publications dealing with childhood acute lymphoblastic leukemia and associated conditions:

- Office of the Director (OD); guidelines consolidated across agencies available at **http://www.nih.gov/health/consumer/conkey.htm**

- National Library of Medicine (NLM); extensive encyclopedia (A.D.A.M., Inc.) with guidelines available at **http://www.nlm.nih.gov/medlineplus/healthtopics.html**

- National Cancer Institute (NCI); guidelines available at **http://cancernet.nci.nih.gov/pdq/pdq_treatment.shtml**

Among the above, the National Cancer Institute (NCI) is particularly noteworthy. The NCI coordinates the National Cancer Program, which conducts and supports research, training, health information dissemination, and other programs with respect to the cause, diagnosis, prevention, and treatment of cancer, rehabilitation from cancer, and the continuing care of cancer patients and the families of cancer patients.[6] Specifically, the Institute:

- Supports and coordinates research projects conducted by universities, hospitals, research foundations, and businesses throughout this country and abroad through research grants and cooperative agreements.

- Conducts research in its own laboratories and clinics.

- Supports education and training in fundamental sciences and clinical disciplines for participation in basic and clinical research programs and treatment programs relating to cancer through career awards, training grants, and fellowships.

- Supports research projects in cancer control.

- Supports a national network of cancer centers.

- Collaborates with voluntary organizations and other national and foreign institutions engaged in cancer research and training activities.

---

[6] This paragraph has been adapted from the NCI: **http://www.nci.nih.gov/**. "Adapted" signifies that a passage has been reproduced exactly or slightly edited for this book.

- Encourages and coordinates cancer research by industrial concerns where such concerns evidence a particular capability for programmatic research.

- Collects and disseminates information on cancer.

- Supports construction of laboratories, clinics, and related facilities necessary for cancer research through the award of construction grants.

The NCI, established under the National Cancer Act of 1937, is the Federal Government's principal agency for cancer research and training. The National Cancer Act of 1971 broadened the scope and responsibilities of the NCI and created the National Cancer Program. Over the years, legislative amendments have maintained the NCI authorities and responsibilities and added new information dissemination mandates as well as a requirement to assess the incorporation of state-of-the-art cancer treatments into clinical practice. Information dissemination is made possible through the NCI Online at **www.cancer.gov**. Cancer.gov offers to the public and physicians up-to-date information on the latest cancer research, current and upcoming clinical trials, statistics, research programs, and research funding.

The following guideline was recently published by the NCI on childhood acute lymphoblastic leukemia.

What Is Childhood Acute Lymphoblastic Leukemia?[7]

Childhood acute lymphoblastic leukemia (also called acute lymphocytic leukemia or ALL) is a disease in which too many underdeveloped infection-fighting white blood cells, called lymphocytes, are found in a child's blood and bone marrow. ALL is the most common form of leukemia in children, and the most common kind of childhood cancer.

Lymphocytes are made by the bone marrow and by other organs of the lymph system. The bone marrow is the spongy tissue inside the large bones in the body. The bone marrow makes red blood cells (which carry oxygen and other materials to all tissues of the body), white blood cells (which fight infection), and platelets (which make the blood clot). Normally, the bone marrow makes cells called blasts that develop (mature) into several different types of blood cells that have specific jobs to do in the body.

The lymph system is made up of thin tubes that branch, like blood vessels, into all parts of the body. Lymph vessels carry lymph, a colorless, watery

---

[7] The following guidelines appeared on the NCI website on Aug. 26, 2002. The text was last modified in April 2002. The text has been adapted for this sourcebook.

fluid that contains lymphocytes. Along the network of vessels are groups of small, bean-shaped organs called lymph nodes. Clusters of lymph nodes are found in the underarm, pelvis, neck, and abdomen. The spleen (an organ in the upper abdomen that makes lymphocytes and filters old blood cells from the blood), the thymus (a small organ beneath the breastbone), and the tonsils (an organ in the throat) are also part of the lymph system.

Lymphocytes fight infection by making substances called antibodies, which attack germs and other harmful bacteria in the body. In ALL, the developing lymphocytes become too numerous and do not mature. These immature lymphocytes are then found in the blood and the bone marrow. They also collect in the lymph tissues and make them swell. Lymphocytes may crowd out other blood cells in the blood and bone marrow. If your child's bone marrow cannot make enough red blood cells to carry oxygen, your child may have anemia. If your child's bone marrow cannot make enough platelets to make the blood clot normally, your child may bleed or bruise easily. The cancerous lymphocytes can also invade other organs, the spinal cord, and the brain.

Leukemia can be acute (progressing quickly with many immature cancer cells) or chronic (progressing slowly with more mature-looking leukemia cells). Acute lymphoblastic leukemia progresses quickly, and can occur in both children and adults. Treatment is different for adults than it is for children.

Early signs of ALL may be similar to those of the flu or other common diseases, such as a fever that won't go away, feeling weak or tired all the time, aching bones or joints, or swollen lymph nodes. If your child has symptoms of leukemia, his or her doctor may order blood tests to count the number of each of the different kinds of blood cells. If the results of the blood tests are not normal, a bone marrow biopsy may be performed. During this test, a needle is inserted into a bone in the hip and a small amount of bone marrow is removed and examined under the microscope, enabling the doctor to determine what kind of leukemia your child has and plan the best treatment.

Your child's doctor may also do a spinal tap, in which a needle is inserted through the back to remove a sample of the fluid that surrounds the brain and spine. The fluid is then examined under a microscope to see if leukemia cells are present.

Your child's chance of recovery (prognosis) depends on your child's age at diagnosis, the number of white blood cells in the blood (the white blood cell count) at diagnosis, how far the disease has spread, the biologic characteristics of the leukemia cells, and how well the leukemia cells respond to treatment.

Stage Information

There is no staging for childhood acute lymphoblastic leukemia. The treatment depends on age, the results of laboratory tests, and whether or not the patient has been previously treated for leukemia.

Untreated

Untreated acute lymphoblastic leukemia (ALL) means that no treatment has been given except to reduce symptoms. There are too many white blood cells in the blood and bone marrow, and there may be other signs and symptoms of leukemia.

In Remission

Remission means that treatment has been given and the number of white blood cells and other blood cells in the blood and bone marrow is normal. There are no signs or symptoms of leukemia.

Recurrent/Refractory

Recurrent disease means that the leukemia has come back (recurred) after going into remission. Refractory disease means that the leukemia failed to go into remission following treatment.

Treatment Option Overview

There are treatments for all patients with childhood acute lymphoblastic leukemia (ALL). The primary treatment for ALL is chemotherapy. Radiation therapy may be used in certain cases. Bone marrow transplantation is being studied in clinical trials.

Chemotherapy uses drugs to kill cancer cells. Chemotherapy drugs may be taken by mouth, or may be put into the body by a needle in a vein or muscle.

Chemotherapy is called a systemic treatment because the drug enters the bloodstream, travels through the body, and can kill cancer cells throughout the body. For ALL, chemotherapy drugs may sometimes be injected (usually through the spine) into the fluid that surrounds the brain and spinal cord; this is known as intrathecal chemotherapy.

Radiation therapy uses x-rays or other high-energy rays to kill cancer cells and shrink tumors. Radiation for ALL usually comes from a machine outside the body (external beam radiation therapy).

Bone marrow transplantation is a newer type of treatment. First, high doses of chemotherapy with or without radiation therapy are given to destroy all of the bone marrow in the body. Healthy marrow is then taken from another person (a donor) whose tissue is the same as or almost the same as the patient's. The donor may be a twin (the best match), a brother or sister, or another person not related to the patient. The healthy marrow from the donor is given to the patient through a needle in a vein, and the marrow replaces the marrow that was destroyed. A bone marrow transplant using marrow from a relative or person not related to the patient is called an allogeneic bone marrow transplant.

An even newer type of bone marrow transplant, called autologous bone marrow transplant, is being studied in clinical trials. During this procedure, bone marrow is taken from the patient and may be treated with drugs to kill any cancer cells. The marrow is frozen to save it. The patient is then given high-dose chemotherapy with or without radiation therapy to destroy all of the remaining marrow. The frozen marrow that was saved is thawed and given through a needle in a vein to replace the marrow that was destroyed.

There are generally 4 phases of treatment for ALL. The first phase, remission induction therapy, uses chemotherapy to kill as many of the leukemia cells as possible to cause the cancer to go into remission.

The second phase, called central nervous system (CNS) prophylaxis, is preventive therapy using intrathecal and/or high-dose systemic chemotherapy to the CNS to kill any leukemia cells present there, or to prevent the spread of cancer cells to the brain and spinal cord even if no cancer has been detected there. Radiation therapy to the brain may also be given, in addition to chemotherapy, for this purpose. CNS prophylaxis is often given in conjunction with consolidation/intensification therapy.

Once a child goes into remission and there are no signs of leukemia, a third phase of treatment called consolidation or intensification therapy, is given.

Consolidation therapy uses high-dose chemotherapy to attempt to kill any remaining leukemia cells.

The fourth phase of treatment, called maintenance therapy, uses chemotherapy for several years to maintain the remission.

Treatment by Stage

Treatment for childhood acute lymphoblastic leukemia depends on the prognostic group to which your child is assigned based primarily on your child's age and white blood cell count at diagnosis.

Your child may receive treatment that is considered standard based on its effectiveness in a number of patients in past studies, or you may choose to have your child take part in a clinical trial. Not all patients are cured with standard therapy and some standard treatments may have more side effects than are desired. For these reasons, clinical trials are designed to test new treatments and to find better ways to treat cancer patients. Clinical trials are ongoing in most parts of the country for most stages of childhood ALL. For more information, call the Cancer Information Service at 1-800-4-CANCER (1-800-422-6237); TTY at 1-800-332-8615.

Untreated Childhood Acute Lymphoblastic Leukemia

Your child's treatment will probably be remission induction chemotherapy to kill cancer cells and cause the leukemia to go into remission. Induction chemotherapy is almost always successful in inducing remission. Intrathecal and/or high-dose systemic chemotherapy, with or without radiation therapy to the brain, may also be given to prevent the spread of cancer cells to the brain and spinal cord. Clinical trials are testing new ways of inducing remission.

Childhood Acute Lymphoblastic Leukemia in Remission

Your child's treatment will probably be intensive chemotherapy to kill any remaining cancer cells. Intrathecal and/or high doses of systemic chemotherapy, with or without radiation therapy to the brain, may also be given during this phase of treatment to prevent the spread of cancer cells to the brain and spinal cord. Following intensification therapy, chemotherapy generally continues until the child has been in continuous remission for several years.

Recurrent Childhood Acute Lymphoblastic Leukemia

Treatment depends on the type of treatment your child received before, how soon the cancer came back following treatment, and whether the leukemia cells are found outside the bone marrow. Your child's treatment will probably be systemic or intrathecal chemotherapy, radiation therapy, or bone marrow transplantation. You may want to consider entering your child into a clinical trial of new chemotherapy drugs or bone marrow transplantation.

To Learn More

Call

For more information, U.S. residents may call the National Cancer Institute's (NCI's) Cancer Information Service toll-free at 1-800-4-CANCER (1-800-422-6237) Monday through Friday from 9:00 a.m. to 4:30 p.m. Deaf and hard-of-hearing callers with TTY equipment may call 1-800-332-8615. The call is free and a trained Cancer Information Specialist is available to answer your questions.

Web Sites and Organizations

The NCI's Cancer.gov Web site (http://cancer.gov) provides online access to information on cancer, clinical trials, and other Web sites and organizations that offer support and resources for cancer patients and their families. There are also many other places where people can get materials and information about cancer treatment and services. Local hospitals may have information on local and regional agencies that offer information about finances, getting to and from treatment, receiving care at home, and dealing with problems associated with cancer treatment.

Publications

The NCI has booklets and other materials for patients, health professionals, and the public. These publications discuss types of cancer, methods of cancer treatment, coping with cancer, and clinical trials. Some publications provide information on tests for cancer, cancer causes and prevention, cancer statistics, and NCI research activities. NCI materials on these and other topics may be ordered online or printed directly from the NCI Publications Locator (**http://cancer.gov/publications**). These materials can also be ordered by telephone from the Cancer Information Service toll-free at 1-800-4-CANCER (1-800-422-6237), TTY at 1-800-332-8615.

LiveHelp

The NCI's LiveHelp service, a program available on several of the Institute's Web sites, provides Internet users with the ability to chat online with an Information Specialist. The service is available from 9:00 a.m. to 7:30 p.m. Eastern time, Monday through Friday. Information Specialists can help Internet users find information on NCI Web sites and answer questions about cancer.

Write

For more information from the NCI, please write to this address:

National Cancer Institute
Office of Communications
31 Center Drive, MSC 2580
Bethesda, MD 20892-2580

About PDQ

PDQ Is a Comprehensive Cancer Database Available on Cancer.gov

PDQ is the National Cancer Institute's (NCI's) comprehensive cancer information database. Most of the information contained in PDQ is available online at Cancer.gov, the NCI's Web site. PDQ is provided as a service of the NCI. The NCI is part of the National Institutes of Health, the federal government's focal point for biomedical research.

PDQ Contains Cancer Information Summaries

The PDQ database contains summaries of the latest published information on cancer prevention, detection, genetics, treatment, supportive care, and complementary and alternative medicine. Most summaries are available in two versions. The health professional versions provide detailed information written in technical language. The patient versions are written in easy-to-understand, non-technical language. Both versions provide current and accurate cancer information.

The PDQ cancer information summaries are developed by cancer experts and reviewed regularly. Editorial Boards made up of experts in oncology and related specialties are responsible for writing and maintaining the cancer information summaries. The summaries are reviewed regularly and changes are made as new information becomes available. The date on each summary ("Date Last Modified") indicates the time of the most recent change.

PDQ Contains Information on Clinical Trials

In the United States, about two-thirds of children with cancer are treated in a clinical trial at some point in their illness. A clinical trial is a study to answer a scientific question, such as whether one treatment is better than another. Trials are based on past studies and what has been learned in the laboratory. Each trial answers certain scientific questions in order to find new and better ways to help cancer patients. During treatment clinical trials, information is collected about new treatments, the risks involved, and how well they do or do not work. If a clinical trial shows that a new treatment is better than one currently being used, the new treatment may become "standard."

Listings of clinical trials are included in PDQ and are available online at Cancer.gov. Descriptions of the trials are available in health professional and patient versions. For additional help in locating a childhood cancer clinical trial, call the Cancer Information Service at 1-800-4-CANCER (1-800-422-6237), TTY at 1-800-332-8615.

The PDQ Database Contains Listings of Groups Specializing in Clinical Trials

The Children's Oncology Group (COG) is the major group that organizes clinical trials for childhood cancers in the United States. Information about contacting COG is available on Cancer.gov or from the Cancer Information Service at 1-800-4-CANCER (1-800-422-6237), TTY at 1-800-332-8615.

The PDQ Database Contains Listings of Cancer Health Professionals and Hospitals with Cancer Programs

Because cancer in children and adolescents is rare, the majority of children with cancer are treated by health professionals specializing in childhood cancers, at hospitals or cancer centers with special facilities to treat them. The PDQ database contains listings of health professionals who specialize in childhood cancer and listings of hospitals with cancer programs. For help locating childhood cancer health professionals or a hospital with cancer programs, call the Cancer Information Service at 1-800-4-CANCER (1-800-422-6237), TTY at 1-800-332-8615.

More Guideline Sources

The previous guideline on childhood acute lymphoblastic leukemia is only one example of the kind of material that you can find online and free of charge. The remainder of this chapter will direct you to other sources which either publish or can help you find additional guidelines on topics related to childhood acute lymphoblastic leukemia. Many of the guidelines listed below address topics that may be of particular relevance to your child's specific situation, while certain guidelines will apply to only some children with childhood acute lymphoblastic leukemia. Due to space limitations these sources are listed in a concise manner. Do not hesitate to consult the following sources by either using the Internet hyperlink provided, or, in cases where the contact information is provided, contacting the publisher or author directly.

Topic Pages: MEDLINEplus

For parents wishing to go beyond guidelines published by specific Institutes of the NIH, the National Library of Medicine has created a vast and parent-oriented healthcare information portal called MEDLINEplus. Within this Internet-based system are "health topic pages." You can think of a health topic page as a guide to patient guides. To access this system, log on to http://www.nlm.nih.gov/medlineplus/healthtopics.html. From there you can either search using the alphabetical index or browse by broad topic areas. Recently, MEDLINEplus listed the following as being relevant to childhood acute lymphoblastic leukemia:

- Guides On Childhood Acute Lymphoblastic Leukemia

  Leukemia, Childhood
  http://www.nlm.nih.gov/medlineplus/leukemiachildhood.html

- Other Guides

  Acute lymphocytic leukemia
  http://www.nlm.nih.gov/medlineplus/ency/article/000541.htm

Within the health topic page dedicated to childhood acute lymphoblastic leukemia, the following was recently recommended to parents:

- General/Overviews

  Acute Lymphoblastic Leukemia in Children
  Source: National Cancer Institute
  http://newscenter.cancer.gov/pressreleases/all3.html

  Leukemia
  http://www.nlm.nih.gov/medlineplus/tutorials/leukemialoader.html

  Leukemia
  Source: Nemours Foundation
  http://kidshealth.org/parent/medical/cancer/cancer_leukemia.html

- Diagnosis/Symptoms

  How is Childhood Leukemia Diagnosed?
  Source: American Cancer Society
  http://www.cancer.org/eprise/main/docroot/CRI/content/CRI_2_4_3X_How_is_leukemia_diagnosed_24?

  Understanding Blood Counts
  Source: Leukemia & Lymphoma Society
  http://www.leukemia-lymphoma.org/all_mat_toc.adp?item_id=9452

- Treatment

    Blood and Marrow Stem Cell Transplantation
    Source: Leukemia & Lymphoma Society
    http://www.leukemia-lymphoma.org/all_mat_toc.adp?item_id=2443

    Blood Transfusion
    Source: Leukemia & Lymphoma Society
    http://www.leukemia-lymphoma.org/all_mat_toc.adp?item_id=17813

    Childhood Acute Lymphocytic Leukemia (PDQ): Treatment
    Source: National Cancer Institute
    http://www.cancer.gov/cancer_information/doc_pdq.aspx?version=patient&viewid=b4293987-e205-4a47-8b28-1120ddaf0a34

    Childhood Acute Myeloid Leukemia / Other Myeloid Malignancies (PDQ): Treatment
    Source: National Cancer Institute
    http://www.cancer.gov/cancer_information/doc_pdq.aspx?version=patient&viewid=277d9e6a-16ac-4592-8294-b855ad5796ff

    Immunotherapy
    Source: Leukemia & Lymphoma Society
    http://www.leukemia-lymphoma.org/all_mat_toc.adp?item_id=9889

    Long Term and Late Effects of Treatment for Blood-Related Cancers
    Source: Leukemia & Lymphoma Society
    http://www.leukemia-lymphoma.org/all_mat_toc.adp?item_id=9965

    New Approaches to Treatment
    Source: Leukemia & Lymphoma Society
    http://www.leukemia-lymphoma.org/all_page?item_id=4702

    Understanding Chemotherapy
    Source: Leukemia & Lymphoma Society
    http://www.leukemia-lymphoma.org/all_mat_toc.adp?item_id=4826

- Alternative Therapy

    Complementary & Alternative Therapies for Leukemia, Lymphoma, Hodgkin's Disease, & Myeloma
    Source: Leukemia & Lymphoma Society
    http://www.leukemia-lymphoma.org/all_mat_toc.adp?item_id=9882

- Nutrition

    Nutrition for Children with Cancer
    Source: American Cancer Society
    http://www.cancer.org/eprise/main/docroot/PED/PED_3_1_nutrition_for_children_with_cancer?

- Coping

    Emotional Aspects of Childhood Leukemia
    Source: Leukemia & Lymphoma Society
    http://www.leukemia-lymphoma.org/all_mat_detail.adp?item_id=28602&sort_order=5&cat_id=

- Specific Conditions/Aspects

    Acute Lymphocytic Leukemia (ALL)
    Source: Leukemia & Lymphoma Society
    http://www.leukemia-lymphoma.org/all_page?item_id=7049

    Acute Myelogenous Leukemia (AML)
    Source: Leukemia & Lymphoma Society
    http://www.leukemia-lymphoma.org/all_page?item_id=8459

    Choosing a Treatment Facility
    Source: Leukemia & Lymphoma Society
    http://www.leukemia-lymphoma.org/all_mat_toc.adp?item_id=9877

    Choosing and Communicating with a Cancer Specialist
    Source: Leukemia & Lymphoma Society
    http://www.leukemia-lymphoma.org/all_mat_toc.adp?item_id=9872

    Chronic Myelomonocytic Leukemias(CMML)
    Source: Leukemia & Lymphoma Society
    http://www.leukemia-lymphoma.org/all_mat_toc.adp?item_id=69974

Facts and Statistics
Source: Leukemia & Lymphoma Society
http://www.leukemia-lymphoma.org/all_page?item_id=12486

What are the Differences Between Cancers in Adults and in Children?
Source: American Cancer Society
http://www.cancer.org/eprise/main/docroot/CRI/content/CRI_2_4_1X_What_are_the_differences_between_cancers_in_adults_and_in_children_31?sitearea=&level=

Young People with Cancer: A Handbook for Parents
Source: National Cancer Institute
http://www.cancer.gov/templates/page_print.aspx?viewid=2944f6e7-996c-47b0-ad4e-23d8fbe9e033

- From the National Institutes of Health

    Questions and Answers About Care for Children and Adolescents with Cancer
    Source: National Cancer Institute
    http://cis.nci.nih.gov/fact/1_21.htm

    What You Need To Know About Leukemia
    Source: National Cancer Institute
    http://www.cancer.gov/cancer_information/doc_wyntk.aspx?viewid=57b3abc6-4b52-41b0-8762-9372062313de

- Organizations

    American Cancer Society
    http://www.cancer.org/

    Leukemia & Lymphoma Society
    http://www.leukemia-lymphoma.org/hm_lls

    National Cancer Institute
    http://www.cancer.gov/

    National Marrow Donor Program
    http://www.marrow.org/

- Statistics

    What Are The Key Statistics About Childhood Leukemia?
    Source: American Cancer Society
    http://www.cancer.org/eprise/main/docroot/CRI/content/CRI_2_4_1X_What_are_the_key_statistics_for_leukemia_24?

If you do not find topics of interest when browsing health topic pages, then you can choose to use the advanced search utility of MEDLINEplus at **http://www.nlm.nih.gov/medlineplus/advancedsearch.html**. This utility is similar to the NIH Search Utility, with the exception that it only includes material linked within the MEDLINEplus system (mostly parent-oriented information). It also has the disadvantage of generating unstructured results. We recommend, therefore, that you use this method only if you have a very targeted search.

The National Guideline Clearinghouse™

The National Guideline Clearinghouse™ offers hundreds of evidence-based clinical practice guidelines published in the United States and other countries. You can search their site located at **http://www.guideline.gov/** by using the keyword "childhood acute lymphoblastic leukemia" or synonyms.

Healthfinder™

Healthfinder™ is an additional source sponsored by the U.S. Department of Health and Human Services which offers links to hundreds of other sites that contain healthcare information. This Web site is located at **http://www.healthfinder.gov**. Again, keyword searches can be used to find guidelines. The following was recently found in this database:

- **AACN Clinical Issues: Advanced Practice in Acute and Critical Care**

    Summary: A quarterly, peer reviewed series of informative volumes designed for advanced practice nurses, case managers, academic and clinical educators, and expert clinicians at the bedside.

    Source: American Association of Critical-Care Nurses

    http://www.healthfinder.gov/scripts/recordpass.asp?RecordType=0&RecordID=5100

The NIH Search Utility

After browsing the references listed at the beginning of this chapter, you may want to explore the NIH Search Utility. This allows you to search for documents on over 100 selected Web sites that comprise the NIH-WEB-SPACE. Each of these servers is "crawled" and indexed on an ongoing basis. Your search will produce a list of various documents, all of which will relate in some way to childhood acute lymphoblastic leukemia. The drawbacks of this approach are that the information is not organized by theme and that the references are often a mix of information for professionals and parents. Nevertheless, a large number of the listed Web sites provide useful background information. We can only recommend this route, therefore, for relatively rare or specific disorders, or when using highly targeted searches. To use the NIH search utility, visit the following Web page: **http://search.nih.gov/index.html**.

Additional Web Sources

A number of Web sites that often link to government sites are available to the public. These can also point you in the direction of essential information. The following is a representative sample:

- AOL: **http://search.aol.com/cat.adp?id=168&layer=&from=subcats**
- drkoop.com®: **http://www.drkoop.com/conditions/ency/index.html**
- Family Village: **http://www.familyvillage.wisc.edu/specific.htm**
- Google: **http://directory.google.com/Top/Health/Conditions_and_Diseases/**
- Med Help International: **http://www.medhelp.org/HealthTopics/A.html**
- Open Directory Project: **http://dmoz.org/Health/Conditions_and_Diseases/**
- Yahoo.com: **http://dir.yahoo.com/Health/Diseases_and_Conditions/**
- WebMD®Health: **http://my.webmd.com/health_topics**

Vocabulary Builder

The material in this chapter may have contained a number of unfamiliar words. The following Vocabulary Builder introduces you to terms used in this chapter that have not been covered in the previous chapter:

Abdomen: The part of the body that contains the pancreas, stomach, intestines, liver, gallbladder, and other organs. [NIH]

Adolescence: The period of life beginning with the appearance of secondary sex characteristics and terminating with the cessation of somatic growth. The years usually referred to as adolescence lie between 13 and 18 years of age. [NIH]

Allogeneic: Taken from different individuals of the same species. [NIH]

Anemia: A condition in which the number of red blood cells is below normal. [NIH]

Autologous: Taken from an individual's own tissues, cells, or DNA. [NIH]

Bacteria: A large group of single-cell microorganisms. Some cause infections and disease in animals and humans. The singular of bacteria is bacterium. [NIH]

Biopsy: The removal of cells or tissues for examination under a microscope. When only a sample of tissue is removed, the procedure is called an incisional biopsy or core biopsy. When an entire tumor or lesion is removed, the procedure is called an excisional biopsy. When a sample of tissue or fluid is removed with a needle, the procedure is called a needle biopsy or fine-needle aspiration. [NIH]

Blasts: Immature blood cells. [NIH]

Blood transfusion: The administration of blood or blood products into a blood vessel. [NIH]

Cell: The individual unit that makes up all of the tissues of the body. All living things are made up of one or more cells. [NIH]

Chemotherapy: Treatment with anticancer drugs. [NIH]

Chronic: A disease or condition that persists or progresses over a long period of time. [NIH]

CNS: Central nervous system. The brain and spinal cord. [NIH]

Immunization: The induction of immunity. [EU]

Immunotherapy: Treatment to stimulate or restore the ability of the immune system to fight infection and disease. Also used to lessen side effects that may be caused by some cancer treatments. Also called biological therapy or biological response modifier (BRM) therapy. [NIH]

Induction: The act or process of inducing or causing to occur, especially the production of a specific morphogenetic effect in the developing embryo through the influence of evocators or organizers, or the production of anaesthesia or unconsciousness by use of appropriate agents. [EU]

Intrathecal: Describes the fluid-filled space between the thin layers of tissue that cover the brain and spinal cord. Drugs can be injected into the fluid or a sample of the fluid can be removed for testing. [NIH]

Leukemia: Cancer of blood-forming tissue. [NIH]

Lymphocyte: A white blood cell. Lymphocytes have a number of roles in the immune system, including the production of antibodies and other substances that fight infection and diseases. [NIH]

Lymphocytic: Referring to lymphocytes, a type of white blood cell. [NIH]

Lymphoma: Cancer that arises in cells of the lymphatic system. [NIH]

Myelogenous: Produced by, or originating in, the bone marrow. [NIH]

Oncology: The study of cancer. [NIH]

Pelvis: The lower part of the abdomen, located between the hip bones. [NIH]

Platelets: A type of blood cell that helps prevent bleeding by causing blood clots to form. Also called thrombocytes. [NIH]

Prophylaxis: An attempt to prevent disease. [NIH]

Prostate: A gland in males that surrounds the neck of the bladder and the urethra. It secretes a substance that liquifies coagulated semen. It is situated in the pelvic cavity behind the lower part of the pubic symphysis, above the deep layer of the triangular ligament, and rests upon the rectum. [NIH]

Refractory: Not readily yielding to treatment. [EU]

Remission: A decrease in or disappearance of signs and symptoms of cancer. In partial remission, some, but not all, signs and symptoms of cancer have disappeared. In complete remission, all signs and symptoms of cancer have disappeared, although there still may be cancer in the body. [NIH]

Sinusitis: Inflammation of a sinus. The condition may be purulent or nonpurulent, acute or chronic. Depending on the site of involvement it is known as ethmoid, frontal, maxillary, or sphenoid sinusitis. [EU]

Spleen: An organ that is part of the lymphatic system. The spleen produces lymphocytes, filters the blood, stores blood cells, and destroys old blood cells. It is located on the left side of the abdomen near the stomach. [NIH]

Staging: Performing exams and tests to learn the extent of the cancer within the body, especially whether the disease has spread from the original site to other parts of the body. [NIH]

Systemic: Affecting the entire body. [NIH]

Thymus: An organ that is part of the lymphatic system, in which T lymphocytes grow and multiply. The thymus is in the chest behind the breastbone. [NIH]

Tonsils: Small masses of lymphoid tissue on either side of the throat. [NIH]

Transplantation: The replacement of an organ with one from another person. [NIH]

Varicella: Chicken pox. [EU]

CHAPTER 2. SEEKING GUIDANCE

Overview

Some parents are comforted by the knowledge that a number of organizations dedicate their resources to helping people with childhood acute lymphoblastic leukemia. These associations can become invaluable sources of information and advice. Many associations offer parent support, financial assistance, and other important services. Furthermore, healthcare research has shown that support groups often help people to better cope with their conditions.[8] In addition to support groups, your child's physician can be a valuable source of guidance and support.

In this chapter, we direct you to resources that can help you find parent organizations and medical specialists. We begin by describing how to find associations and parent groups that can help you better understand and cope with your child's condition. The chapter ends with a discussion on how to find a doctor that is right for your child.

There are a number of directories that list additional medical associations that you may find useful. While not all of these directories will provide different information, by consulting all of them, you will have nearly exhausted all sources for parent associations.

The National Cancer Institute (NCI)

The National Cancer Institute (NCI) has complied a list of national organizations that offer services to people with cancer and their families. To

---

[8] Churches, synagogues, and other houses of worship might also have groups that can offer you the social support you need.

view the list, see the NCI fact sheet online at the following Web address: **http://cis.nci.nih.gov/fact/8_1.htm**. The name of each organization is accompanied by its contact information and a brief explanation of its services. Information on a number of organizations specializing in children's issues is also available.

The National Health Information Center (NHIC)

The National Health Information Center (NHIC) offers a free referral service to help people find organizations that provide information about childhood acute lymphoblastic leukemia. For more information, see the NHIC's Web site at **http://www.health.gov/NHIC/** or contact an information specialist by calling 1-800-336-4797.

DIRLINE

A comprehensive source of information on associations is the DIRLINE database maintained by the National Library of Medicine. The database comprises some 10,000 records of organizations, research centers, and government institutes and associations which primarily focus on health and biomedicine. DIRLINE is available via the Internet at the following Web site: **http://dirline.nlm.nih.gov**. Simply type in "childhood acute lymphoblastic leukemia" (or a synonym) or the name of a topic, and the site will list information contained in the database on all relevant organizations.

The Combined Health Information Database

Another comprehensive source of information on healthcare associations is the Combined Health Information Database. Using the "Detailed Search" option, you will need to limit your search to "Organizations" and "childhood acute lymphoblastic leukemia". Type the following hyperlink into your Web browser: **http://chid.nih.gov/detail/detail.html**. To find associations, use the drop boxes at the bottom of the search page where "You may refine your search by." For publication date, select "All Years." Then, select your preferred language and the format option "Organization Resource Sheet." By making these selections and typing in "childhood acute lymphoblastic leukemia" (or synonyms) into the "For these words:" box, you will only receive results on organizations dealing with childhood acute lymphoblastic leukemia. You should check back periodically with this database since it is updated every 3 months.

The National Organization for Rare Disorders, Inc.

The National Organization for Rare Disorders, Inc. has prepared a Web site that provides, at no charge, lists of associations organized by specific medical conditions. You can access this database at the following Web site: **http://www.rarediseases.org/cgi-bin/nord/searchpage**. Select the option called "Organizational Database (ODB)" and type "childhood acute lymphoblastic leukemia" (or a synonym) in the search box.

Cancer Support Groups[9]

People diagnosed with cancer and their families face many challenges that may leave them feeling overwhelmed, afraid, and alone. It can be difficult to cope with these challenges or to talk to even the most supportive family members and friends. Often, support groups can help people affected by cancer feel less alone and can improve their ability to deal with the uncertainties and challenges that cancer brings. Support groups give people who are affected by similar diseases an opportunity to meet and discuss ways to cope with the illness.

How Can Support Groups Help?

People who have been diagnosed with cancer sometimes find they need assistance coping with the emotional as well as the practical aspects of their disease. In fact, attention to the emotional burden of cancer is sometimes part of a patient's treatment plan. Cancer support groups are designed to provide a confidential atmosphere where cancer patients or cancer survivors can discuss the challenges that accompany the illness with others who may have experienced the same challenges. For example, people gather to discuss the emotional needs created by cancer, to exchange information about their disease—including practical problems such as managing side effects or returning to work after treatment—and to share their feelings. Support groups have helped thousands of people cope with these and similar situations.

---

[9] This section has been adapted from the NCI: **http://cis.nci.nih.gov/fact/8_8.htm**.

Can Family Members and Friends Participate in Support Groups?

Family and friends are affected when cancer touches someone they love, and they may need help in dealing with stresses such as family disruptions, financial worries, and changing roles within relationships. To help meet these needs, some support groups are designed just for family members of people diagnosed with cancer; other groups encourage families and friends to participate along with the cancer patient or cancer survivor.

How Can People Find Support Groups?

Many organizations offer support groups for people diagnosed with cancer and their family members or friends. The NCI fact sheet *National Organizations That Offer Services to People With Cancer and Their Families* lists many cancer-concerned organizations that can provide information about support groups. This fact sheet is available at **http://cis.nci.nih.gov/fact/8_1.htm** on the Internet, or can be ordered from the Cancer Information Service at 1–800–4–CANCER (1–800–422–6237). Some of these organizations provide information on their Web sites about contacting support groups.

Doctors, nurses, or hospital social workers who work with cancer patients may also have information about support groups, such as their location, size, type, and how often they meet. Most hospitals have social services departments that provide information about cancer support programs. Additionally, many newspapers carry a special health supplement containing information about where to find support groups.

What Types of Support Groups Are Available?

Several kinds of support groups are available to meet the individual needs of people at all stages of cancer treatment, from diagnosis through follow-up care. Some groups are general cancer support groups, while more specialized groups may be for teens or young adults, for family members, or for people affected by a particular disease. Support groups may be led by a professional, such as a psychiatrist, psychologist, or social worker, or by cancer patients or survivors. In addition, support groups can vary in approach, size, and how often they meet. Many groups are free, but some require a fee (people can contact their health insurance company to find out whether their plan will cover the cost). It is important for people to find an atmosphere that is comfortable and meets their individual needs.

Online Support Groups

In addition to support groups, commercial Internet service providers offer forums and chat rooms to discuss different illnesses and conditions. WebMD®, for example, offers such a service at their Web site: **http://boards.webmd.com/roundtable**. These online communities can help you connect with a network of people whose concerns are similar to yours. Online support groups are places where people can talk informally. If you read about a novel approach, consult with your child's doctor or other healthcare providers, as the treatments or discoveries you hear about may not be scientifically proven to be safe and effective.

The Cancer Information Service[10]

The Cancer Information Service (CIS) is a program of the National Cancer Institute (NCI), the Nation's lead agency for cancer research. As a resource for information and education about cancer, the CIS is a leader in helping people become active participants in their own health care by providing the latest information on cancer in understandable language. Through its network of regional offices, the CIS serves the United States, Puerto Rico, the U.S. Virgin Islands, and the Pacific Islands.

For 25 years, the Cancer Information Service has provided the latest and most accurate cancer information to patients and families, the public, and health professionals by:

- Interacting with people one-on-one through its Information Service,
- Working with organizations through its Partnership Program,
- Participating in research efforts to find the best ways to help people adopt healthier behaviors,
- Providing access to NCI information over the Internet.

How Does the CIS Assist the Public?

Through the CIS toll-free telephone service (1-800-4-CANCER), callers speak with knowledgeable, caring staff who are experienced at explaining medical information in easy-to-understand terms. CIS information specialists answer calls in English and Spanish. They also provide cancer information to deaf and hard of hearing callers through the toll-free TTY number (1-800-

---

[10] This section has been adapted from the NCI: **http://cis.nci.nih.gov/fact/2_5.htm**.

332-8615). CIS staff have access to comprehensive, accurate information from the NCI on a range of cancer topics, including the most recent advances in cancer treatment. They take as much time as each caller needs, provide thorough and personalized attention, and keep all calls confidential.

The CIS also provides live, online assistance to users of NCI Web sites through LiveHelp, an instant messaging service that is available from 9:00 a.m. to 7:30 p.m. Eastern time, Monday through Friday. Through LiveHelp, information specialists provide answers to questions about cancer and help in navigating Cancer.gov, the NCI's Web site.

Through the telephone numbers or LiveHelp service, CIS users receive:

- Answers to their questions about cancer, including ways to prevent cancer, symptoms and risks, diagnosis, current treatments, and research studies;

- Written materials from the NCI;

- Referrals to clinical trials and cancer-related services, such as treatment centers, mammography facilities, or other cancer organizations;

- Assistance in quitting smoking from information specialists trained in smoking cessation counseling.

What Kind of Assistance Does the CIS Partnership Program Offer?

Through its Partnership Program, the CIS collaborates with established national, state, and regional organizations to reach minority and medically underserved audiences with cancer information. Partnership Program staff provide assistance to organizations developing programs that focus on breast and cervical cancer, clinical trials, tobacco control, and cancer awareness for special populations. To reach those in need, the CIS:

- Helps bring cancer information to people who do not traditionally seek health information or who may have difficulties doing so because of educational, financial, cultural, or language barriers;

- Provides expertise to organizations to help strengthen their ability to inform people they serve about cancer; and

- Links organizations with similar goals and helps them plan and evaluate programs, develop coalitions, conduct training on cancer-related topics, and use NCI resources.

How Do CIS Research Efforts Assist the Public?

The CIS plays an important role in research by studying the most effective ways to communicate with people about healthy lifestyles; health risks; and options for preventing, diagnosing, and treating cancer. The ability to conduct health communications research is a unique aspect of the CIS. Results from these research studies can be applied to improving the way the CIS communicates about cancer and can help other programs communicate more effectively.

How Do People Reach the Cancer Information Service?

- To speak with a CIS information specialist call 1-800-4-CANCER (1-800-422-6237), 9:00 a.m. to 4:30 p.m. local time, Monday through Friday. Deaf or hard of hearing callers with TTY equipment may call 1-800-332-8615.

- To obtain online assistance visit the NCI's Cancer Information Web site at **http://cancer.gov/cancer_information** and click on the LiveHelp link between 9:00 a.m. and 7:30 p.m. Eastern time, Monday through Friday.

- For information 24 hours a day, 7 days a week call 1-800-4-CANCER and select option 4 to hear recorded information at any time.

- Visit NCI's Web site at **http://cancer.gov** on the Internet.

- Visit the CIS Web site at **http://cancer.gov/cis** on the Internet.

Finding Cancer Resources in Your Community[11]

When your child has cancer or is undergoing cancer treatment, there are places in your community to turn to for help. There are many local organizations throughout the country that offer a variety of practical and support services to children with cancer and their families. However, parents often don't know about these services or are unable to find them. National cancer organizations can assist you in finding these resources, and there are a number of things you can do for yourself.

Whether you are looking for a support group, counseling, advice, financial assistance, transportation for your child to and from treatment, or information about cancer, most neighborhood organizations, local health care providers, or area hospitals are a good place to start. Often, the hardest part of looking for help is knowing the right questions to ask.

---

[11] Adapted from the NCI: **http://cis.nci.nih.gov/fact/8_9.htm**.

What Kind of Help Can I Get?

Until now, you probably never thought about the many issues and difficulties that arise with a diagnosis of cancer. There are support services to help you deal with almost any type of problem that might occur. The first step in finding the help you need is knowing what types of services are available. The following pages describe some of these services and how to find them.

- **Information on Cancer.** Most national cancer organizations provide a range of information services, including materials on different types of cancer, treatments, and treatment-related issues.

- **Counseling.** While some parents are reluctant to seek counseling, studies show that having someone to talk to reduces stress. Counseling can also provide emotional support to children with cancer and help them better understand their illness. Different types of counseling include individual, group, family, self-help (sometimes called peer counseling), bereavement, patient-to-patient, and sexuality.

- **Medical Treatment Decisions.** Often, parents need to make complicated medical decisions. Many organizations provide hospital and physician referrals for second opinions and information on clinical trials, which may expand treatment options.

- **Home Health Care.** Home health care assists patients who no longer need to stay in a hospital, but still require professional medical help. Skilled nursing care, physical therapy, social work services, and nutrition counseling are all available at home.

- **Hospice Care.** Hospice is care focused on the special needs of terminally ill cancer patients. Sometimes called palliative care, it centers around providing comfort, controlling physical symptoms, and giving emotional support to patients who can no longer benefit from curative treatment. Hospice programs provide services in various settings, including the patient's home, hospice centers, hospitals, or skilled nursing facilities. Your child's doctor or social worker can provide a referral for these services.

- **Rehabilitation.** Rehabilitation services help people adjust to the effects of cancer and its treatment. Physical rehabilitation focuses on recovery from the physical effects of surgery or the side effects associated with chemotherapy.

- **Advocacy.** Advocacy is a general term that refers to promoting or protecting the rights and interests of a certain group, such as cancer patients. Advocacy groups may offer services to assist with legal, ethical, medical, employment, legislative, or insurance issues, among others. For instance, if you feel your insurance company has not handled your child's claim fairly, you may want to advocate for a review of its decision.

- **Financial.** Treating cancer can be a tremendous financial burden. There are programs sponsored by the government and nonprofit organizations to help parents of cancer patients with problems related to medical billing, insurance coverage, and reimbursement issues. There are also sources for financial assistance.

- **Housing/Lodging.** Some organizations provide lodging for the family of a patient undergoing treatment, especially if it is a child who is ill and the parents are required to accompany the child to treatment.

- **Children's Services.** A number of organizations provide services for children with cancer, including summer camps, make-a-wish programs, and help for parents seeking child care.

How to Find These Services

Often, the services that people with cancer are looking for are right in their own neighborhood or city. The following is a list of places where you can begin your search for help.

- Your child's hospital, clinic, or medical center should be able to give you information. The doctor or nurse may be able to tell you about your child's specific medical condition, pain management, rehabilitation services, home nursing, or hospice care.

- Most hospitals also have a social work, home care, or discharge planning department. This department may be able to help you find a support group or a nonprofit agency that helps people who have cancer and their families. While your child is undergoing treatment, be sure to ask the hospital about transportation, practical assistance, or even temporary child care. Talk to a hospital financial counselor in the business office about developing a monthly payment plan if you need help with hospital expenses.

- The public library is an excellent source of information, as are patient libraries at many cancer centers. A librarian can help you find books and articles through a literature search.

- A local church, synagogue, YMCA or YWCA, or fraternal order may provide financial assistance, or may have volunteers who can help with transportation and home care. Catholic Charities, the United Way, or the American Red Cross may also operate local offices. Some of these organizations may provide home care, and the United Way's information and referral service can refer you to an agency that provides financial help. To find the United Way serving your community, visit their online directory at **http://www.unitedway.org** on the Internet or look in the White Pages of your local telephone book.

- Local or county government agencies may offer low-cost transportation (sometimes called para-transit) to individuals unable to use public transportation. The Federal government runs the Hill-Burton program (1-800-638-0742), which funds certain medical facilities and hospitals to provide children with cancer with free or low-cost care if their families are in financial need.

Getting the Most From a Service: What To Ask

No matter what type of help you are looking for, the only way to find resources to fit your needs is to ask the right questions. When you are calling an organization for information, it is important to think about what questions you are going to ask before you call. Many people find it helpful to write out their questions in advance, and to take notes during the call. Another good tip is to ask the name of the person with whom you are speaking in case you have follow-up questions. Below are some of the questions you may want to consider if you are calling or visiting a new agency and want to learn about how they can help:

- How do I apply [for this service]?
- Are there eligibility requirements? What are they?
- Is there an application process? How long will it take? What information will I need to complete the application process? Will I need anything else to get the service?
- Do you have any other suggestions or ideas about where I can find help?

The most important thing to remember is that you will rarely receive help unless you ask for it. In fact, asking can be the hardest part of getting help. Don't be afraid or ashamed to ask for assistance. Cancer is a very difficult disease, but there are people and services that can ease your burdens and help you focus on your child's treatment and recovery.

Finding Doctors Who Specialize in Cancer Care[12]

A common way to find a doctor who specializes in cancer care is to ask for a referral from your child's primary care physician. Sometimes, you may know a specialist yourself, or through the experience of a family member, coworker, or friend.

The following resources may also be able to provide you with names of doctors who specialize in treating specific diseases or conditions. However, these resources may not have information about the quality of care that the doctors provide.

- Your local hospital or its patient referral service may be able to provide you with a list of specialists who practice at that hospital.

- Your nearest National Cancer Institute (NCI)-designated cancer center can provide information about doctors who practice at that center. The NCI fact sheet *The National Cancer Institute Cancer Centers Program* describes and gives contact information, including Web sites, for NCI-designated cancer treatment centers around the country. Many of the cancer centers' Web sites have searchable directories of physicians who practice at each facility. The NCI's fact sheet is available at **http://cis.nci.nih.gov/fact/1_2.htm** on the Internet, or by calling the Cancer Information Service (CIS) at 1-800-4-CANCER (1-800-422-6237).

- The American Board of Medical Specialties (ABMS) publishes a list of board-certified physicians. The *Official ABMS Directory of Board Certified Medical Specialists* lists doctors' names along with their specialty and their educational background. This resource is available in most public libraries. The ABMS also has a Web site that can be used to verify whether a specific physician is board-certified. This free service is located at **http://www.abms.org/newsearch.asp** on the Internet. Verification of a physician's board certification can also be obtained by calling the ABMS at 1-866-275-2267 (1-866-ASK-ABMS).

- The American Medical Association (AMA) provides an online service called AMA Physician Select that offers basic professional information on virtually every licensed physician in the United States and its possessions. The database can be searched by doctor's name or by medical specialty. The AMA Physician Select service is located at **http://www.ama-assn.org/aps/amahg.htm** on the Internet.

- The American Society of Clinical Oncologists (ASCO) provides an online list of doctors who are members of ASCO. The member database has the

---

[12] Adapted from the NCI: **http://cis.nci.nih.gov/fact/7_47.htm**.

names and affiliations of over 15,000 oncologists worldwide. It can be searched by doctor's name, institution's name, location, and/or type of board certification. This service is located at **http://www.asco.org/people/db/html/m_db.htm** on the Internet.

- The American College of Surgeons (ACOS) Fellowship Database is an online list of surgeons who are Fellows of the ACOS. The list can be searched by doctor's name, geographic location, or medical specialty. This service is located at **http://web.facs.org/acsdir/default.htm** on the Internet. The ACOS can be contacted at 633 North Saint Clair Street, Chicago, IL 60611-3211; or by telephone at 312-202-5000.

- Local medical societies may maintain lists of doctors in each specialty.

- Public and medical libraries may have print directories of doctors' names, listed geographically by specialty.

- Your local Yellow Pages may have doctors listed by specialty under "Physicians."

The Agency for Healthcare Research and Quality (AHRQ) offers *Your Guide to Choosing Quality Health Care*, which has information for consumers on choosing a health plan, a doctor, a hospital, or a long-term care provider. The Guide includes suggestions and checklists that you can use to determine which doctor or hospital is best for you. This resource is available at **http://www.ahrq.gov/consumer/qntool.htm** on the Internet. You can also order the Guide by calling the AHRQ Publications Clearinghouse at 1-800-358-9295.

If you are a member of a health insurance plan, your choice may be limited to doctors who participate in your plan. Your insurance company can provide you with a list of participating primary care doctors and specialists. It is important to ask your insurance company if the doctor you choose is accepting new patients through your health plan. You also have the option of seeing a doctor outside your health plan and paying the costs yourself. If you have a choice of health insurance plans, you may first wish to consider which doctor or doctors you would like to use, then choose a plan that includes your chosen physician(s).

The National Comprehensive Cancer Network (NCCN) Physician Directory lists specialists who practice in the NCCN's 19 member institutions across the U.S. To access the directory, go to **http://www.nccn.org/** and click on "Physician Directory". To use this service, you will be required to scroll to the bottom of the page and select "I agree." Enter your search criteria and select "Find" at the bottom of the page. To obtain more information on a physician or institution, contact the institution's Physician Referral Department or the NCCN Patient Information and Referral Service at 1-888-909-NCCN or **patientinformation@nccn.org**.

If the previous sources did not meet your needs, you may want to log on to the Web site of the National Organization for Rare Disorders (NORD) at **http://www.rarediseases.org/**. NORD maintains a database of doctors with expertise in various rare diseases. The Metabolic Information Network (MIN), 800-945-2188, also maintains a database of physicians with expertise in various metabolic diseases.

Selecting Your Child's Doctor[13]

There are many factors to consider when choosing a doctor. To make the most informed decision, you may wish to speak with several doctors before choosing one. When you meet with each doctor, you might want to consider the following:

- Does the doctor have the education and training to meet my child's needs?
- Does the doctor use the hospital that I have chosen?
- Does the doctor explain things clearly and encourage me to ask questions?
- What are the doctor's office hours?
- Who covers for the doctor when he or she is unavailable? Will that person have access to my medical records?
- How long does it take to get an appointment with the doctor?

If you are choosing a surgeon, you may wish to ask additional questions about the surgeon's background and experience with specific procedures. These questions may include:

- Is the surgeon board-certified?[14]
- Has the surgeon been evaluated by a national professional association of surgeons, such as the American College of Surgeons (ACOS)?
- At which treatment facility or facilities does the surgeon practice?

---

[13] This section has been adapted from the AHRQ: www.ahrq.gov/consumer/qntascii/qntdr.htm.

[14] While board certification is a good measure of a doctor's knowledge, it is possible to receive quality care from doctors who are not board certified.

- How often does the surgeon perform the type of surgery that my child needs?
- How many of these procedures has the surgeon performed? What was the success rate?

It is important for you and your child to feel comfortable with the specialist that you choose, because you will be working closely with that person to make decisions about your child's cancer treatment. Trust your own observations and feelings when deciding on a doctor for your child's medical care.

Other health professionals and support services may also be important during cancer treatment. The National Cancer Institute fact sheet *Your Health Care Team: Your Doctor Is Only the Beginning* has information about these providers and services, and how to locate them. This fact sheet is located at **http://cis.nci.nih.gov/fact/8_10.htm** on the Internet, or can be obtained by calling the CIS at 1–800–4–CANCER (1–800–422–6237).

Working with Your Child's Doctor[15]

Research has shown that parents who have good relationships with their children's doctors tend to be more satisfied with their children's care. Here are some tips to help you and your child's doctor become partners:

- You know important things about your child's symptoms and health history. Tell the doctor what you think he or she needs to know.
- Always bring any medications your child is currently taking with you to the appointment, or you can bring a list of your child's medications including dosage and frequency information. Talk about any allergies or reactions your child has had to medications.
- Tell your doctor about any natural or alternative medicines your child is taking.
- Bring other medical information, such as x-ray films, test results, and medical records.
- Ask questions. If you don't, the doctor will assume that you understood everything that was said.
- Write down your questions before the doctor's visit. List the most important ones first to make sure that they are addressed.

---

[15] This section has been adapted from the AHRQ: **www.ahrq.gov/consumer/qntascii/qntdr.htm**.

- Ask the doctor to draw pictures if you think that this will help you and your child understand.

- Take notes. Some doctors do not mind if you bring a tape recorder to help you remember things, but always ask first.

- Take information home. Ask for written instructions. Your child's doctor may also have brochures and audio and videotapes on childhood acute lymphoblastic leukemia.

By following these steps, you will enhance the relationship you and your child have with the physician.

Getting a Second Opinion[16]

Once you have chosen a doctor and discussed a diagnosis and treatment plan, but before treatment has started, you may want to get a second opinion - that is, you may want to ask a different doctor to review the diagnosis and plan. Some insurance companies require a second opinion; some may pay for it if you ask. A second opinion may also be obtained during the course of treatment if it is not working as hoped. Most doctors support a parent's decision to get a second opinion and many even suggest you do so. To find specialists to get a second opinion, you might:

- Ask your child's doctor to suggest a specialist for a second opinion.

- Get the names of doctors who specialize in treating childhood cancer from the local medical society, a nearby hospital, or a medical school. You can find the telephone numbers for these organizations in your telephone directory or the Yellow Pages.

- Contact an NCI Comprehensive Cancer Center for a second opinion and possible treatment. Considered "Centers of Excellence," these cancer centers' programs have been reviewed and selected by NCI. They offer the most up-todate diagnosis and treatment of cancer and are devoted to both basic and clinical research. To obtain information about the location of the different cancer centers, call the CIS at 1-800-4-CANCER (1-800-422-6237) or TTY at 1-800-332-8615.

- Contact the Pediatric Oncology Branch, NCI, located in Bethesda, Maryland, to ask for a second opinion appointment. They can be reached at 1-877-624-4878.

---

[16] This section was adapted from the NCI:
http://www.cancer.gov/CancerInformation/youngpeople.

Finding a Cancer Treatment Facility[17]

Choosing a treatment facility is another important consideration for getting the best medical care possible. Although you may not be able to choose which hospital treats your child in an emergency, you can choose a facility for scheduled and ongoing care. If you have already found a doctor for your child's cancer treatment, you may need to choose a facility based on where the doctor practices. The doctor may be able to recommend a facility that provides quality care. You may wish to ask the following questions when considering a treatment facility:

- Has the facility had experience and success in treating my child's condition?

- Has the facility been rated by state, consumer, or other groups for its quality of care?

- How does the facility check and work to improve its quality of care?

- Has the facility been approved by a nationally recognized accrediting body, such as the American College of Surgeons (ACOS) and/or the Joint Commission on Accredited Healthcare Organizations (JCAHO)?

- Does the facility explain patients' rights and responsibilities? Are copies of this information available to patients?

- Does the treatment facility offer support services, such as social workers and resources to help me find financial assistance if I need it?

- Is the facility conveniently located?

If you are a member of a health insurance plan, your choice of treatment facilities may be limited to those that participate in your plan. Your insurance company can provide you with a list of approved facilities. Although the costs of cancer treatment can be very high, you have the option of paying out-of-pocket if you want to use a treatment facility that is not covered by your insurance plan. If you are considering paying for treatment yourself, you may wish to discuss the potential costs with your child's doctor beforehand. You may also want to speak with the person who does the billing for the treatment facility. In some instances, nurses and social workers can provide you with more information about coverage, eligibility, and insurance issues.

---

[17] Adapted from the NCI: **http://cis.nci.nih.gov/fact/7_47.htm**. At this Web site, information on how to find treatment facilities is also available for patients living outside the U.S.

The following resources may help you find a treatment facility for your child's care:

- The NCI fact sheet *The National Cancer Institute Cancer Centers Program* describes and gives contact information for NCI-designated cancer treatment centers around the country.

- The ACOS accredits cancer programs at hospitals and other treatment facilities. More than 1,400 programs in the United States have been designated by the ACOS as Approved Cancer Programs. The ACOS Web site offers a searchable database of these programs at **http://web.facs.org/cpm/default.htm** on the Internet. The ACOS can be contacted at 633 North Saint Clair Street, Chicago, IL 60611-3211; or by telephone at 312-202-5000.

- The JCAHO is an independent, not-for-profit organization that evaluates and accredits health care organizations and programs in the United States. It also offers information for the general public about choosing a treatment facility. The JCAHO Web site is located at **http://www.jcaho.org** on the Internet. The JCAHO is located at One Renaissance Boulevard, Oakbrook Terrace, IL 60181-4294. The telephone number is 630-792-5800.

- The JCAHO offers an online Quality Check service that parents can use to determine whether a specific facility has been accredited by the JCAHO and view the organization's performance reports. This service is located at **http://www.jcaho.org/qualitycheck/directry/directry.asp** on the Internet.

- The AHRQ publication *Your Guide To Choosing Quality Health Care* has suggestions and checklists for choosing the treatment facility that is right for you.

Questions and Answers about Children's Cancer Centers[18]

Survival rates for childhood cancer have risen sharply over the past 20 years. In the United States, more than 75 percent of children with cancer are now alive 5 years after diagnosis, compared with about 60 percent in the mid-1970s. Much of this dramatic improvement is due to the development of improved therapies at children's cancer centers, where the majority of children with cancer have their treatment.

---

[18] This section has been adapted from the NCI: **http://cis.nci.nih.gov/fact/1_21.htm**.

What Are Children's Cancer Centers?

Children's cancer centers are hospitals or units in hospitals that specialize in the diagnosis and treatment of cancer in children and adolescents. Most children's, or pediatric, cancer centers treat patients up to the age of 20.

Are There Standards for Children's Cancer Centers?

The following groups have established standards for children's cancer centers or programs:

- The National Cancer Institute (NCI)-sponsored Children's Oncology Group (COG), formerly known as the Children's Cancer Group (CCG) and the Pediatric Oncology Group (POG), is a network of children's cancer centers that meet strict quality assurance standards.
- The American Academy of Pediatrics (AAP) published Guidelines for the Pediatric Cancer Center and Role of such Centers in Diagnosis and Treatment in 1986 and 1997.
- The American Society of Pediatric Hematology/Oncology (ASPH/O) established standard requirements for programs treating children with cancer and blood disorders.

These groups agree that a childhood cancer center should be staffed by trained pediatric oncologists (doctors who specialize in childhood cancer) and other specialists who work as a team. Other members of the health professional team usually include pediatric surgeons, specialist surgeons (for instance neurosurgeons and urologic surgeons), radiation oncologists, pathologists, nurses, consulting pediatric specialists, psychiatrists, oncology social workers, nutritionists, and home health care professionals—all with expertise in treating children and adolescents with cancer. Together, these professionals offer comprehensive care.

What Are the Advantages of a Specialized Children's Cancer Center?

Because childhood cancer is relatively rare, it is important to seek treatment in centers that specialize in the treatment of children with cancer. Specialized cancer programs at comprehensive, multidisciplinary cancer centers follow established protocols (step-by-step guidelines for treatment). These protocols are carried out using a team approach. The team of health professionals is involved in designing the appropriate treatment and support program for the child and the child's family. In addition, these centers participate in specially designed and monitored research studies that help develop more effective treatments and address issues of long-term childhood cancer survival.

Can Children with Cancer Be Treated at the National Cancer Institute?

The Pediatric Oncology Branch (POB) of the National Cancer Institute conducts clinical trials for a wide variety of childhood cancers at the Warren Grant Magnuson Clinical Center, which is located at the National Institutes of Health in Bethesda, Maryland. There is no charge to patients for services provided at the Clinical Center.

Children, teenagers, and young adults with newly diagnosed or recurrent cancer (cancer that has come back) may be referred to the POB. To refer a patient with cancer, the patient's doctor should call the POB's toll-free number at 1-877-624-4878 between the hours of 8:30 a.m. and 5:00 p.m. and ask for the attending physician. The attending physician will discuss the case with the patient's doctor, determine whether the patient is eligibile for treatment at NCI, and help arrange the referral. The POB can also be reached at **http://www-dcs.nci.nih.gov/branches/pedonc/index.html** on the Internet.

POB attending physicians also are available to provide a second opinion about a patient. The patient, family, or physician can contact the POB to arrange for a second opinion. POB staff can offer assistance in cases where a diagnosis is difficult and also can aid in developing an appropriate treatment plan.

Finding a Children's Cancer Center

A family's pediatrician or family doctor often can provide a referral to a comprehensive children's cancer center. Families and health professionals also can call the NCI's Cancer Information Service (CIS) at 1-800-4-CANCER to learn about children's cancer centers that belong to the Children's Cancer Study Group and the Pediatric Oncology Group. All of the cancer centers that participate in these Groups have met strict standards of excellence for childhood cancer care.

Additional Cancer Support Information

In addition to the references above, the NCI has set up guidance Web sites that offers information on issues relating to cancer. These include:

- Facing Forward - A Guide for Cancer Survivors:
  http://www.cancer.gov/cancer_information/doc_img.aspx?viewid=cc93a843-6fc0-409e-8798-5c65afc172fe

- Taking Time: Support for People With Cancer and the People Who Care About Them:
  http://www.cancer.gov/cancer_information/doc_img.aspx?viewid=21a46445-a5c8-4fee-95a3-d9d0d665077a

- When Cancer Recurs: Meeting the Challenge:
  http://www.cancer.gov/cancer_information/doc_img.aspx?viewid=9e13d0d2-b7de-4bd6-87da-5750300a0dab

- Your Health Care Team: Your Doctor Is Only the Beginning:
  http://cis.nci.nih.gov/fact/8_10.htm

- When Someone in Your Family Has Cancer:
  http://www.cancer.gov/CancerInformation/whensomeoneinyourfamily

Vocabulary Builder

The following vocabulary builder provides definitions of words used in this chapter that have not been defined in previous chapters:

Bereavement: Refers to the whole process of grieving and mourning and is associated with a deep sense of loss and sadness. [NIH]

Cervical: Relating to the neck, or to the neck of any organ or structure. Cervical lymph nodes are located in the neck; cervical cancer refers to cancer of the uterine cervix, which is the lower, narrow end (the "neck") of the uterus. [NIH]

Charities: Social welfare organizations with programs designed to assist individuals in times of need. [NIH]

Curative: Tending to overcome disease and promote recovery. [EU]

Hematology: A subspecialty of internal medicine concerned with morphology, physiology, and pathology of the blood and blood-forming tissues. [NIH]

Mammography: The use of x-rays to create a picture of the breast. [NIH]

Neurosurgeon: A doctor who specializes in surgery on the brain, spine, and other parts of the nervous system. [NIH]

Oncologist: A doctor who specializes in treating cancer. Some oncologists specialize in a particular type of cancer treatment. For example, a radiation oncologist specializes in treating cancer with radiation. [NIH]

Palliative: 1. affording relief, but not cure. 2. an alleviating medicine. [EU]

Pathologist: A doctor who identifies diseases by studying cells and tissues under a microscope. [NIH]

Pediatrics: A medical specialty concerned with maintaining health and providing medical care to children from birth to adolescence. [NIH]

CHAPTER 3. CLINICAL TRIALS AND CHILDHOOD ACUTE LYMPHOBLASTIC LEUKEMIA

Overview

Very few medical conditions have a single treatment. The basic treatment guidelines that your child's physician has discussed with you, or those that you have found using the techniques discussed in Chapter 1, may provide you with all that you will require. For some patients, current treatments can be enhanced with new or innovative techniques currently under investigation. In this chapter, we will describe how clinical trials work and show you how to keep informed of trials concerning childhood acute lymphoblastic leukemia.

What Is a Clinical Trial?[19]

Clinical trials involve the participation of people in medical research. Most medical research begins with studies in test tubes and on animals. Treatments that show promise in these early studies may then be tried with people. The only sure way to find out whether a new treatment is safe, effective, and better than other treatments for childhood acute lymphoblastic leukemia is to try it on patients in a clinical trial.

---

[19] The discussion in this chapter has been adapted from the NIH and the NEI: www.nei.nih.gov/netrials/ctivr.htm.

What Kinds of Clinical Trials Are There?

Clinical trials are carried out in three phases:

- **Phase I.** Researchers first conduct Phase I trials with small numbers of patients and healthy volunteers. If the new treatment is a medication, researchers also try to determine how much of it can be given safely.
- **Phase II.** Researchers conduct Phase II trials in small numbers of patients to find out the effect of a new treatment on childhood acute lymphoblastic leukemia.
- **Phase III.** Finally, researchers conduct Phase III trials to find out how new treatments for childhood acute lymphoblastic leukemia compare with standard treatments already being used. Phase III trials also help to determine if new treatments have any side effects. These trials--which may involve hundreds, perhaps thousands, of people--can also compare new treatments with no treatment.

How Is a Clinical Trial Conducted?

Various organizations support clinical trials at medical centers, hospitals, universities, and doctors' offices across the United States. The "principal investigator" is the researcher in charge of the study at each facility participating in the clinical trial. Most clinical trial researchers are medical doctors, academic researchers, and specialists. The "clinic coordinator" knows all about how the study works and makes all the arrangements for your child's visits.

All doctors and researchers who take part in the study on childhood acute lymphoblastic leukemia carefully follow a detailed treatment plan called a protocol. This plan fully explains how the doctors will treat your child in the study. The "protocol" ensures that all patients are treated in the same way, no matter where they receive care.

Clinical trials are controlled. This means that researchers compare the effects of the new treatment with those of the standard treatment. In some cases, when no standard treatment exists, the new treatment is compared with no treatment. Patients who receive the new treatment are in the treatment group. Patients who receive a standard treatment or no treatment are in the "control" group. In some clinical trials, patients in the treatment group get a new medication while those in the control group get a placebo. A placebo is a harmless substance, a "dummy" pill, that has no effect on childhood acute lymphoblastic leukemia. In other clinical trials, where a new surgery or device (not a medicine) is being tested, patients in the control group may receive a "sham treatment." This treatment, like a placebo, has no effect on childhood acute lymphoblastic leukemia and will not harm your child.

Researchers assign patients "randomly" to the treatment or control group. This is like flipping a coin to decide which patients are in each group. If you choose to have your child participate in a clinical trial, you will not know which group he or she will be appointed to. The chance of any patient getting the new treatment is about 50 percent. You cannot request that your child receive the new treatment instead of the placebo or "sham" treatment. Often, you will not know until the study is over whether your child has been in the treatment group or the control group. This is called a "masked" study. In some trials, neither doctors nor patients know who is getting which treatment. This is called a "double masked" study. These types of trials help to ensure that the perceptions of the participants or doctors will not affect the study results.

Natural History Studies

Unlike clinical trials in which patient volunteers may receive new treatments, natural history studies provide important information to researchers on how childhood acute lymphoblastic leukemia develops over time. A natural history study follows patient volunteers to see how factors such as age, sex, race, or family history might make some people more or less at risk for childhood acute lymphoblastic leukemia. A natural history study may also tell researchers if diet, lifestyle, or occupation affects how a medical condition develops and progresses. Results from these studies provide information that helps answer questions such as: How fast will a medical condition usually progress? How bad will the condition become? Will treatment be needed?

What Is Expected of Your Child in a Clinical Trial?

Not everyone can take part in a clinical trial for a specific medical condition. Each study enrolls patients with certain features or eligibility criteria. These criteria may include the type and stage of the condition, as well as, the age and previous treatment history of the patient. You or your child's doctor can contact the sponsoring organization to find out more about specific clinical trials and their eligibility criteria. If you would like your child to participate in a clinical trial, your child's doctor must contact one of the trial's investigators and provide details about his or her diagnosis and medical history.

When participating in a clinical trial, your child may be required to have a number of medical tests. Your child may also need to take medications and/or undergo surgery. Depending upon the treatment and the examination procedure, your child may be required to receive inpatient hospital care. He or she may have to return to the medical facility for follow-up examinations. These exams help find out how well the treatment is working. Follow-up studies can take months or years. However, the success of the clinical trial often depends on learning what happens to patients over a long period of time. Only patients who continue to return for follow-up examinations can provide this important long-term information.

Recent Trials on Childhood Acute Lymphoblastic Leukemia

The National Institutes of Health and other organizations sponsor trials on various medical conditions. Because funding for research goes to the medical areas that show promising research opportunities, it is not possible for the NIH or others to sponsor clinical trials for every medical condition at all times. The following lists recent trials dedicated to childhood acute lymphoblastic leukemia.[20] If the trial listed by the NIH is still recruiting, your child may be eligible. If it is no longer recruiting or has been completed, then you can contact the sponsors to learn more about the study and, if published, the results. Further information on the trial is available at the Web site indicated. Please note that some trials may no longer be recruiting patients or are otherwise closed. Before contacting sponsors of a clinical trial, consult with your child's physician who can help you determine if your child might benefit from participation.

- **Chemotherapy Followed by Donor White Blood Cells Plus Interleukin-2 in Treating Patients With Acute Myeloid or Lymphocytic Leukemia**

  Condition(s): recurrent adult acute myeloid leukemia; recurrent childhood acute myeloid leukemia; recurrent adult acute lymphoblastic leukemia; recurrent childhood acute lymphoblastic leukemia

  Study Status: This study is currently recruiting patients.

  Sponsor(s): National Cancer Institute (NCI); Fred Hutchinson Cancer Research Center

  Purpose - Excerpt: RATIONALE: Drugs used in chemotherapy use different ways to stop cancer cells from dividing so they stop growing or

---

[20] These are listed at **www.ClinicalTrials.gov**.

die. Interleukin-2 may stimulate a person's white blood cells to kill leukemia cells. Treating donor white blood cells with interleukin-2 in the laboratory may help them kill more cancer cells. PURPOSE: Phase I/II trial to study the effectiveness of chemotherapy plus donor white blood cells treated with interleukin-2 in treating patients who have acute myeloid leukemia or acute lymphoid leukemia.

Phase(s): Phase I; Phase II

Study Type: Treatment

Contact(s): Washington; Fred Hutchinson Cancer Research Center, Seattle, Washington, 98109-1024, United States; Recruiting; Mary E. D. Flowers 206-667-6557. Study chairs or principal investigators: Mary E. D. Flowers, Study Chair; Fred Hutchinson Cancer Research Center

Web Site: http://clinicaltrials.gov/ct/gui/show/NCT00005802;jsessionid=88607F5B0637D034AB4D6A3C20254C79

- **Clofarabine in Treating Children With Acute Lymphoblastic Leukemia**

    Condition(s): L2 childhood acute lymphoblastic leukemia; non-T, non-B, cALLa negative childhood acute lymphoblastic leukemia; L1 childhood acute lymphoblastic leukemia; B-cell childhood acute lymphoblastic leukemia; non-T, non-B, cALLa positive, pre-B childhood acute lymphoblastic leukemia; TdT positive childhood acute lymphoblastic leukemia; T-cell childhood acute lymphoblastic leukemia; TdT negative childhood acute lymphoblastic leukemia; recurrent childhood acute lymphoblastic leukemia; L3 childhood acute lymphoblastic leukemia; non-T, non-B, cALLa positive childhood acute lymphoblastic leukemia

    Study Status: This study is currently recruiting patients.

    Sponsor(s): National Cancer Institute (NCI); Memorial Sloan-Kettering Cancer Center

    Purpose - Excerpt: RATIONALE: Drugs used in chemotherapy use different ways to stop cancer cells from dividing so they stop growing or die. PURPOSE: Phase II trial to study the effectiveness of clofarabine in treating children who have refractory or relapsed acute lymphoblastic leukemia.

    Phase(s): Phase II

    Study Type: Treatment

    Contact(s): California; Jonsson Comprehensive Cancer Center, UCLA, Los Angeles, California, 90095-1781, United States; Recruiting; Kathleen Sakamoto 310-825-6447; New York; Memorial Sloan-Kettering Cancer Center, New York, New York, 10021, United States; Recruiting; Peter G.

Steinherz 212-639-7951. Study chairs or principal investigators: Peter G. Steinherz, Study Chair; Memorial Sloan-Kettering Cancer Center

Web Site: http://clinicaltrials.gov/ct/gui/show/NCT00045656;jsessionid=88607F5B0637D034AB4D6A3C20254C79

- **Combination Chemotherapy and Bone Marrow Transplantation in Treating Infants With Newly Diagnosed Acute Lymphocytic Leukemia**

  Condition(s): acute undifferentiated leukemia; untreated childhood acute lymphoblastic leukemia

  Study Status: This study is currently recruiting patients.

  Sponsor(s): National Cancer Institute (NCI); Children's Oncology Group

  Purpose - Excerpt: RATIONALE: Drugs used in chemotherapy use different ways to stop cancer cells from dividing so they stop growing or die. Combining bone marrow transplantation with chemotherapy may allow the doctor to give higher doses of chemotherapy drugs and kill more cancer cells. PURPOSE: Phase II trial to study the effectiveness of combination chemotherapy and bone marrow transplantation in treating infants with newly diagnosed acute lymphocytic leukemia.

  Phase(s): Phase II

  Study Type: Treatment

  Contact(s): see Web site below

  Web Site: http://clinicaltrials.gov/ct/gui/show/NCT00002756;jsessionid=88607F5B0637D034AB4D6A3C20254C79

- **Combination Chemotherapy and Total-Body Irradiation Followed by Peripheral Stem Cell or Bone Marrow Transplantation in Treating Patients With Acute Lymphoblastic Leukemia**

  Condition(s): adult acute lymphoblastic leukemia in remission; childhood acute lymphoblastic leukemia in remission

  Study Status: This study is currently recruiting patients.

  Sponsor(s): National Cancer Institute (NCI); Fred Hutchinson Cancer Research Center

  Purpose - Excerpt: RATIONALE: Drugs used in chemotherapy use different ways to stop cancer cells from dividing so they stop growing or die. Peripheral stem cell transplantation may be able to replace immune cells that were destroyed by chemotherapy and radiation therapy. Sometimes the transplanted cells are rejected by the body's normal tissues. Mycophenolate mofetil and donor white blood cells may prevent this from happening. PURPOSE: Phase I/II trial to determine the effectiveness of combination chemotherapy and total-body irradiation followed by peripheral stem cell transplantation in treating patients who have acute lymphoblastic leukemia.

Phase(s): Phase I; Phase II

Study Type: Treatment

Contact(s): Washington; Fred Hutchinson Cancer Research Center, Seattle, Washington, 98109-1024, United States; Recruiting; Frederick R. Appelbaum 206-288-1024. Study chairs or principal investigators: Lyle Feinstein, Study Chair; Fred Hutchinson Cancer Research Center

Web Site: http://clinicaltrials.gov/ct/gui/show/NCT00027547;jsessionid=88607F5B0637D034AB4D6A3C20254C79

- **Combination Chemotherapy Followed by Peripheral Stem Cell Transplantation and Interleukin-2 in Treating Patients With Acute Leukemia**

    Condition(s): childhood acute myeloid leukemia in remission; adult acute lymphoblastic leukemia in remission; recurrent adult acute myeloid leukemia; adult acute myeloid leukemia in remission; recurrent childhood acute myeloid leukemia; recurrent adult acute lymphoblastic leukemia; secondary acute myeloid leukemia; recurrent childhood acute lymphoblastic leukemia; childhood acute lymphoblastic leukemia in remission

    Study Status: This study is currently recruiting patients.

    Sponsor(s): National Cancer Institute (NCI); Herbert Irving Comprehensive Cancer Center

    Purpose - Excerpt: RATIONALE: Drugs used in chemotherapy use different ways to stop cancer cells from dividing so they stop growing or die. Combining chemotherapy with peripheral stem cell transplantation may allow the doctor to give higher doses of chemotherapy drugs and kill more cancer cells. Interleukin-2 may stimulate a person's white blood cells to kill leukemia cells. PURPOSE: Phase II trial to study the effectiveness of combination chemotherapy followed by peripheral stem cell transplantation and interleukin-2 in treating patients who have acute leukemia.

    Phase(s): Phase II

    Study Type: Treatment

Contact(s): New York; Herbert Irving Comprehensive Cancer Center, New York, New York, 10032, United States; Recruiting; James H. Garvin, Jr. 212-305-9770. Study chairs or principal investigators: Charles S. Hesdorffer, Study Chair; Herbert Irving Comprehensive Cancer Center

Web Site: http://clinicaltrials.gov/ct/gui/show/NCT00008190;jsessionid=88607F5B0637D034AB4D6A3C20254C79

- **Combination Chemotherapy in Treating Children With Acute Lymphoblastic Leukemia**

  Condition(s): B-cell childhood acute lymphoblastic leukemia; childhood acute lymphoblastic leukemia in remission

  Study Status: This study is currently recruiting patients.

  Sponsor(s): National Cancer Institute (NCI); Pediatric Oncology Group

  Purpose - Excerpt: RATIONALE: Drugs used in chemotherapy use different ways to stop cancer cells from dividing so they stop growing or die. Combining more than one chemotherapy drug may kill more cancer cells. It is not yet known which combination chemotherapy regimen is more effective for acute lymphoblastic leukemia. PURPOSE: Phase III trial to determine the effectiveness of combination chemotherapy in treating children who have newly diagnosed acute lymphoblastic leukemia.

  Phase(s): Phase III

  Study Type: Treatment

  Contact(s): see Web site below

  Web Site: http://clinicaltrials.gov/ct/gui/show/NCT00005603;jsessionid=88607F5B0637D034AB4D6A3C20254C79

- **Combination Chemotherapy in Treating Children With Acute Lymphoblastic Leukemia, Osteosarcoma, or Non-Hodgkin's Lymphoma**

  Condition(s): recurrent childhood large cell lymphoma; recurrent childhood small noncleaved cell lymphoma; recurrent osteosarcoma; recurrent childhood lymphoblastic lymphoma; recurrent childhood acute lymphoblastic leukemia

  Study Status: This study is currently recruiting patients.

  Sponsor(s): Memorial Sloan-Kettering Cancer Center

Purpose - Excerpt: RATIONALE: Drugs used in chemotherapy use different ways to stop cancer cells from dividing so they stop growing or die. Combining more than one drug may kill more cancer cells. PURPOSE: Phase II trial to study the effectiveness of combination chemotherapy consisting of trimetrexate glucuronate plus leucovorin in treating children who have recurrent acute lymphoblastic leukemia, recurrent osteosarcoma, or refractory non-Hodgkin's lymphoma.

Phase(s): Phase II

Study Type: Treatment

Contact(s): New York; Memorial Sloan-Kettering Cancer Center, New York, New York, 10021, United States; Recruiting; Tanya Trippett 212-639-8267. Study chairs or principal investigators: Tanya Trippett, Study Chair; Memorial Sloan-Kettering Cancer Center

Web Site: http://clinicaltrials.gov/ct/gui/show/NCT00002738;jsessionid=88607F5B0637D034AB4D6A3C20254C79

- **Combination Chemotherapy in Treating Children With Newly Diagnosed Acute Lymphoblastic Leukemia**

  Condition(s): untreated childhood acute lymphoblastic leukemia

  Study Status: This study is currently recruiting patients.

  Sponsor(s): National Cancer Institute (NCI); Pediatric Oncology Group

  Purpose - Excerpt: RATIONALE: Drugs used in chemotherapy use different ways to stop cancer cells from dividing so they stop growing or die. Combining more than one drug may kill more cancer cells. It is not yet known which regimen of chemotherapy is more effective for acute lymphoblastic leukemia. PURPOSE: Randomized phase III trial to compare the effectiveness of four regimens of combination chemotherapy in treating children who have newly diagnosed acute lymphoblastic leukemia.

  Phase(s): Phase III

  Study Type: Treatment

  Contact(s): see Web site below

  Web Site: http://clinicaltrials.gov/ct/gui/show/NCT00005596;jsessionid=88607F5B0637D034AB4D6A3C20254C79

- **Combination Chemotherapy in Treating Patients With Newly Diagnosed Acute Lymphoblastic Leukemia**

    Condition(s): untreated childhood acute lymphoblastic leukemia; T-cell childhood acute lymphoblastic leukemia

    Study Status: This study is currently recruiting patients.

    Sponsor(s): National Cancer Institute (NCI); Children's Oncology Group

    Purpose - Excerpt: RATIONALE: Drugs used in chemotherapy use different ways to stop cancer cells from dividing so they stop growing or die. Combining more than one drug may kill more cancer cells. PURPOSE: Phase II trial to study the effectiveness of different combination chemotherapy regimens in treating patients who have newly diagnosed acute lymphoblastic leukemia.

    Phase(s): Phase II

    Study Type: Treatment

    Contact(s): see Web site below

    Web Site: http://clinicaltrials.gov/ct/gui/show/NCT00016302;jsessionid=88607F5B0637D034AB4D6A3C20254C79

- **Combination Chemotherapy in Treating Patients With Non-Hodgkin's Lymphoma or Acute Lymphocytic Leukemia**

    Condition(s): L3 adult acute lymphoblastic leukemia; stage IV adult diffuse small noncleaved cell/Burkitt's lymphoma; Burkitt's lymphoma; stage IV childhood small noncleaved cell lymphoma; B-cell childhood acute lymphoblastic leukemia; stage III adult diffuse small noncleaved cell/Burkitt's lymphoma; B-cell adult acute lymphoblastic leukemia; L3 childhood acute lymphoblastic leukemia; stage III childhood small noncleaved cell lymphoma

    Study Status: This study is currently recruiting patients.

    Sponsor(s): National Cancer Institute (NCI); Pediatric Oncology Group

    Purpose - Excerpt: RATIONALE: Drugs used in chemotherapy use different ways to stop cancer cells from dividing so they stop growing or die. Combining more than one drug may kill more cancer cells. PURPOSE: Phase II trial to study the effectiveness of combination chemotherapy in treating patients who have non-Hodgkin's lymphoma or acute lymphocytic leukemia.

    Phase(s): Phase III

    Study Type: Treatment

Contact(s): see Web site below

Web Site: http://clinicaltrials.gov/ct/gui/show/NCT00005977;jsessionid=88607F5B0637D034AB4D6A3C20254C79

- **Combination Chemotherapy Plus Steroid Therapy in Treating Children With Acute Lymphoblastic Leukemia or Lymphoblastic Non-Hodgkin's Lymphoma**

   Condition(s): L2 childhood acute lymphoblastic leukemia; untreated childhood acute lymphoblastic leukemia; stage III childhood lymphoblastic lymphoma; L1 childhood acute lymphoblastic leukemia; acute undifferentiated leukemia; B-cell childhood acute lymphoblastic leukemia; stage IV childhood lymphoblastic lymphoma; T-cell childhood acute lymphoblastic leukemia; stage I childhood lymphoblastic lymphoma; stage II childhood lymphoblastic lymphoma

   Study Status: This study is currently recruiting patients.

   Sponsor(s): EORTC Children's Leukemia Cooperative Group

   Purpose - Excerpt: RATIONALE: Drugs used in chemotherapy use different ways to stop tumor cells from dividing so they stop growing or die. Combining more than one drug may kill more tumor cells. It is not yet known which regimen of combination chemotherapy plus steroid therapy is more effective for acute lymphoblastic leukemia or lymphoblastic non-Hodgkin's lymphoma. PURPOSE: Randomized phase III trial to compare the effectiveness of different regimens of combination chemotherapy plus steroid therapy in treating children who have acute lymphoblastic leukemia or lymphoblastic non-Hodgkin's lymphoma.

   Phase(s): Phase III

   Study Type: Treatment

   Contact(s): see Web site below

   Web Site: http://clinicaltrials.gov/ct/gui/show/NCT00003728;jsessionid=88607F5B0637D034AB4D6A3C20254C79

- **Comparison of Different Combination Chemotherapy Regimens in Treating Children With Acute Lymphoblastic Leukemia**

   Condition(s): L2 childhood acute lymphoblastic leukemia; untreated childhood acute lymphoblastic leukemia; L1 childhood acute lymphoblastic leukemia

   Study Status: This study is currently recruiting patients.

Sponsor(s): National Cancer Institute (NCI); Children's Cancer Group

Purpose - Excerpt: RATIONALE: Drugs used in chemotherapy use different ways to stop cancer cells from dividing so they stop growing or die. Combining more than one drug may kill more cancer cells. It is not yet known which combination chemotherapy regimen is most effective for childhood acute lymphoblastic leukemia. PURPOSE: Randomized phase III trial to compare the effectiveness of different combination chemotherapy regimens in treating children who have acute lymphoblastic leukemia.

Phase(s): Phase III

Study Type: Treatment

Contact(s): see Web site below

Web Site: http://clinicaltrials.gov/ct/gui/show/NCT00005945;jsessionid=88607F5B0637D034AB4D6A3C20254C79

- **Comparison of Different Combination Chemotherapy Regimens in Treating Infants With Acute Lymphoblastic Leukemia**

  Condition(s): untreated childhood acute lymphoblastic leukemia; graft versus host disease

  Study Status: This study is currently recruiting patients.

  Sponsor(s): International Coordination Unit

  Purpose - Excerpt: RATIONALE: Drugs used in chemotherapy use different ways to stop cancer cells from dividing so they stop growing or die. Combining more than one drug may kill more cancer cells. It is not yet known which combination chemotherapy regimen is most effective for treating infants with acute lymphoblastic leukemia. PURPOSE: Randomized phase III trial to compare the effectiveness of different combination chemotherapy regimens in treating infants who have newly diagnosed acute lymphoblastic leukemia.

  Phase(s): Phase III

  Study Type: Treatment

  Contact(s): see Web site below

  Web Site: http://clinicaltrials.gov/ct/gui/show/NCT00015873;jsessionid=88607F5B0637D034AB4D6A3C20254C79

- **Diagnostic Study of Gene Alterations in Children Who Have Been Treated for Relapsed Acute Lymphocytic Leukemia**

    Condition(s): recurrent childhood acute lymphoblastic leukemia

    Study Status: This study is currently recruiting patients.

    Sponsor(s): National Cancer Institute (NCI); Children's Cancer Group

    Purpose - Excerpt: RATIONALE: Diagnostic procedures, such as genetic testing, may improve the ability to detect acute lymphocytic leukemia and determine the extent of disease. PURPOSE: Diagnostic study to try to detect changes in the genes of children who have been treated for relapsed acute lymphocytic leukemia.

    Study Type: Diagnostic

    Contact(s): see Web site below

    Web Site: http://clinicaltrials.gov/ct/gui/show/NCT00003933;jsessionid=88607F5B0637D034AB4D6A3C20254C79

- **Docetaxel in Treating Children With Relapsed or Refractory Leukemia**

    Condition(s): recurrent childhood acute myeloid leukemia; childhood acute promyelocytic leukemia (M3); recurrent childhood acute lymphoblastic leukemia

    Study Status: This study is currently recruiting patients.

    Sponsor(s): National Cancer Institute (NCI); Children's Oncology Group

    Purpose - Excerpt: RATIONALE: Drugs used in chemotherapy use different ways to stop cancer cells from dividing so they stop growing or die. PURPOSE: Phase II trial to study the effectiveness of docetaxel in treating children who have relapsed or refractory leukemia.

    Phase(s): Phase II

    Study Type: Treatment

    Contact(s): see Web site below

    Web Site: http://clinicaltrials.gov/ct/gui/show/NCT00021242;jsessionid=88607F5B0637D034AB4D6A3C20254C79

- **Donor Peripheral Stem Cell Transplantation in Treating Patients With Acute Lymphoblastic Leukemia**

    Condition(s): adult acute lymphoblastic leukemia in remission; childhood acute lymphoblastic leukemia in remission

Study Status: This study is currently recruiting patients.

Sponsor(s): National Cancer Institute (NCI); Fred Hutchinson Cancer Research Center

Purpose - Excerpt: RATIONALE: Peripheral stem cell transplantation may be able to replace immune cells that were destroyed by chemotherapy or radiation therapy. Sometimes the transplanted cells are rejected by the body's tissues. Mycophenolate mofetil, cyclosporine, and donor white blood cells may prevent this rejection. PURPOSE: Phase I/II trial to study the effectiveness of donor peripheral stem cell transplantation in treating patients who have acute lymphoblastic leukemia.

Phase(s): Phase I; Phase II

Study Type: Treatment

Contact(s): see Web site below

Web Site: http://clinicaltrials.gov/ct/gui/show/NCT00031655;jsessionid=88607F5B0637D034AB4D6A3C20254C79

- **Filgrastim-Treated Donor Peripheral Stem Cell Transplantation in Treating Patients With Acute Leukemia</p>**

    Condition(s): adult acute lymphoblastic leukemia in remission; recurrent adult acute myeloid leukemia; acute undifferentiated leukemia; recurrent childhood acute myeloid leukemia; recurrent adult acute lymphoblastic leukemia; secondary acute myeloid leukemia; recurrent childhood acute lymphoblastic leukemia; childhood acute lymphoblastic leukemia in remission

    Study Status: This study is currently recruiting patients.

    Sponsor(s): National Cancer Institute (NCI); Fred Hutchinson Cancer Research Center

    Purpose - Excerpt: RATIONALE: Transplanted peripheral stem cells can sometimes be rejected by the body's tissues. Treating donor peripheral stem cells with filgrastim may increase the number of donor white blood cells. This may help to decrease the rejection of the transplanted cells in patients receiving them as treatment for acute leukemia. PURPOSE: Phase II trial to study the effectiveness of filgrastim-treated donor peripheral stem cells in treating patients with acute leukemia who are undergoing peripheral stem cell transplantation.

    Phase(s): Phase II

    Study Type: Treatment

Contact(s): Washington; Fred Hutchinson Cancer Research Center, Seattle, Washington, 98109-1024, United States; Recruiting; Claudio Anasetti 206-667-7115. Study chairs or principal investigators: Claudio Anasetti, Study Chair; Fred Hutchinson Cancer Research Center

Web Site: http://clinicaltrials.gov/ct/gui/show/NCT00025545;jsessionid=88607F5B0637D034AB4D6A3C20254C79

- **Fludarabine and Total-Body Irradiation Followed By Donor Peripheral Stem Cell Transplantation in Treating Patients With Acute Lymphoblastic Leukemia or Chronic Myelogenous Leukemia That Has Responded to Treatment With Imatinib Mesylate**

    Condition(s): Philadelphia chromosome positive chronic myelogenous leukemia; recurrent adult acute lymphoblastic leukemia; recurrent childhood acute lymphoblastic leukemia; blastic phase chronic myelogenous leukemia

    Study Status: This study is currently recruiting patients.

    Sponsor(s): National Cancer Institute (NCI); Fred Hutchinson Cancer Research Center

    Purpose - Excerpt: RATIONALE: Imatinib mesylate may stop the growth of cancer cells by blocking the enzymes necessary for cancer cell growth. Peripheral stem cell transplantation may be able to replace immune cells that were destroyed by chemotherapy and radiation therapy used to kill cancer cells. Combining imatinib mesylate with fludarabine and total-body irradiation followed by donor peripheral stem cell transplantation may kill more cancer cells. PURPOSE: Phase II trial to study the effectiveness of fludarabine and total-body irradiation followed by donor peripheral stem cell transplantation in treating patients who have acute lymphoblastic leukemia or chronic myelogenous leukemia that has responded to previous treatment with imatinib mesylate.

    Phase(s): Phase II

    Study Type: Treatment

    Contact(s): see Web site below

    Web Site: http://clinicaltrials.gov/ct/gui/show/NCT00036738;jsessionid=88607F5B0637D034AB4D6A3C20254C79

- **Gemcitabine in Treating Children With Relapsed or Refractory Acute Lymphoblastic Leukemia or Acute Myelogenous Leukemia**

    Condition(s): recurrent childhood acute myeloid leukemia; recurrent childhood acute lymphoblastic leukemia

    Study Status: This study is currently recruiting patients.

    Sponsor(s): National Cancer Institute (NCI); Children's Oncology Group

    Purpose - Excerpt: RATIONALE: Drugs used in chemotherapy use different ways to stop tumor cells from dividing so they stop growing or die. PURPOSE: Phase II trial to study the effectiveness of gemcitabine in treating children who have relapsed or refractory acute lymphoblastic leukemia or acute myelogenous leukemia.

    Phase(s): Phase II

    Study Type: Treatment

    Contact(s): see Web site below

    Web Site: http://clinicaltrials.gov/ct/gui/show/NCT00006462;jsessionid=88607F5B0637D034AB4D6A3C20254C79

- **Gene Mutations in Children With Newly Diagnosed Acute Lymphoblastic Leukemia**

    Condition(s): untreated childhood acute lymphoblastic leukemia; B-cell childhood acute lymphoblastic leukemia; T-cell childhood acute lymphoblastic leukemia

    Study Status: This study is currently recruiting patients.

    Sponsor(s): National Cancer Institute (NCI); Children's Cancer Group

    Purpose - Excerpt: RATIONALE: The identification of gene mutations may allow doctors to better determine the prognosis of children with acute lymphoblastic leukemia. PURPOSE: Clinical trial to study the relationship between gene mutations and cancer prognosis in children with newly diagnosed acute lymphoblastic leukemia.

    Study Type: Diagnostic

    Contact(s): New Jersey; Saint Peter's University Hospital, New Brunswick, New Jersey, 08901-1780, United States; Recruiting; Lawrence J. Ettinger 732-745-6674; Australia, Western Australia; Division of Children's Leukaemia and Cancer Research, West Perth, Western Australia, 6872, Australia; Recruiting; Ursula Kees 618-9340-8827. Study chairs or principal investigators: Ursula Kees, Study Chair; Children's Cancer Group

Web Site: http://clinicaltrials.gov/ct/gui/show/NCT00003291;jsessionid=88607F5B0637D034AB4D6A3C20254C79

- **Hormone Therapy Plus Chemotherapy in Treating Children With Acute Lymphocytic Leukemia**

    Condition(s): untreated childhood acute lymphoblastic leukemia; recurrent childhood acute lymphoblastic leukemia

    Study Status: This study is currently recruiting patients.

    Sponsor(s): Medical Research Council

    Purpose - Excerpt: RATIONALE: Hormone therapy may stop the growth of cancer cells. Drugs used in chemotherapy use different ways to stop tumor cells from dividing so they stop growing or die. Combining hormone therapy with chemotherapy may kill more tumor cells. It is not yet known which hormone therapy and chemotherapy regimen is most effective for acute lymphocytic leukemia. PURPOSE: Randomized phase III trial to compare the effectiveness of different steroids and chemotherapy drugs in treating children who have acute lymphocytic leukemia.

    Phase(s): Phase III

    Study Type: Treatment

    Contact(s): United Kingdom, England; Oxford Radcliffe Hospital, Oxford, England, 0X3 9DU, United Kingdom; Recruiting; C. Mitchell +44 1865 221066. Study chairs or principal investigators: C. Mitchell, Study Chair; Medical Research Council

    Web Site: http://clinicaltrials.gov/ct/gui/show/NCT00003437;jsessionid=88607F5B0637D034AB4D6A3C20254C79

- **STI571 in Treating Patients With Recurrent Leukemia**

    Condition(s): relapsing chronic myelogenous leukemia; Philadelphia chromosome positive chronic myelogenous leukemia; recurrent childhood acute myeloid leukemia; recurrent childhood acute lymphoblastic leukemia

    Study Status: This study is currently recruiting patients.

    Sponsor(s): National Cancer Institute (NCI); Children's Cancer Group; Pediatric Oncology Group

    Purpose - Excerpt: RATIONALE: STI571 may interfere with the growth of cancer cells and may be an effective treatment for leukemia. PURPOSE:

Phase I trial to study the effectiveness of STI571 in treating patients who have recurrent leukemia.

Phase(s): Phase I

Study Type: Treatment

Contact(s): see Web site below

Web Site: http://clinicaltrials.gov/ct/gui/show/NCT00004932;jsessionid=88607F5B0637D034AB4D6A3C20254C79

- **TITLE:Less Intensive Therapy for Children With Non-Hodgkin's Lymphoma**

  Condition(s): stage IV childhood small noncleaved cell lymphoma; stage III childhood large cell lymphoma; stage IV childhood large cell lymphoma; untreated childhood acute lymphoblastic leukemia; stage I childhood large cell lymphoma; stage II childhood large cell lymphoma; Burkitt's lymphoma; stage I childhood small noncleaved cell lymphoma; stage II childhood small noncleaved cell lymphoma; L3 childhood acute lymphoblastic leukemia; stage III childhood small noncleaved cell lymphoma

  Study Status: This study is currently recruiting patients.

  Sponsor(s): National Cancer Institute (NCI); Societe Francaise Oncologie Pediatrique; United Kingdom Children's Cancer Study Group; Children's Cancer Group

  Purpose - Excerpt: RATIONALE: Less intensive therapy may attain in the same results as intensive therapy in children with non-Hodgkin's lymphoma. PURPOSE: Randomized phase III trial to study the effectiveness of less intensive therapy for children who have non-Hodgkin's lymphoma.

  Phase(s): Phase III

  Study Type: Treatment

  Contact(s): France; Institut Gustave Roussy, Villejuif, F-94805, France; Recruiting; Catherine Patte 33-1-42-11-41-80; United Kingdom, England; Children's Hospital - Sheffield, Sheffield, England, S10 2TH, United Kingdom; Recruiting; Mary P. Gerrard 00-44-0114-271-7229. Study chairs or principal investigators: W. Archie Bleyer, Study Chair; Children's Cancer Group; Catherine Patte, Study Chair; Mary P. Gerrard, Study Chair

Web Site: http://clinicaltrials.gov/ct/gui/show/NCT00002757;jsessionid=88607F5B0637D034AB4D6A3C20254C79

- **Total-Body Irradiation Plus Chemotherapy Followed By Donor Bone Marrow Transplantation in Treating Children With Hematologic Cancer**

    Condition(s): accelerated phase chronic myelogenous leukemia; recurrent childhood small noncleaved cell lymphoma; relapsing chronic myelogenous leukemia; childhood acute myeloid leukemia in remission; de novo myelodysplastic syndromes; chronic phase chronic myelogenous leukemia; recurrent childhood lymphoblastic lymphoma; recurrent childhood large cell lymphoma; secondary myelodysplastic syndromes; secondary acute myeloid leukemia; previously treated myelodysplastic syndromes; childhood acute lymphoblastic leukemia in remission

    Study Status: This study is currently recruiting patients.

    Sponsor(s): National Cancer Institute (NCI); Memorial Sloan-Kettering Cancer Center

    Purpose - Excerpt: RATIONALE: Radiation therapy uses high-energy x-rays to damage cancer cells. Drugs used in chemotherapy use different ways to stop cancer cells from dividing so they stop growing or die. Bone marrow transplantation may be able to replace immune cells that were destroyed by chemotherapy and radiation therapy used to kill cancer cells. Sometimes the transplanted cells from a donor can make an immune response against the body's normal cells. Eliminating the T cells from the donor cells before transplanting them may prevent this from happening. PURPOSE: Phase II trial to study the effectiveness of total-body irradiation and chemotherapy followed by T-cell depleted donor bone marrow transplantation in treating children who have hematologic cancer.

    Phase(s): Phase II

    Study Type: Treatment

    Contact(s): New York; Memorial Sloan-Kettering Cancer Center, New York, New York, 10021, United States; Recruiting; Nancy A. Kernan 212-639-7250. Study chairs or principal investigators: Nancy A. Kernan, Study Chair; Memorial Sloan-Kettering Cancer Center

    Web Site: http://clinicaltrials.gov/ct/gui/show/NCT00028730;jsessionid=88607F5B0637D034AB4D6A3C20254C79

- **Vaccine Therapy in Preventing Flu in Children With Acute Lymphoblastic Leukemia**

  Condition(s): infection; childhood acute lymphoblastic leukemia in remission

  Study Status: This study is currently recruiting patients.

  Sponsor(s): National Cancer Institute (NCI); Roswell Park Cancer Institute

  Purpose - Excerpt: RATIONALE: Flu vaccine may help the body build an immune response and decrease the occurrence of flu in children who are receiving chemotherapy for acute lymphoblastic leukemia. PURPOSE: Clinical trial to study the effectiveness of vaccine therapy in preventing flu in children who have acute lymphoblastic leukemia.

  Study Type: Supportive Care

  Contact(s): New Jersey; Hackensack University Medical Center, Hackensack, New Jersey, 07601, United States; Recruiting; Burton Eloit Appel 201-996-5437; New York; Roswell Park Cancer Institute, Buffalo, New York, 14263-0001, United States; Recruiting; Martin L. Brecher 716-845-2333. Study chairs or principal investigators: Martin L. Brecher, Study Chair; Roswell Park Cancer Institute

  Web Site: http://clinicaltrials.gov/ct/gui/show/NCT00022035;jsessionid=88607F5B0637D034AB4D6A3C20254C79

- **Vaccine Therapy in Treating Patients With Acute Lymphoblastic Leukemia**

  Condition(s): B-cell childhood acute lymphoblastic leukemia; recurrent adult acute lymphoblastic leukemia; recurrent childhood acute lymphoblastic leukemia; B-cell adult acute lymphoblastic leukemia

  Study Status: This study is currently recruiting patients.

  Sponsor(s): National Cancer Institute (NCI); Dana-Farber/Harvard Cancer Center

  Purpose - Excerpt: RATIONALE: Vaccines made from cancer cells may make the body build an immune response to kill cancer cells. PURPOSE: Phase I trial to study the effectiveness of vaccine therapy in treating patients who have acute lymphoblastic leukemia.

  Phase(s): Phase I

  Study Type: Treatment

  Contact(s): Massachusetts; Dana-Farber Cancer Institute, Boston, Massachusetts, 02115, United States; Recruiting; Daniel DeAngelo 617-

632-2645; Massachusetts General Hospital Cancer Center, Boston, Massachusetts, 02114, United States; Recruiting; Philip Crawford Amrein 617-726-8748. Study chairs or principal investigators: W. Nicholas Haining, Study Chair; Dana-Farber/Harvard Cancer Center

Web Site: http://clinicaltrials.gov/ct/gui/show/NCT00020670;jsessionid=88607F5B0637D034AB4D6A3C20254C79

- **Combination Chemotherapy With or Without Donor Bone Marrow Transplantation in Treating Infants With Previously Untreated Acute Lymphoblastic Leukemia**

  Condition(s): L2 childhood acute lymphoblastic leukemia; untreated childhood acute lymphoblastic leukemia; L1 childhood acute lymphoblastic leukemia; acute undifferentiated leukemia

  Study Status: This study is not yet open for patient recruitment.

  Sponsor(s): National Cancer Institute (NCI); Children's Oncology Group

  Purpose - Excerpt: RATIONALE: Drugs used in chemotherapy use different ways to stop cancer cells from dividing so they stop growing or die. Giving the drugs in different combinations may kill more cancer cells. Bone marrow transplantation allows the doctor to give higher doses of chemotherapy and kill more cancer cells. PURPOSE: Phase II trial to compare the effectiveness of combination chemotherapy with or without donor bone marrow transplantation in treating infants who have previously untreated acute lymphoblastic leukemia.

  Phase(s): Phase II

  Study Type: Treatment

  Contact(s): Gregory H. Reaman 202-884-2147. Study chairs or principal investigators: Gregory H. Reaman, Study Chair; Children's Oncology Group

  Web Site: http://clinicaltrials.gov/ct/gui/show/NCT00022126;jsessionid=88607F5B0637D034AB4D6A3C20254C79

- **Combination Chemotherapy With or Without Peripheral Stem Cell Transplantation in Treating Children With Acute Lymphoblastic Leukemia**

  Condition(s): recurrent childhood acute lymphoblastic leukemia; childhood acute lymphoblastic leukemia in remission

  Study Status: This study is not yet open for patient recruitment.

Sponsor(s): National Cancer Institute (NCI); Children's Oncology Group

Purpose - Excerpt: RATIONALE: Drugs used in chemotherapy use different ways to stop tumor cells from dividing so they stop growing or die. Peripheral stem cell transplantation may allow the doctor to give higher doses of chemotherapy drugs and kill more cancer cells. PURPOSE: Phase II pilot study to determine the effectiveness of combination chemotherapy with or without donor peripheral stem cell transplantation in treating children who have acute lymphoblastic leukemia.

Phase(s): Phase II

Study Type: Treatment

Contact(s): Gregory H. Reaman 202-884-2147. Study chairs or principal investigators: Gregory H. Reaman, Study Chair; Children's Oncology Group

Web Site: http://clinicaltrials.gov/ct/gui/show/NCT00022737;jsessionid=88607F5B0637D034AB4D6A3C20254C79

- **Decitabine in Treating Children With Relapsed or Refractory Acute Myeloid Leukemia or Acute Lymphoblastic Leukemia**

  Condition(s): recurrent childhood acute myeloid leukemia; childhood acute promyelocytic leukemia (M3); secondary acute myeloid leukemia; recurrent childhood acute lymphoblastic leukemia; childhood acute myeloblastic leukemia with maturation (M2)

  Study Status: This study is not yet open for patient recruitment.

  Sponsor(s): National Cancer Institute (NCI); Children's Oncology Group

  Purpose - Excerpt: RATIONALE: Drugs used in chemotherapy use different ways to stop tumor cells from dividing so they stop growing or die. PURPOSE: Phase I trial to study the effectiveness of decitabine in treating children who have relapsed or refractory acute myeloid leukemia or acute lymphoblastic leukemia.

  Phase(s): Phase I

  Study Type: Treatment

  Contact(s): Gregory H. Reaman 202-884-2147. Study chairs or principal investigators: Gregory H. Reaman, Study Chair; Children's Oncology Group

  Web Site: http://clinicaltrials.gov/ct/gui/show/NCT00042796;jsessionid=88607F5B0637D034AB4D6A3C20254C79

Benefits and Risks[21]

What Are the Benefits of Participating in a Clinical Trial?

If you are considering a clinical trial, it is important to realize that your child's participation can bring many benefits:

- A new treatment could be more effective than the current treatment for childhood acute lymphoblastic leukemia. Although only half of the participants in a clinical trial receive the experimental treatment, if the new treatment is proved to be more effective and safer than the current treatment, then those patients who did not receive the new treatment during the clinical trial may be among the first to benefit from it when the study is over.
- If the treatment is effective, then it may improve your child's health.
- Clinical trial patients receive the highest quality of medical care. Experts watch them closely during the study and may continue to follow them after the study is over.
- People who take part in trials contribute to scientific discoveries that may help others with childhood acute lymphoblastic leukemia. In cases where certain medical conditions run in families, your child's participation may lead to better care or prevention for you and other family members.

The Informed Consent

Once you agree to have your child take part in a clinical trial, you will be asked to sign an "informed consent." This document explains a clinical trial's risks and benefits, the researcher's expectations of you and your child, and your child's rights as a patient.

What Are the Risks?

Clinical trials may involve risks as well as benefits. Whether or not a new treatment will work cannot be known ahead of time. There is always a chance that a new treatment may not work better than a standard treatment. There is also the possibility that it may be harmful. The treatment your child

---

[21] This section has been adapted from ClinicalTrials.gov, a service of the National Institutes of Health:
http://www.clinicaltrials.gov/ct/gui/c/a1r/info/whatis?JServSessionIdzone_ct=9jmun6f291.

receives may cause side effects that are serious enough to require medical attention.

How Is Your Child's Safety Protected?

Clinical trials can raise fears of the unknown. Understanding the safeguards that protect your child can ease some of these fears. Before a clinical trial begins, researchers must get approval from their hospital's Institutional Review Board (IRB), an advisory group that makes sure a clinical trial is designed to protect your child's safety. During a clinical trial, doctors will closely watch your child to see if the treatment is working and if he or she is experiencing any side effects. All the results are carefully recorded and reviewed. In many cases, experts from the Data and Safety Monitoring Committee carefully monitor each clinical trial and can recommend that a study be stopped at any time. Your child will only be asked to participate in a clinical trial as a volunteer with your informed consent.

What Are Your Child's Rights in a Clinical Trial?

If your child is eligible for a clinical trial, you will be given information to help you decide whether or not you want him or her to participate. You and your child have the right to:

- Information on all known risks and benefits of the treatments in the study.
- Know how the researchers plan to carry out the study, for how long, and where.
- Know what is expected of your child.
- Know any costs involved for you or your child's insurance provider.
- Know before any of your child's medical or personal information is shared with other researchers involved in the clinical trial.
- Talk openly with doctors and ask any questions.

After your child joins a clinical trial, you and your child have the right to:

- Leave the study at any time. Participation is strictly voluntary.
- Receive any new information about the new treatment.
- Continue to ask questions and get answers.
- Maintain your child's privacy. Your child's name will not appear in any reports based on the study.

- Know whether your child participated in the treatment group or the control group (once the study has been completed).

What Questions Should You Ask before Your Child Participates in a Clinical Trial?

Questions you should ask when deciding whether or not to enroll your child in a clinical trial include the following:

- What is the purpose of the clinical trial?
- What are the standard treatments for childhood acute lymphoblastic leukemia? Why do researchers think the new treatment may be better? What is likely to happen to my child with or without the new treatment?
- What tests and treatments will my child need? Will my child need surgery? Medication? Hospitalization?
- How long will the treatment last? How often will my child have to come back for follow-up exams?
- What are the treatment's possible benefits to my child's condition? What are the short- and long-term risks? What are the possible side effects?
- Will the treatment be uncomfortable? Will it make my child sick? If so, for how long?
- How will my child's health be monitored?
- Where will my child need to go for the clinical trial?
- How much will it cost to participate in the study? What costs are covered by the study? How much will my child's health insurance cover?
- Who will be in charge of my child's care?
- Will taking part in the study affect my child's daily life?
- How does my child feel about taking part in a clinical trial? Will other family members benefit from my child's contributions to new medical knowledge?

Clinical Trials and Insurance Coverage[22]

As you consider enrolling your child in a clinical trial, you will face the critical issue of how to cover the costs of care. Even if you have health

---

[22] Adapted from the NCI:
http://www.cancer.gov/clinical_trials/doc_header.aspx?viewid=1d92be79-8748-4bda-8005-2a56d332463b.

insurance, your coverage may not include some or all of the patient care costs associated with a clinical trial. This is because some health plans define clinical trials as "experimental" or "investigational" procedures.

Because lack of coverage for these costs can keep prospective participants from enrolling in trials, the National Cancer Institute is working with major health plans and managed care groups to find solutions. In the meantime, there are strategies that may help you deal with cost and coverage barriers. This section answers frequently asked questions about insurance coverage for clinical trial participation and directs you to additional information resources.

The material here is mainly concerned with treatment clinical trials, since other types of trials (prevention, screening, etc.) are newer and generally not covered by health insurance at all. However, this guide may become more relevant for prevention and other types of trials as these trials grow more common.

If you do not have any health insurance, you may find this section helpful for understanding some of the costs that trials involve.

What Costs Do Trials Involve? Who Is Usually Responsible for Paying Them?

There are two types of costs associated with a trial: patient care costs and research costs. Patient care costs fall into two categories:

- Usual care costs, such as doctor visits, hospital stays, clinical laboratory tests, x-rays, etc., which occur whether you are participating in a trial or receiving standard treatment. These costs have usually been covered by a third-party health plan, such as Medicare or private insurance.

- Extra care costs associated with clinical trial participation, such as the additional tests that may or may not be fully covered by the clinical trial sponsor and/or research institution.

The sponsor and the participant's health plan need to resolve coverage of these costs for particular trials.

Research costs are those associated with conducting the trial, such as data collection and management, research physician and nurse time, analysis of results, and tests purely performed for research purposes. Such costs are usually covered by the sponsoring organization, such as NCI or a pharmaceutical company.

Criteria Used by Health Plans to Make Reimbursement Decisions about Trials

Health insurance companies and managed care companies decide which health care services they will pay for by developing coverage policy regarding the specific services. In general, the most important factor determining whether something is covered is a health plan's judgment as to whether the service is established or investigational. Health plans usually designate a service as established if there is a certain amount of scientific data to show that it is safe and effective. If the health plan does not think that such data exist in sufficient quantity, the plan may label the service as investigational.

Health care services delivered within the setting of a clinical trial are very often categorized as investigational and not covered. This is because the health plan thinks that the major reason to perform the clinical trial is that there is not enough data to establish the safety and effectiveness of the service being studied. Thus, for some health plans, any mention of the fact that your child is involved in a clinical trial results in a denial of payment.

Your health plan may define specific criteria that a trial must meet before extending coverage, such as the following:

Sponsorship

Some plans may only cover costs of trials sponsored by organizations whose review and oversight of the trial is careful and scientifically rigorous, according to standards set by the health plan.

Trial Phase and Type

Some plans may cover patient care costs only for the clinical trials they judge to be "medically necessary" on a case-by-case basis. Trial phase may also affect coverage; for example, while a plan may be willing to cover costs associated with Phase III trials, which include treatments that have already been successful with a certain number of people, the plan may require some documentation of effectiveness before covering a Phase I or II trial.

While health plans are interested in efforts to improve prevention and screening, they currently seem less likely to have a review process in place for these trials. Therefore, it may be more difficult to get coverage for the care costs associated with them.

Some plans, especially smaller ones, will not cover any costs associated with a clinical trial. Policies vary widely, but in most cases your best bet is to have your child's doctor initiate discussions with the health plan.

Cost "Neutrality"

Some health plans may limit coverage to trials they consider cost-neutral (i.e., not significantly more expensive than the treatments considered standard).

Lack of Standard Therapy

Some plans limit coverage of trials to situations in which no standard therapy is available.

Facility and Personnel Qualifications

A health plan may require that the facility and medical staff meet specific qualifications to conduct a trial involving unique services, especially intensive therapy such as a bone marrow transplant (high-dose chemotherapy with bone marrow/ stem cell rescue).

Increasing the Likelihood of Insurance Coverage for Trials[23]

There are several steps you can follow to deal with coverage issues up front when deciding to enroll your child in a clinical trial. Along the way, enlist the help of family members and your child's doctor or other health professionals. You may find the following checklist useful:

---

[23] This section has been adapted from the NCI:
http://www.cancer.gov/clinical_trials/doc_header.aspx?viewid=1d92be79-8748-4bda-8005-2a56d332463b&docid=0df4397a-eccb-465f-bd33-a89e7a708c46.

Understand the Costs Associated with the Trial

Ask your child's doctor or the trial's contact person about the costs that must be covered by you or your health plan. Are these costs significantly higher than those associated with standard care? Also, inquire about the experience of other patients in the trial. Have their plans paid for their care? Have there been any persistent problems with coverage? How often have the trial's administrators been successful in getting plans to cover patient care costs?

Understand Your Health Plan

Be sure you know what's in your policy; request and carefully review the actual contract language. If there's a specific exclusion for "experimental treatment," look closely at the policy to see how the plan defines such treatment and under what conditions it might be covered. If it is not clearly defined, call the plan's customer service line, consult their Web site, and/or write to them. Ask for specific information about clinical trials coverage.

Work Closely with Your Child's Doctor

Talk with the doctor about the paperwork he or she submits to your health plan. If there have been problems with coverage in the past, you might ask the doctor or the hospital to send an information package to the plan that includes studies supporting the procedure's safety, benefits, and medical appropriateness. This package might include:

- Publications from peer-reviewed literature about the proposed therapy that demonstrate patient benefits;
- A letter that uses the insurance contract's own language to explain why the treatment, screening method, or preventive measure should be covered;
- Letters from researchers that explain the clinical trial;
- Support letters from patient advocacy groups.

Be sure to keep your own copy of any materials that the doctor sends to your health plan for future reference.

Work Closely with Your Company's Benefits Manager

This person may be helpful in enlisting the support of your employer to request coverage for your child by the health plan.

Give Your Health Plan a Deadline

Ask the hospital or cancer center to set a target date for the therapy. This will help to ensure that coverage decisions are made promptly.

Know Your Child's Rights[24]

A number of state governments are addressing the question of whether insurance companies ought to cover the costs associated with patients' participation in clinical trials. Lack of such coverage is a significant barrier to many patients who might otherwise benefit from enrolling in a trial. Lack of coverage also makes it harder for researchers to successfully conduct trials that could improve prevention and treatment options. Information on State initiatives and legislation concerning cancer-related clinical trials is available at **http://www.cancer.gov/ClinicalTrials/insurancelaws**. By conducting your own research and learning about your child's rights, you may increase the likelihood that your insurance company will cover the costs of a trial.

If Your Insurance Claim Is Denied after the Trial Has Begun

If a claim is denied, read your policy to find out what steps you can follow to make an appeal. In "What Cancer Survivors Need to Know about Health Insurance", the National Coalition for Cancer Survivorship suggests that you and your doctor demonstrate to the health plan that:

- The therapy in the trial is not just a research study, but also a valid procedure that benefits patients;
- Your child's situation is similar to that of other patients who are participating in clinical trials as part of a covered benefit;
- Possible complications have been anticipated and can be handled effectively.

---

[24] Adapted from Cancer.gov: **http://www.cancer.gov/ClinicalTrials/insurancelaws**.

You also may wish to contact your state insurance counseling hotline or insurance department for more help, or write your state insurance commissioner describing the problem.

Where Else Can I Turn for Assistance?

It's never easy to deal with financial issues when a loved one faces cancer. Unfortunately, costs can present a significant barrier to clinical trials participation. The range of insurance issues and health plan contracts makes it impossible to deal with all of them here. You may wish to consult this partial list of publications, organizations, and Web sites for more information:

Publications

What Cancer Survivors Need to Know about Health Insurance
National Coalition of Cancer Survivorship
1010 Wayne Avenue, 5th floor
Silver Spring, MD 20910
(301) 650-8868
http://www.cansearch.org/

Cancer Treatments Your Insurance Should Cover
The Association of Community Cancer Centers
11600 Nebel Street, Suite 201
Rockville, MD 20852
(301) 984-9496
http://www.accc-cancer.org/main2001.shtml

The Managed Care Answer Guide
Patient Advocate Foundation
739 Thimble Shoals Boulevard, Suite 704
Newport News, VA 23606
(757) 873-6668
E-mail: **ndepaf@pinn.net**

1998 Guide to Health Insurance for People with Medicare, The Medicare Handbook
Medicare Helpline: 1-800-444-4606
Health Care Financing Administration: **http://www.hcfa.gov/**
New Medicare site: **http://www.medicare.gov/**

Assistance Programs

Candlelighters Childhood Cancer Foundation
Ombudsman Program
910 Woodmont Avenue, #4607
Bethesda, MD 20814
(301) 657-8401; 1-800-366-2223 (toll-free)
E-mail: **info@candlelighters.org**
http://www.candlelighters.org
The Ombudsman Program helps families of children with cancer and survivors of childhood cancer resolve a range of problems, including insurance coverage difficulties. Local groups appoint a Parent Advocate who works with the treatment center on behalf of families.

Medical Care Management Corporation
5272 River Road, Suite 650
Bethesda, MD 20816-1405
(301) 652-1818
email: mcman@mcman.com
http://www.mcman.com/
Working for a range of clients, including health plans, employers, and patients, MCMC conducts independent, objective reviews of high-technology medical care cases to assist in decision-making. While it does charge for its services, MCMC also offers a volunteer program for those who cannot afford to pay.

More Information Resources

OncoLink
A service of the University of Pennsylvania Cancer Center.
http://www.oncolink.com/
In addition to general cancer information, this web site features a section on financial information for patients. Among the topics: viatical settlements, life insurance, a glossary of financial and medical terms, and news about billing and insurance.

American Association of Health Plans
1129 20th Street, NW, Suite 600
Washington, DC 20036-3421
(202) 778-3200
http://www.aahp.org/
The Web site section "For Consumers" includes a fact sheet on clinical research that describes various health plans' efforts to support research initiatives and collaborate with academic health centers and universities.

Health Insurance Association of America
555 13th Street, NW
Washington, DC 20004
(202) 824-1600

- Home page: **http://www.hiaa.org/**

- Consumer Information: **http://www.hiaa.org/consumer/**

- Insurance Counseling Hotlines by State:
  http://www.hiaa.org/consumer/insurance_counsel.cfm

- State Insurance Departments:
  http://www.hiaa.org/consumer/state_insurance.cfm

Government Initiatives to Expand Insurance Coverage for Trials[25]

The good news is that there has been a recent effort in the U.S. to assure clinical trials coverage, with NCI involved in several new initiatives as described below:

NCI-Department of Defense Agreement

An innovative 1996 agreement between NCI and the Department of Defense (DoD) has given thousands of DoD cancer patients more options for care and greater access to state-of-the-art treatments. Patients who are beneficiaries of TRICARE/CHAMPUS, the DoD's health program, are covered for NCI-sponsored Phase II and Phase III clinical treatment trials. NCI and DoD are refining a system that allows physicians and patients to determine quickly what current trials meet their needs and where they are taking place.

---

[25] Adapted from the NCI:
http://www.cancer.gov/clinical_trials/doc_header.aspx?viewid=1d92be79-8748-4bda-8005-2a56d332463b&docid=d8092601-daf9-4794-8536-3be2712eb6b9.

NCI-Department of Veterans Affairs Agreement

A 1997 agreement with the Department of Veterans Affairs provides coverage for eligible veterans of the armed services to participate in NCI-sponsored prevention, diagnosis, and treatment studies nationwide. For additional information, see the VA/DoD Beneficiaries Digest Page at **http://www.va.gov/cancer.htm**.

Midwest Health Plans Agreement

Some NCI Cooperative Groups have reached agreements with several insurers in Wisconsin and Minnesota to provide more than 200,000 people with coverage. The coverage is designated for patient care costs if they participate in a cooperative group-sponsored trial.

Pediatric Cancer Care Network

This network, a cooperative agreement among the Children's Cancer Group, the Pediatric Oncology Group, and the Blue Cross Blue Shield System Association (BCBS) nationwide, will ensure that children of BCBS subscribers receive care at designated centers of cancer care excellence and may promote the enrollment of children in Cooperative Group clinical trials.

Keeping Current on Clinical Trials

Various government agencies maintain databases on trials. The U.S. National Institutes of Health, through the National Library of Medicine, has developed ClinicalTrials.gov to provide the public and physicians with current information about clinical research across the broadest number of medical conditions.

The site was launched in February 2000 and currently contains approximately 5,700 clinical studies in over 59,000 locations worldwide, with most studies being conducted in the United States. ClinicalTrials.gov receives about 2 million hits per month and hosts approximately 5,400 visitors daily. To access this database, simply go to their Web site (**www.clinicaltrials.gov**) and search by "childhood acute lymphoblastic leukemia" (or synonyms).

While ClinicalTrials.gov is the most comprehensive listing of NIH-supported clinical trials available, not all trials are in the database. The database is updated regularly, so clinical trials are continually being added. The following is a list of specialty databases affiliated with the National Institutes of Health that offer additional information on trials:

- For clinical studies at the Warren Grant Magnuson Clinical Center located in Bethesda, Maryland, visit their Web site:
  http://clinicalstudies.info.nih.gov/

- For clinical studies conducted at the Bayview Campus in Baltimore, Maryland, visit their Web site:
  http://www.jhbmc.jhu.edu/studies/index.html

- For cancer trials, visit the National Cancer Institute:
  http://cancertrials.nci.nih.gov/

General References

The following references describe clinical trials and experimental medical research. They have been selected to ensure that they are likely to be available from your local or online bookseller or university medical library. These references are usually written for healthcare professionals, so you may consider consulting with a librarian or bookseller who might recommend a particular reference. The following includes some of the most readily available references (sorted alphabetically by title; hyperlinks provide rankings, information and reviews at Amazon.com):

- **A Guide to Patient Recruitment: Today's Best Practices & Proven Strategies** by Diana L. Anderson; Paperback - 350 pages (2001), CenterWatch, Inc.; ISBN: 1930624115;
  http://www.amazon.com/exec/obidos/ASIN/1930624115/icongroupinterna

- **A Step-By-Step Guide to Clinical Trials** by Marilyn Mulay, R.N., M.S., OCN; Spiral-bound - 143 pages Spiral edition (2001), Jones & Bartlett Pub; ISBN: 0763715697;
  http://www.amazon.com/exec/obidos/ASIN/0763715697/icongroupinterna

- **The CenterWatch Directory of Drugs in Clinical Trials** by CenterWatch; Paperback - 656 pages (2000), CenterWatch, Inc.; ISBN: 0967302935;
  http://www.amazon.com/exec/obidos/ASIN/0967302935/icongroupinterna

- **The Complete Guide to Informed Consent in Clinical Trials** by Terry Hartnett (Editor); Paperback - 164 pages (2000), PharmSource Information Services, Inc.; ISBN: 0970153309;
  http://www.amazon.com/exec/obidos/ASIN/0970153309/icongroupinterna

- **Dictionary for Clinical Trials** by Simon Day; Paperback - 228 pages (1999), John Wiley & Sons; ISBN: 0471985961;
  http://www.amazon.com/exec/obidos/ASIN/0471985961/icongroupinterna
- **Extending Medicare Reimbursement in Clinical Trials** by Institute of Medicine Staff (Editor), et al; Paperback 1st edition (2000), National Academy Press; ISBN: 0309068886;
  http://www.amazon.com/exec/obidos/ASIN/0309068886/icongroupinterna
- **Handbook of Clinical Trials** by Marcus Flather (Editor); Paperback (2001), Remedica Pub Ltd; ISBN: 1901346293;
  http://www.amazon.com/exec/obidos/ASIN/1901346293/icongroupinterna

Vocabulary Builder

The following vocabulary builder gives definitions of words used in this chapter that have not been defined in previous chapters:

506U78: An anticancer drug that belongs to the family of drugs called antimetabolites. [NIH]

Chromosome: Part of a cell that contains genetic information. Except for sperm and eggs, all human cells contain 46 chromosomes. [NIH]

Cyclosporine: A drug used to help reduce the risk of rejection of organ and bone marrow transplants by the body. It is also used in clinical trials to make cancer cells more sensitive to anticancer drugs. [NIH]

Decitabine: An anticancer drug that belongs to the family of drugs called antimetabolites. [NIH]

Docetaxel: An anticancer drug that belongs to the family of drugs called mitotic inhibitors. [NIH]

Enzyme: A protein that speeds up chemical reactions in the body. [NIH]

Filgrastim: A colony-stimulating factor that stimulates the production of neutrophils (a type of white blood cell). It is a cytokine that belongs to the family of drugs called hematopoietic (blood-forming) agents. Also called granulocyte colony-stimulating factor (G-CSF). [NIH]

Fludarabine: An anticancer drug that belongs to the family of drugs called antimetabolites. [NIH]

Gemcitabine: An anticancer drug that belongs to the family of drugs called antimetabolites. [NIH]

Graft: Healthy skin, bone, or other tissue taken from one part of the body and used to replace diseased or injured tissue removed from another part of the body. [NIH]

Leucovorin: A drug used to protect normal cells from high doses of the anticancer drug methotrexate. It is also used to increase the antitumor effects of fluorouracil and tegafur-uracil, an oral treatment alternative to intravenous fluorouracil. [NIH]

Leukaemia: An acute or chronic disease of unknown cause in man and other warm-blooded animals that involves the blood-forming organs, is characterized by an abnormal increase in the number of leucocytes in the tissues of the body with or without a corresponding increase of those in the circulating blood, and is classified according of the type leucocyte most prominently involved. [EU]

Lymphoid: Referring to lymphocytes, a type of white blood cell. Also refers to tissue in which lymphocytes develop. [NIH]

Osteosarcoma: A cancer of the bone that affects primarily children and adolescents. Also called osteogenic sarcoma. [NIH]

Randomized: Describes an experiment or clinical trial in which animal or human subjects are assigned by chance to separate groups that compare different treatments. [NIH]

Regimen: A treatment plan that specifies the dosage, the schedule, and the duration of treatment. [NIH]

Screening: Checking for disease when there are no symptoms. [NIH]

Steroids: Drugs used to relieve swelling and inflammation. [NIH]

STI571: A drug that is being studied for its ability to inhibit the growth of certain cancers. It interferes with a portion of the protein produced by the bcr/abl oncogene. [NIH]

Trimetrexate: A nonclassical folic acid inhibitor through its inhibition of the enzyme dihydrofolate reductase. It is being tested for efficacy as an antineoplastic agent and as an antiparasitic agent against Pneumocystis carinii pneumonia in AIDS patients. Myelosuppression is its dose-limiting toxic effect. [NIH]

Vaccine: A substance or group of substances meant to cause the immune system to respond to a tumor or to microorganisms, such as bacteria or viruses. [NIH]

PART II: ADDITIONAL RESOURCES AND ADVANCED MATERIAL

ABOUT PART II

In Part II, we introduce you to additional resources and advanced research on childhood acute lymphoblastic leukemia. All too often, parents who conduct their own research are overwhelmed by the difficulty in finding and organizing information. The purpose of the following chapters is to provide you an organized and structured format to help you find additional information resources on childhood acute lymphoblastic leukemia. In Part II, as in Part I, our objective is not to interpret the latest advances on childhood acute lymphoblastic leukemia or render an opinion. Rather, our goal is to give you access to original research and to increase your awareness of sources you may not have already considered. In this way, you will come across the advanced materials often referred to in pamphlets, books, or other general works. Once again, some of this material is technical in nature, so consultation with a professional familiar with childhood acute lymphoblastic leukemia is suggested.

CHAPTER 4. STUDIES ON CHILDHOOD ACUTE LYMPHOBLASTIC LEUKEMIA

Overview

Every year, academic studies are published on childhood acute lymphoblastic leukemia or related conditions. Broadly speaking, there are two types of studies. The first are peer reviewed. Generally, the content of these studies has been reviewed by scientists or physicians. Peer-reviewed studies are typically published in scientific journals and are usually available at medical libraries. The second type of studies is non-peer reviewed. These works include summary articles that do not use or report scientific results. These often appear in the popular press, newsletters, or similar periodicals.

In this chapter, we will show you how to locate peer-reviewed references and studies on childhood acute lymphoblastic leukemia. We will begin by discussing research that has been summarized and is free to view by the public via the Internet. We then show you how to generate a bibliography on childhood acute lymphoblastic leukemia and teach you how to keep current on new studies as they are published or undertaken by the scientific community.

The Combined Health Information Database

The Combined Health Information Database summarizes studies across numerous federal agencies. To limit your investigation to research studies and childhood acute lymphoblastic leukemia, you will need to use the advanced search options. First, go to **http://chid.nih.gov/index.html**. From there, select the "Detailed Search" option (or go directly to that page with the following hyperlink: **http://chid.nih.gov/detail/detail.html**). The trick in extracting studies is found in the drop boxes at the bottom of the search page where "You may refine your search by." Select the dates and language you prefer, and the format option "Journal Article." At the top of the search form, select the number of records you would like to see (we recommend 100) and check the box to display "whole records." We recommend that you type in "childhood acute lymphoblastic leukemia" (or synonyms) into the "For these words:" box. Consider using the option "anywhere in record" to make your search as broad as possible. If you want to limit the search to only a particular field, such as the title of the journal, then select this option in the "Search in these fields" drop box. The following is a sample of what you can expect from this type of search:

- **Parental Smoking, CYP1A1 Genetic Polymorphisms and Childhood Leukemia (Quebec, Canada)**

  Source: Cancer Causes and Control. 11(6):547-553, July 2000.

  Summary: In order to evaluate the effect of parental smoking on childhood acute lymphoblastic leukemia and to determine if it is modified by child genetic polymorphisms, Canadian researchers carried out a case-control study in Quebec, Canada, including 491 incident cases age 0 to 9 years and as many healthy controls matched on age and sex. Each parent was interviewed separately with respect to smoking habits during and after pregnancy. Researchers conducted an additional case-only substudy with 158 cases classified according to the presence or absence of alleles in the CYP1A1 gene. The findings indicated there were small risk increases with maternal smoking during the later trimesters. Interaction odds ratios were increased (although often not significantly) for the CYP1A14 allele at high levels of maternal smoking in the last trimester and at low levels of paternal postnatal smoking, and decreased for the CYP1A12B allele. The latter appeared to confer a protective advantage at low levels for maternal prenatal smoking and at high levels for paternal postnatal smoking. The authors conclude that reported smoking habits showed no association with leukemia. Risks for genetic polymorphisms lacked precision but indicated that the effect of paternal smoking could be modified by variant alleles in the CYP141 gene. 3 tables, 35 references.

Federally-Funded Research on Childhood Acute Lymphoblastic Leukemia

The U.S. Government supports a variety of research studies relating to childhood acute lymphoblastic leukemia and associated conditions. These studies are tracked by the Office of Extramural Research at the National Institutes of Health.[26] CRISP (Computerized Retrieval of Information on Scientific Projects) is a searchable database of federally-funded biomedical research projects conducted at universities, hospitals, and other institutions. Visit the site at **http://commons.cit.nih.gov/crisp3/CRISP.Generate_Ticket**. You can perform targeted searches by various criteria including geography, date, as well as topics related to childhood acute lymphoblastic leukemia and related conditions.

For most of the studies, the agencies reporting into CRISP provide summaries or abstracts. As opposed to clinical trial research using patients, many federally-funded studies use animals or simulated models to explore childhood acute lymphoblastic leukemia and related conditions. In some cases, therefore, it may be difficult to understand how some basic or fundamental research could eventually translate into medical practice. The following sample is typical of the type of information found when searching the CRISP database for childhood acute lymphoblastic leukemia:

- **Project Title: Bone Density in Survivors of Pediatric Acute Lymphoblastic Leukemia**

    Principal Investigator & Institution: Kadan-Lottick, Nina; University of Colorado Hlth Sciences Ctr 4200 E 9Th Ave Denver, Co 80262

    Timing: Fiscal Year 2000

    Summary: We investigated whether previous reports of reduced bone mineral density after treatment for childhood acute lymphoblastic leukemia (chALL) are confirmed in a more recent cohort. In a cross-sectional study, 75 subjects diagnosed with chALL between 1/1/91 - 12/31/97 (69% standard, 31% high risk) at Denver Children's Hospital, with no history of relapse, secondary malignancy, or transplant underwent whole body areal bone mineral densitometry (BMDA expressed as age- and sex- standardized z-scores), a food frequency questionnaire, and a weight-bearing activity survey.

---

[26] Healthcare projects are funded by the National Institutes of Health (NIH), Substance Abuse and Mental Health Services (SAMHSA), Health Resources and Services Administration (HRSA), Food and Drug Administration (FDA), Centers for Disease Control and Prevention (CDCP), Agency for Healthcare Research and Quality (AHRQ), and Office of Assistant Secretary of Health (OASH).

Website: http://commons.cit.nih.gov/crisp3/CRISP.Generate_Ticket

- **Project Title: Detection and Therapy of Residual Leukemia in Children**

   Principal Investigator & Institution: Campana, Dario; Member; St. Jude Children's Research Hospital 332 N Lauderdale St Memphis, Tn 38105

   Timing: Fiscal Year 2000; Project Start 1-SEP-1993; Project End 1-JAN-2002

   Summary: (Applicant's Abstract) Despite advancing cure rates in childhood acute lymphoblastic leukemia (ALL), 25-30% of all patients eventually succumb to their disease. The long-term objective of the proposed research is to improve clinical outcome in this subset of patients. By early identification of patients who are likely to relapse, it should be possible to instigate potentially curative therapy in a more timely manner, thus boosting the proportion of long term survivors. This goal will be pursued through three interrelated projects. In the first, overexpression of WT1 and BCL-2 genes will be assessed as markers of minimal residual disease (MRD) in childhood ALL patients. The underlying hypothesis is that these two indicators are more widely associated with leukemia than current markers, and will significantly expand capabilities for prospective identification of high risk patients. Specific Aim 2 seeks to expand results obtained during the previous period of support, suggesting that immunologic monitoring of MRD has clinical utility in the assessment of childhood ALL patients. Immunologic findings in sequential bone marrow samples from patients with B- and T-lineage ALL will be compared with event free survival, as well as presenting clinical and biologic risk features, to establish the independent predictive strength of this assay. The data will also provide opportunities for cross comparisons with results of WT1 and BCL-2 screening in Specific Aim 1. Based on encouraging preliminary results, studies in Specific Aim 3 seek to assess the clinical utility of MRD investigations using peripheral blood instead of bone marrow. Success in this endeavor will radically improve remission studies in patients with ALL, by overcoming the practical and ethical constraints posed by sequential bone marrow aspirations in children. The clinical significance of MRD has been in doubt because of the lack of prospective studies in a large group of uniformly treated patients. The studies proposed in this application should meet that need and demonstrate the feasibility of clinical management decisions based on MRD detection in children with ALL.

   Website: http://commons.cit.nih.gov/crisp3/CRISP.Generate_Ticket

- **Project Title: Enhancing Treatment Outcomes in Childhood Acute Lymphocytic Leukemia**

    Principal Investigator & Institution: Sallan, Stephen E.; Professor; Dana-Farber Cancer Institute 44 Binney St Boston, Ma 02115

    Timing: Fiscal Year 2000

    Summary: (Applicant's Description) Childhood acute lymphoblastic leukemia (ALL) is a model of a curable malignancy. The best therapies to date have resulted in cure for 75-80 percent of childhood ALL, although only 35 percent for adult ALL. Most survivors of childhood ALL have sequelae of treatment. The goal of Project 4 is to maximize the therapeutic index (the efficacy:toxicity balance) in the treatment of ALL. We seek to increase the proportion of patients cured, assess the long-term outcome of anti-leukemia therapy, and augment the usual event-free survival comparisons of treatment programs by use of methods to adjust survival for its quality. In a randomized clinical trial, we will determine the relative efficacy of an augmented intensification regimen and a conventional intensification regimen (Core 9001). We will also extend our program to adult patients (ages 18-40 years) and assess biological (Projects 4, 7, 8, 9) and outcome differences of adults compared to children with ALL. Specific Aim 1 will determine the efficacy and toxicity of pharmacokinetically-based, individualized dosing of E.coli asparaginase - a pillar of our successful program. Specific Aim 2 will test the hypothesis that L-carnitine can decrease late doxorubicin-induced cardiomyopathy. (We will continue our long-term assessment of the value of serial cardiac monitoring during doxorubicin therapy, as well as the long-term natural history of doxorubicin-induced cardiomyopathy, continuous infusions of doxorubicin, and cardioprotection with dexrazoxane). Specific Aim 3 will define the efficacy and neuropsychologic morbidity of either intensive intrathecal therapy or radiation therapy. In Specific Aim 4 quality-adjusted analyses using Q-TWiST and QALY methods will evaluate the trade-off between the benefit of improved cure rates and the cost in terms of treatment-related toxicity. We seek to determine the most effective, least toxic therapies for ALL, balancing health-related quality of life against the proportion of patients cured, thus maximizing the therapeutic index.

    Website: http://commons.cit.nih.gov/crisp3/CRISP.Generate_Ticket

- **Project Title: Functional Analysis of MDM2 Overexpression**

    Principal Investigator & Institution: Haines, Dale S.; Fels Inst/Cancer Res/Mol Biol; Temple University Broad St and Montgomery Ave Philadelphia, Pa 19122

Timing: Fiscal Year 2000; Project Start 1-SEP-1997; Project End 1-AUG-2002

Summary: (adapted from the investigator's abstract) The experiments presented and outlined in this proposal are designed to improve the understanding of molecular checkpoint pathways that are altered in chemo-resistant human tumors. Work by the applicant's laboratory, as well as by others, has provided strong evidence which suggests that mdm2 onco-protein overexpression may play a key role in affecting clinical outcome by altering the response of tumor cells to chemotherapeutic agents. The overexpression of mdm2 has been associated with a number of tumors of poor prognosis and has been associated with early treatment failure in childhood acute lymphoblastic leukemia (ALL). It is now accepted that one mechanism by which mdm2 overexpression may provide a selective growth advantage to chemo-treated tumor cells is through its ability to block p53 controlled checkpoint responses. Experimental overexpression of mdm2 has been shown to block the transactivation, cell cycle arrest and apoptotic functions of p53. New data generated by his laboratory suggests that mdm2 overexpression may affect p53 independent pathways mediating chemosensitivity. P53 null cells that have been transfected with an mdm2 expression construct and express elevated levels of mdm2 protein display marked differences in their ability to respond to the chemotherapeutic drug cisplatin when compared to vector alone transfected cells. Furthermore, we have identified that mdm2 can interact with a novel DNA damage checkpoint molecule, DNA polymerase epsilon (DNA pol E). Based on these observations, we hypothesize that mdm2 protein overexpression can alter the response of transformed cells by chemotherapeutic drugs by affecting p53 dependent and independent checkpoint pathways. To test this hypothesis and to identify these p53 independent checkpoint pathways, the following aims are proposed: 1) To determine whether experimental overexpression of mdm2 in p53 null cells alters the response of human tumor cells to chemotherapeutic agents in a drug or tissue specific manner, 2) To determine whether mdm2 protein is overexpressed in primary leukemic cells from relapsed patients harboring p53 gene mutations, 3) To determine whether mdm2 and DNA pol E interact during a DNA damage response and to identify amino acids of both mdm2 and DNA pol E that are required for association and 4) To determine whether mdm2 overexpression can block a DNA pol E mediated checkpoint response to DNA damage. These studies will not only improve the understanding of mdm2 activities in checkpoint pathways, but will also be important for understanding how altered expression of mdm2 affects the response of tumor cells to chemotherapeutic agents. Understanding these processes will hopefully lead to novel therapeutic strategies restoring chemosensitivity to chemo-resistant tumors that overexpress mdm2.

Website: http://commons.cit.nih.gov/crisp3/CRISP.Generate_Ticket

- **Project Title: Fusion Genes in Leukemia--Determining Significance**

  Principal Investigator & Institution: Loh, Mignon L.; Pediatrics; University of California San Francisco 500 Parnassus Ave San Francisco, Ca 94122

  Timing: Fiscal Year 2000; Project Start 6-JUL-1999; Project End 0-JUN-2004

  Summary: With recent advances in molecular biology, it is now possible to identify genetic events that lead to malignancy. In particular, chromosomal translocations that result in the expression of novel leukemogenic fusion proteins have been identified, and the genes encoding these proteins have been cloned from patients with leukemia. Ultimately, these gene rearrangements may serve as targets for novel therapies. Additionally, fusion genes arising, from somatic mutations may be used a markers of malignancy that allow clinical investigators to monitor patients' response to therapy. Thus, these gene rearrangements might therefore be used to identify and follow groups of patients who could benefit from a specific treatment. This project will create a paradigm for exploring the integration of molecular genetics into clinical investigation using the two most commonly occurring gene rearrangements in childhood acute lymphoblastic leukemia. The first specific aim of this proposal is to prospectively determine the prognostic significance of TEL/AML1 in patients treated on DFCI-ALL Consortium protocols. TEL/AML1 is the most common fusion gene known to occur in any pediatric malignancy. Though initially reported to confer a favorable prognosis, recent analyses from Europe indicate that the TEL/AML1 fusion occurs with the same frequency at relapse as it dose at initial diagnosis. There is thus controversy over the prognostic significance of the TEL/AML1 gene rearrangement. The second specific aim of this proposal is to use quantitative RT-PCR techniques on serial samples to determine the prognostic significance of TEL/AML1 transcript copy number. The third specific aim is to apply quantitative RT-PCR techniques to pediatric leukemias associated with the E2A/PBX1 gene rearrangement. The second and third specific aims are based on the premise developed in analysis of other leukemias that fusion transcript copy number is a predictor of clinical outcome. Advances in molecular technology are heralding an era when genetic testing will become routine for many diseases. It is an ideal time to develop simple and efficient quantitative approaches to minimal residual disease detection; we can capitalize on the growing number of discoveries in molecular genetics and thereby maximize the treatment of childhood acute lymphoblastic leukemia.

Website: http://commons.cit.nih.gov/crisp3/CRISP.Generate_Ticket

- **Project Title: Mutual Regulation of P53, MDM2 and NFKB**

  Principal Investigator & Institution: Zhou, Muxiang; Pediatrics; Emory University 1380 S Oxford Rd Atlanta, Ga 30322

  Timing: Fiscal Year 2000; Project Start 1-APR-2000; Project End 1-MAR-2005

  Summary: (Applicant's Abstract) Despite substantial advances in the treatment of childhood acute lymphoblastic leukemia (ALL), approximately 25-35% of children with this disease will relapse or fail induction therapy. Failure to respond to treatment may result from development of resistance to apoptosis induced by chemotherapeutic agents. In the applicant's studies of pediatric ALL in relapse, he has found that leukemic cells expressing a mutant p53 gene or overexpressing the p53-inhibitory MDM2 oncogene express constitutively high levels of activated Nuclear Factor kappa B (NFkB), which has been linked to resistance to apoptosis following DNA damage. Conversely, ALL cells expressing wild type (wt)-p53 typically show either no or very low levels of activated NFkB. Since wt-p53 function is induced in cells following DNA damage, and since this function is lost in cells expressing a mut-p53 allele or overexpressing MDM2, the applicant hypothesizes that an important apoptosis-inducing effect of wt-p53 may be inhibition of NFkB activity. Accordingly, expression of mut-p53 or high levels of MDM2 would increase the level of activated NFkB by suppressing the NFkB-inhibitory function of wt-p53. Thus, in normal cells, p53 and NFkB would mutually interact in response to DNA damage to permit apoptosis in cells sustaining irreparable DNA damage; loss of this mutual regulation by either p53 mutation or MDM2 overexpression would result in resistance to apoptosis-inducing agents. To test his hypothesis, he will study the potential upregulation of NFkB activity by either mutant p53 or MDM2 in ALL cells. Importantly, he will examine the cellular consequences of directly inhibiting MDM2 and NFkB activation. These studies may have direct clinical application in suggesting ways to inhibit NFkB-mediated therapy resistance in leukemia and other malignancies. The specific aims of this study are 1) To evaluate the ability of mutant p53 and overexpressed MDM2 to activate NFkB by transcriptionally regulating NFkB/p65 gene expression, including identification of possible p53- or MDM2-binding and response elements in the p65/RelA promoter; 2) To investigate the ability of mutp53 and MDM2 proteins to activate NFkB by enhancing turnover of the NFkB inhibitor IkBa and 3) To evaluate the effect of blocking MDM2 overexpression and augmenting IkB levels on sensitivity to apoptosis utilizing anti-MDM2 antisense and proteasome inhibitors, respectively.

Website: http://commons.cit.nih.gov/crisp3/CRISP.Generate_Ticket

- **Project Title: P450 Metabolism of Epipodophyllotoxins in Children**

Principal Investigator & Institution: Relling, Mary V.; Associate Member; St. Jude Children's Research Hospital 332 N Lauderdale St Memphis, Tn 38105

Timing: Fiscal Year 2000; Project Start 1-APR-1990; Project End 8-FEB-2002

Summary: The epipodophyllotoxins, teniposide and etoposide, are among the most effective drugs for the treatment of childhood acute lymphoblastic leukemia (ALL) and other cancers. Although ALL is curable in 70% of patients, therapy is complicated by the development of a secondary acute myeloid leukemia (AML) in up to 12% of children who have been cured of their primary ALL. Currently, it is not possible to identify those patients at highest risk for this fatal secondary AML. Epipodophyllotoxin- induced AML is a distinct clinical and biologic entity, characterized by a unique mechanism: illegitimate site-specific recombination of the MLL (mixed lineage leukemia) gene on chromosome 11 (region q23) with one of a number of partner genes, resulting in the leukemic phenotype and accompanied by translocations of 11q23. The distinctive molecular signature of illegitimately acting V(D)J recombinase has been found at the translocation breakpoints, indicating an ill-fated cellular attempt at inappropriate DNA recombination secondary to the epipodophyllotoxins' inhibition of normal recombination. There have been no prior attempts to determine whether epipodophyllotoxins or their metabolites induce site- specific illegitimate V(D)J-recombination, either in vivo or in vitro. We will define the quantitative relationship between epipodophyllotoxins or their metabolites and illegitimate recombination. We demonstrated that cytochrome P450 3A4 (CYP3A4) O-demethylates teniposide and etoposide in human liver. O-demethylation is important not only because it may represent a major route of elimination, but also because it indicates oxidative activation to reactive catechols. We have demonstrated 10-fold interpatient variability in the systemic clearance of the epipodophyllotoxins and in the formation of catechol metabolites in children. Our hypotheses are that this interpatient variability in CYP3A4-mediated O-demethylation accounts for variability in the overall disposition of epipodophyllotoxins, and that high systemic exposure to etoposide, its catechol, or both is the principal determinant of the mutagenic recombination caused by the epipodophyllotoxins. We will use in vivo pharmacokinetic studies in children with ALL to determine whether O- demethylation determines the clearance of the epipodophyllotoxins. We will evaluate whether high systemic exposure to etoposide, its catechol, or both are significantly related to the frequency of illegitimate V(D)J recombinase-mediated mutations in serial samples of children's leukocyte HPRT DNA, a specific marker of the biologically relevant mechanism of leukemogenesis in vivo. We have also developed in vitro model systems to determine whether illegitimate recombinase activity in specific cell lines is related to epipodophyllotoxin parent drug or metabolite concentrations and/or to the duration of exposure. Together, these laboratory and clinical studies will elucidate the contribution of pharmacokinetic and metabolic variability as determinants of the disposition and leukemogenic effects of the epipodophyllotoxins in children with cancer.

Website: http://commons.cit.nih.gov/crisp3/CRISP.Generate_Ticket

- **Project Title: Pharmacodynamics of Antileukemic Agents in Children**

  Principal Investigator & Institution: Evans, William E.; Professor and Chairman; St. Jude Children's Research Hospital 332 N Lauderdale St Memphis, Tn 38105

  Timing: Fiscal Year 2000; Project Start 1-JUN-1998; Project End 1-MAR-2003

  Summary: Methotrexate (MTX) is one of the most active and widely used drugs for the treatment of childhood acute lymphoblastic leukemia (ALL), yet there remains considerable uncertainty about the optimal dosage and schedule of MTX, with doses ranging from 0.04 gm/m2 to 8 gm/m2 currently in clinical use. The rationale for high-dose MTX (HDMTX) has been questioned on the basis of in vitro studies demonstrating saturable membrane transport and polyglutamylation, indicating that HDMTX would not achieve higher concentrations in ALL blasts. However, the PI has established that HDMTX achieves higher lymphoblast concentrations of the active polyglutamylated metabolites (MTXPG) in patients (JCI 94:1996-2001, 1994), and that this is associated with greater antileukemic effects (JCI, 97:73-80, 1996). These studies also revealed significantly greater MTXPG accumulation in B-lineage vs. T-lineage blasts, and in hyperdiploid vs. non-hyperdiploid lymphoblasts. Our more recent studies suggest that MTXPG accumulation is eventually saturable but that higher MTX plasma concentrations (Cpss) may be required to achieve maximum MTXPG in T-lineage lymphoblasts. It is clinically important to establish the optimal MTX dosage for leukemia of different lineages and ploidy, to avoid unnecessarily high dosages that can induce encephalopathy and other serious toxicities. Therefore, aims of the current studies are: (Aim 1) to define in vivo, the MTX Cpss producing maximum accumulation of MTXPG in leukemic lymphoblasts of children and whether there are significant differences among leukemic subtypes (phenotype and genotype), (Aim 2) to define the relation between MTXPG concentrations in leukemic blasts and the antileukemic effects of MTX and whether there are significant differences among leukemic subtypes, (Aim 3) to determine whether high MTX Cpss is associated with a (paradoxical) decrease in lymphoblast accumulation of long-chain MTXPG in vivo, and (Aim 4) to determine the mechanism(s) underlying phenotypic and genotypic differences in MTXPG accumulation in ALL blasts. Collectively, these integrated clinical and laboratory studies will provide important new insights for the rational design of future treatment protocols for childhood ALL.

Website: http://commons.cit.nih.gov/crisp3/CRISP.Generate_Ticket

- **Project Title: Prognosis in Childhood ALL**

Principal Investigator & Institution: Kees, Ursula R.; Tvw Telethon Institute-Child Health Res for Child Health Research Subiaco,

Timing: Fiscal Year 2002; Project Start 9-JUN-2002; Project End 0-APR-2004

Summary: (provided by applicant) Despite the high rate of cure, resistant forms of childhood acute lymphoblastic leukemia (ALL) constitute a leading cause of cancer-related deaths in children. We propose to study childhood ALL patients in order to arrive at a better risk stratification, based on gene expression profiles measured in microarray studies which allow simultaneous testing of the expression levels of thousands of genes. The primary aim of the study is to characterise the profiles of relapsing and non-relapsing patients in order to identity features with prognostic value. This will be achieved by studying complementary sets of patient specimens banked at our own institution. The quality of this set of more than 130 patient specimens makes them particularly suited for microarray studies. They allow us to ask very specific questions. (1) Which genes are expressed in leukemia specimens from patients who will relapse because their disease is resistant to chemotherapy, while not expressed (or expressed at lower levels) in patients who will respond to therapy? (2) Which genes are expressed at low levels in specimens from relapsing patients? (3) Are the same genes differentially expressed in the leukemia cells at relapse, compared to the time of diagnosis? The answers to these three questions will provide the basis for the selection of a panel of suitable prognostic marker genes. The aim of the project is to establish tests to measure expression levels of these candidate prognostic markers by realtime quantitative polymerase chain reaction (PCR). These will subsequently be studied in a separate cohort of patients who have received uniform treatment to verify that they are indeed of prognostic significance. The overall goal is to develop a prognostic test to be used at the time of diagnosing a child with ALL to determine whether the patient is likely to be successfully treated on current therapy protocols or has a high risk of relapse, hence, should be receiving more intensive therapy.

Website: http://commons.cit.nih.gov/crisp3/CRISP.Generate_Ticket

- **Project Title: TNF-Alpha and Its Receptors in Pediatric Acute Leukemia**

  Principal Investigator & Institution: Findley, Harry W.; Pediatrics; Emory University 1380 S Oxford Rd Atlanta, Ga 30322

  Timing: Fiscal Year 2000; Project Start 1-JUL-1996; Project End 0-JUN-2001

  Summary: Despite substantial advances in the treatment of childhood acute lymphoblastic leukemia (ALL), approximately 35 percent of children with this disease will relapse or fail induction therapy. The applicant has observed that endogenous production of tumor necrosis factor-alpha (TNF) by pediatric ALL cells may be linked to refractory disease. Growth of leukemic cells by the majority of patients tested was inhibited by TNF in a dose-dependent manner and was accompanied by apoptosis. In contrast, cells from a subset of patients produced TNF and were resistant to the inhibitory effects of exogenous TNF. Leukemic cell lines derived from TNF-producing, TNF-resistant (TNF+) cells and from TNF-nonproducing, TNF sensitive (TNF-) cells retained the responsiveness of the primary cells to exogenous TNF. Both TNF+ and TNF- lines expressed p60 and p80 TNF receptors (TNFrs), suggesting that phenotypic differences in TNF response between these lines are not due to altered expression of TNFrs. Preliminary experiments indicate marked differences between TNF+ and TNF-cells in the regulation of certain apoptosis/survival associated genes after genotoxic treatments. Moreover, clinical data suggest that the TNF+ phenotype is associated with refractory disease and poor prognosis: The percentage of patients remaining in complete remission at one year post-diagnosis was 20 percent for TNF+ ALL cells vs 89 percent for TNF- ALL. He hypothesizes that endogenous TNF acts as a survival factor for TNF+ ALL cells, protecting these cells from apoptosis. To test the hypothesis, he proposes the following specific aims: 1) To further investigate the response of TNF+ and TNF- ALL cell lines to exogenous TNF, adriamycin, and IR by examining differences in expression of apoptosis vs. survival genes following DNA damage; 2) To determine if blockade of endogenous TNF production (using a TNF-antisense expression construct) affects the response of TNF+ ALL cell lines to exogenous TNF, adriamycin, and IR; 3) To investigate the effects of induction of endogenous TNF (using a TNF expression vector) on the response of TNF- ALL cell lines to these agents; 4) To examine primary leukemic cells fro pediatric ALL patients for expression of TNF and TNF receptors, and to correlate this data with clinical response and in vitro response to genotoxic agents; 5) To determine the cytotoxicity of a recombinant TNF-Pseudomonas endotoxin (TNF-PE) for TNFR+ ALL cells in vitro as well as in the SCID model for engrafted leukemia.

Website: http://commons.cit.nih.gov/crisp3/CRISP.Generate_Ticket

E-Journals: PubMed Central[27]

PubMed Central (PMC) is a digital archive of life sciences journal literature developed and managed by the National Center for Biotechnology Information (NCBI) at the U.S. National Library of Medicine (NLM).[28] Access to this growing archive of e-journals is free and unrestricted.[29] To search, go to **http://www.pubmedcentral.nih.gov/index.html#search**, and type "childhood acute lymphoblastic leukemia" (or synonyms) into the search box. This search gives you access to full-text articles. The following is a sample of items found for childhood acute lymphoblastic leukemia in the PubMed Central database:

- **AF5q31, a newly identified AF4-related gene, is fused to MLL in infant acute lymphoblastic leukemia with ins(5;11)(q31;q13q23)** by Tomohiko Taki, Hirotsugu Kano, Masafumi Taniwaki, Masahiro Sako, Masayoshi Yanagisawa, and Yasuhide Hayashi; 1999 December 7
http://www.pubmedcentral.nih.gov/articlerender.fcgi?artid=24471

---

[27] Adapted from the National Library of Medicine: http://www.pubmedcentral.nih.gov/about/intro.html.
[28] With PubMed Central, NCBI is taking the lead in preservation and maintenance of open access to electronic literature, just as NLM has done for decades with printed biomedical literature. PubMed Central aims to become a world-class library of the digital age.
[29] The value of PubMed Central, in addition to its role as an archive, lies the availability of data from diverse sources stored in a common format in a single repository. Many journals already have online publishing operations, and there is a growing tendency to publish material online only, to the exclusion of print.

- **Acrophialophora fusispora Brain Abscess in a Child with Acute Lymphoblastic Leukemia: Review of Cases and Taxonomy** by I. Z. Al-Mohsen, D. A. Sutton, L. Sigler, E. Almodovar, N. Mahgoub, H. Frayha, S. Al-Hajjar, M. G. Rinaldi, and T. J. Walsh; 2000 December
  http://www.pubmedcentral.nih.gov/articlerender.fcgi?artid=87638

- **Disseminated Invasive Infection Due to Metarrhizium anisopliae in an Immunocompromised Child** by David Burgner, Gillian Eagles, Margaret Burgess, Peter Procopis, Maureen Rogers, David Muir, Robert Pritchard, Ailsa Hocking, and Michael Priest; 1998 April
  http://www.pubmedcentral.nih.gov/articlerender.fcgi?artid=104710

- **Fusion of the TEL Gene on 12p13 to the AML1 Gene on 21q22 in Acute Lymphoblastic Leukemia** by TR Golub, GF Barker, SK Bohlander, SW Hiebert, DC Ward, P Bray-Ward, E Morgan, SC Raimondi, JD Rowley, and DG Gilliland; 1995 May 23
  http://www.pubmedcentral.nih.gov/articlerender.fcgi?rendertype=abstract&artid=41818

- **Methylenetetrahydrofolate reductase (MTHFR) polymorphisms and risk of molecularly defined subtypes of childhood acute leukemia** by Joseph L. Wiemels, Rosalyn N. Smith, G. Malcolm Taylor, Osborn B. Eden, Freda E. Alexander, Mel F. Greaves, and United Kingdom Childhood Cancer Study Investigators; 2001 March 27
  http://www.pubmedcentral.nih.gov/articlerender.fcgi?artid=31169

- **Tumor necrosis factor and lymphotoxin-alpha genetic polymorphisms and risk of relapse in childhood B-cell precursor acute lymphoblastic leukemia: a case-control study of patients treated with BFM therapy** by Martin Stanulla, Andre Schrauder, Karl Welte, and Martin Schrappe; 2001
  http://www.pubmedcentral.nih.gov/articlerender.fcgi?artid=32163

The National Library of Medicine: PubMed

One of the quickest and most comprehensive ways to find academic studies in both English and other languages is to use PubMed, maintained by the National Library of Medicine. The advantage of PubMed over previously mentioned sources is that it covers a greater number of domestic and foreign references. It is also free to the public.[30] If the publisher has a Web site that offers full text of its journals, PubMed will provide links to that site, as well as to sites offering other related data. User registration, a subscription fee, or some other type of fee may be required to access the full text of articles in some journals.

To generate your own bibliography of studies dealing with childhood acute lymphoblastic leukemia, simply go to the PubMed Web site at **www.ncbi.nlm.nih.gov/pubmed**. Type "childhood acute lymphoblastic leukemia" (or synonyms) into the search box, and click "Go." The following is the type of output you can expect from PubMed for "childhood acute lymphoblastic leukemia" (hyperlinks lead to article summaries):

- **Deletion of chromosomal region 13q14.3 in childhood acute lymphoblastic leukemia.**
  Author(s): Cave H, Avet-Loiseau H, Devaux I, Rondeau G, Boutard P, Lebrun E, Mechinaud F, Vilmer E, Grandchamp B.
  Source: Leukemia : Official Journal of the Leukemia Society of America, Leukemia Research Fund, U.K. 2001 March; 15(3): 371-6.
  http://www.ncbi.nlm.nih.gov:80/entrez/query.fcgi?cmd=Retrieve&db=PubMed&list_uids=11237059&dopt=Abstract

- **Diagnostic X-rays and ultrasound exposure and risk of childhood acute lymphoblastic leukemia by immunophenotype.**
  Author(s): Shu XO, Potter JD, Linet MS, Severson RK, Han D, Kersey JH, Neglia JP, Trigg ME, Robison LL.

---

[30] PubMed was developed by the National Center for Biotechnology Information (NCBI) at the National Library of Medicine (NLM) at the National Institutes of Health (NIH). The PubMed database was developed in conjunction with publishers of biomedical literature as a search tool for accessing literature citations and linking to full-text journal articles at Web sites of participating publishers. Publishers that participate in PubMed supply NLM with their citations electronically prior to or at the time of publication.

Source: Cancer Epidemiology, Biomarkers & Prevention : a Publication of the American Association for Cancer Research, Cosponsored by the American Society of Preventive Oncology. 2002 February; 11(2): 177-85.
http://www.ncbi.nlm.nih.gov:80/entrez/query.fcgi?cmd=Retrieve&db=PubMed&list_uids=11867505&dopt=Abstract

- **Early child-care and preschool experiences and the risk of childhood acute lymphoblastic leukemia.**
  Author(s): Rosenbaum PF, Buck GM, Brecher ML.
  Source: American Journal of Epidemiology. 2000 December 15; 152(12): 1136-44.
  http://www.ncbi.nlm.nih.gov:80/entrez/query.fcgi?cmd=Retrieve&db=PubMed&list_uids=11130619&dopt=Abstract

- **Early resistance to therapy during induction in childhood acute lymphoblastic leukemia.**
  Author(s): Brisco MJ, Sykes PJ, Dolman G, Hughes E, Neoh SH, Peng L, Snell LE, Toogood IR, Rice MS, Morley AA.
  Source: Cancer Research. 2000 September 15; 60(18): 5092-6.
  http://www.ncbi.nlm.nih.gov:80/entrez/query.fcgi?cmd=Retrieve&db=PubMed&list_uids=11016634&dopt=Abstract

- **Effect of protracted high-dose L-asparaginase given as a second exposure in a Berlin-Frankfurt-Munster-based treatment: results of the randomized 9102 intermediate-risk childhood acute lymphoblastic leukemia study--a report from the Associazione Italiana Ematologia Oncologia Pediatrica.**
  Author(s): Rizzari C, Valsecchi MG, Arico M, Conter V, Testi A, Barisone E, Casale F, Lo Nigro L, Rondelli R, Basso G, Santoro N, Masera G.
  Source: Journal of Clinical Oncology : Official Journal of the American Society of Clinical Oncology. 2001 March 1; 19(5): 1297-303.
  http://www.ncbi.nlm.nih.gov:80/entrez/query.fcgi?cmd=Retrieve&db=PubMed&list_uids=11230471&dopt=Abstract

- **Effects of high-dose methotrexate on the hemostatic system in childhood acute lymphoblastic leukemia.**
  Author(s): Totan M, Dagdemir A, Ak AR, Albayrak D, Kucukoduk S.
  Source: Medical and Pediatric Oncology. 2001 April; 36(4): 429-33.
  http://www.ncbi.nlm.nih.gov:80/entrez/query.fcgi?cmd=Retrieve&db=PubMed&list_uids=11260565&dopt=Abstract

- **Epstein-Barr virus-related lymphoproliferative disease complicating childhood acute lymphoblastic leukemia: no recurrence after unrelated donor bone marrow transplantation.**
  Author(s): Pondarre C, Kebaili K, Dijoud F, Basset T, Philippe N, Bertrand Y.
  Source: Bone Marrow Transplantation. 2001 January; 27(1): 93-5.
  http://www.ncbi.nlm.nih.gov:80/entrez/query.fcgi?cmd=Retrieve&db=PubMed&list_uids=11244444&dopt=Abstract

- **Expression of myeloid-specific genes in childhood acute lymphoblastic leukemia - a cDNA array study.**
  Author(s): Niini T, Vettenranta K, Hollmen J, Larramendy ML, Aalto Y, Wikman H, Nagy B, Seppanen JK, Ferrer Salvador A, Mannila H, Saarinen-Pihkala UM, Knuutila S.
  Source: Leukemia : Official Journal of the Leukemia Society of America, Leukemia Research Fund, U.K. 2002 November; 16(11): 2213-2221.
  http://www.ncbi.nlm.nih.gov:80/entrez/query.fcgi?cmd=Retrieve&db=PubMed&list_uids=12399964&dopt=Abstract

- **Expression of the multidrug transporter P-glycoprotein is highly correlated with clinical outcome in childhood acute lymphoblastic leukemia: results of a long-term prospective study.**
  Author(s): Dhooge C, De Moerloose B, Laureys G, Ferster A, De Bacquer D, Philippe J, Leroy J, Benoit Y.
  Source: Leukemia & Lymphoma. 2002 February; 43(2): 309-14.
  http://www.ncbi.nlm.nih.gov:80/entrez/query.fcgi?cmd=Retrieve&db=PubMed&list_uids=11999562&dopt=Abstract

- **Extremely low-frequency magnetic fields and childhood acute lymphoblastic leukemia: an exploratory analysis of alternative exposure metrics.**
  Author(s): Auvinen A, Linet MS, Hatch EE, Kleinerman RA, Robison LL, Kaune WT, Misakian M, Niwa S, Wacholder S, Tarone RE.
  Source: American Journal of Epidemiology. 2000 July 1; 152(1): 20-31.
  http://www.ncbi.nlm.nih.gov:80/entrez/query.fcgi?cmd=Retrieve&db=PubMed&list_uids=10901326&dopt=Abstract

- **Fasting hypoglycemia is common during maintenance therapy for childhood acute lymphoblastic leukemia.**
  Author(s): Halonen P, Salo MK, Makipernaa A.

Source: The Journal of Pediatrics. 2001 March; 138(3): 428-31.
http://www.ncbi.nlm.nih.gov:80/entrez/query.fcgi?cmd=Retrieve&db=PubMed&list_uids=11241057&dopt=Abstract

- **Genetic susceptibility to childhood acute lymphoblastic leukemia.**
  Author(s): Sinnett D, Krajinovic M, Labuda D.
  Source: Leukemia & Lymphoma. 2000 August; 38(5-6): 447-62. Review.
  http://www.ncbi.nlm.nih.gov:80/entrez/query.fcgi?cmd=Retrieve&db=PubMed&list_uids=10953966&dopt=Abstract

- **Germline mutation of the p27/Kip1 gene in childhood acute lymphoblastic leukemia.**
  Author(s): Takeuchi C, Takeuchi S, Ikezoe T, Bartram CR, Taguchi H, Koeffler HP.
  Source: Leukemia : Official Journal of the Leukemia Society of America, Leukemia Research Fund, U.K. 2002 May; 16(5): 956-8. No Abstract Available.
  http://www.ncbi.nlm.nih.gov:80/entrez/query.fcgi?cmd=Retrieve&db=PubMed&list_uids=11986963&dopt=Abstract

- **Glutathione S-transferase genotypes, genetic susceptibility, and outcome of therapy in childhood acute lymphoblastic leukemia.**
  Author(s): Davies SM, Bhatia S, Ross JA, Kiffmeyer WR, Gaynon PS, Radloff GA, Robison LL, Perentesis JP.
  Source: Blood. 2002 July 1; 100(1): 67-71.
  http://www.ncbi.nlm.nih.gov:80/entrez/query.fcgi?cmd=Retrieve&db=PubMed&list_uids=12070010&dopt=Abstract

- **High level resistance to glucocorticoids, associated with a dysfunctional glucocorticoid receptor, in childhood acute lymphoblastic leukemia cells selected for methotrexate resistance.**
  Author(s): Catts VS, Farnsworth ML, Haber M, Norris MD, Lutze-Mann LH, Lock RB.
  Source: Leukemia : Official Journal of the Leukemia Society of America, Leukemia Research Fund, U.K. 2001 June; 15(6): 929-35.
  http://www.ncbi.nlm.nih.gov:80/entrez/query.fcgi?cmd=Retrieve&db=PubMed&list_uids=11417479&dopt=Abstract

- **Household solvent exposures and childhood acute lymphoblastic leukemia.**
  Author(s): Freedman DM, Stewart P, Kleinerman RA, Wacholder S, Hatch EE, Tarone RE, Robison LL, Linet MS.

Source: American Journal of Public Health. 2001 April; 91(4): 564-7.
http://www.ncbi.nlm.nih.gov:80/entrez/query.fcgi?cmd=Retrieve&db=PubMed&list_uids=11291366&dopt=Abstract

- **Immunosuppression in childhood acute lymphoblastic leukemia after remission induction therapy concerns B not T lymphocytes.**
  Author(s): Luczynski W, Krawczuk-Rybak M, Muszynska-Roslan K, Stasiak-Barmuta A, Zak J.
  Source: Medical and Pediatric Oncology. 2002 August; 39(2): 147-8. No Abstract Available.
  http://www.ncbi.nlm.nih.gov:80/entrez/query.fcgi?cmd=Retrieve&db=PubMed&list_uids=12116070&dopt=Abstract

- **Importance of using comparative genomic hybridization to improve detection of chromosomal changes in childhood acute lymphoblastic leukemia.**
  Author(s): Jarosova M, Holzerova M, Jedlickova K, Mihal V, Zuna J, Stary J, Pospisilova D, Zemanova Z, Trka J, Blazek J, Pikalova Z, Indrak K.
  Source: Cancer Genetics and Cytogenetics. 2000 December; 123(2): 114-22.
  http://www.ncbi.nlm.nih.gov:80/entrez/query.fcgi?cmd=Retrieve&db=PubMed&list_uids=11156736&dopt=Abstract

- **Incidence, clinical characteristics and early treatment outcome in Indian patients of childhood acute lymphoblastic leukemia with ALL 1 gene rearrangement.**
  Author(s): Sazawal S, Gurbuxani S, Bhatia K, Khattar A, Raina V, Arya LS, Vats T, Magrath I, Bhargava M.
  Source: Leukemia Research. 2001 August; 25(8): 693-8.
  http://www.ncbi.nlm.nih.gov:80/entrez/query.fcgi?cmd=Retrieve&db=PubMed&list_uids=11397475&dopt=Abstract

- **Increased incidence of spontaneous apoptosis in the bone marrow of hyperdiploid childhood acute lymphoblastic leukemia.**
  Author(s): Zhang Y, Lu J, van den Berghe J, Lee SH.
  Source: Experimental Hematology. 2002 April; 30(4): 333-9.
  http://www.ncbi.nlm.nih.gov:80/entrez/query.fcgi?cmd=Retrieve&db=PubMed&list_uids=11937268&dopt=Abstract

- **Initial P-glycoprotein expression in childhood acute lymphoblastic leukemia: no evidence of prognostic impact in follow-up.**
  Author(s): Kanerva J, Tiirikainen MI, Makipernaa A, Riikonen P, Mottonen M, Salmi TT, Krusius T, Saarinen-Pihkala UM.

Source: Pediatric Hematology and Oncology. 2001 January-February; 18(1): 27-36.
http://www.ncbi.nlm.nih.gov:80/entrez/query.fcgi?cmd=Retrieve&db=PubMed&list_uids=11205837&dopt=Abstract

- **International Childhood Acute Lymphoblastic Leukemia Workshop: Sausalito, CA, 30 November-1 December 2000.**
Author(s): Pui CH, Sallan S, Relling MV, Masera G, Evans WE.
Source: Leukemia : Official Journal of the Leukemia Society of America, Leukemia Research Fund, U.K. 2001 May; 15(5): 707-15. No Abstract Available.
http://www.ncbi.nlm.nih.gov:80/entrez/query.fcgi?cmd=Retrieve&db=PubMed&list_uids=11368430&dopt=Abstract

- **Langerhans cell histiocytosis following childhood acute lymphoblastic leukemia.**
Author(s): Raj A, Bendon R, Moriarty T, Suarez C, Bertolone S.
Source: American Journal of Hematology. 2001 December; 68(4): 284-6.
http://www.ncbi.nlm.nih.gov:80/entrez/query.fcgi?cmd=Retrieve&db=PubMed&list_uids=11754419&dopt=Abstract

- **Late relapse of childhood acute lymphoblastic leukemia and pcr-monitoring of minimal residual disease: how much time can elapse between "molecular" and clinical relapse?**
Author(s): Arico M, Germano G, del Giudice L, Ziino O, Locatelli F, Basso G.
Source: Haematologica. 2002 April; 87(4): Elt19. No Abstract Available.
http://www.ncbi.nlm.nih.gov:80/entrez/query.fcgi?cmd=Retrieve&db=PubMed&list_uids=11940504&dopt=Abstract

- **Long-term follow-up of childhood acute lymphoblastic leukemia in Tokyo Children's Cancer Study Group 1981-1995.**
Author(s): Tsuchida M, Ikuta K, Hanada R, Saito T, Isoyama K, Sugita K, Toyoda Y, Manabe A, Koike K, Kinoshita A, Maeda M, Ishimoto K, Sato T, Okimoto Y, Kaneko T, Kajiwara M, Sotomatsu M, Hayashi Y, Yabe H, Hosoya R, Hoshi Y, Ohira M, Bessho F, Tsunematsu Y, Tsukimoto I, Nakazawa S.
Source: Leukemia : Official Journal of the Leukemia Society of America, Leukemia Research Fund, U.K. 2000 December; 14(12): 2295-306.
http://www.ncbi.nlm.nih.gov:80/entrez/query.fcgi?cmd=Retrieve&db=PubMed&list_uids=11187921&dopt=Abstract

- **Long-term results of large prospective trials in childhood acute lymphoblastic leukemia.**
  Author(s): Schrappe M, Camitta B, Pui CH, Eden T, Gaynon P, Gustafsson G, Janka-Schaub GE, Kamps W, Masera G, Sallan S, Tsuchida M, Vilmer E.
  Source: Leukemia : Official Journal of the Leukemia Society of America, Leukemia Research Fund, U.K. 2000 December; 14(12): 2193-4. No Abstract Available.
  http://www.ncbi.nlm.nih.gov:80/entrez/query.fcgi?cmd=Retrieve&db=PubMed&list_uids=11187910&dopt=Abstract

- **Long-term results of three randomized trials (58831, 58832, 58881) in childhood acute lymphoblastic leukemia: a CLCG-EORTC report. Children Leukemia Cooperative Group.**
  Author(s): Vilmer E, Suciu S, Ferster A, Bertrand Y, Cave H, Thyss A, Benoit Y, Dastugue N, Fournier M, Souillet G, Manel AM, Robert A, Nelken B, Millot F, Lutz P, Rialland X, Mechinaud F, Boutard P, Behar C, Chantraine JM, Plouvier E, Laureys G, Brock P, Uyttebroeck A, Margueritte G, Plantaz D, Norton L, Francotte N, Gyselinck J, Waterkeyn C, Solbu G, Philippe N, Otten J.
  Source: Leukemia : Official Journal of the Leukemia Society of America, Leukemia Research Fund, U.K. 2000 December; 14(12): 2257-66.
  http://www.ncbi.nlm.nih.gov:80/entrez/query.fcgi?cmd=Retrieve&db=PubMed&list_uids=11187917&dopt=Abstract

- **Long-term results of Total Therapy studies 11, 12 and 13A for childhood acute lymphoblastic leukemia at St Jude Children's Research Hospital.**
  Author(s): Pui CH, Boyett JM, Rivera GK, Hancock ML, Sandlund JT, Ribeiro RC, Rubnitz JE, Behm FG, Raimondi SC, Gajjar A, Razzouk B, Campana D, Kun LE, Relling MV, Evans WE.
  Source: Leukemia : Official Journal of the Leukemia Society of America, Leukemia Research Fund, U.K. 2000 December; 14(12): 2286-94.
  http://www.ncbi.nlm.nih.gov:80/entrez/query.fcgi?cmd=Retrieve&db=PubMed&list_uids=11187920&dopt=Abstract

- **Long-term results of treatment studies for childhood acute lymphoblastic leukemia: Pediatric Oncology Group studies from 1986-1994.**
  Author(s): Maloney KW, Shuster JJ, Murphy S, Pullen J, Camitta BA.

Source: Leukemia : Official Journal of the Leukemia Society of America, Leukemia Research Fund, U.K. 2000 December; 14(12): 2276-85.
http://www.ncbi.nlm.nih.gov:80/entrez/query.fcgi?cmd=Retrieve&db=PubMed&list_uids=11187919&dopt=Abstract

- **Loss at 12p detected by comparative genomic hybridization (CGH): association with TEL-AML1 fusion and favorable prognostic features in childhood acute lymphoblastic leukemia (ALL). A multi-institutional study.**
  Author(s): Kanerva J, Niini T, Vettenranta K, Riikonen P, Makipernaa A, Karhu R, Knuutila S, Saarinen-Pihkala UM.
  Source: Medical and Pediatric Oncology. 2001 November; 37(5): 419-25.
  http://www.ncbi.nlm.nih.gov:80/entrez/query.fcgi?cmd=Retrieve&db=PubMed&list_uids=11745869&dopt=Abstract

- **Loss of X chromosome in childhood acute lymphoblastic leukemia.**
  Author(s): Riesch M, Niggli FK, Leibundgut K, Caflisch U, Betts DR.
  Source: Cancer Genetics and Cytogenetics. 2001 February; 125(1): 27-9.
  http://www.ncbi.nlm.nih.gov:80/entrez/query.fcgi?cmd=Retrieve&db=PubMed&list_uids=11297764&dopt=Abstract

- **Low-dose daunorubicin in induction treatment of childhood acute lymphoblastic leukemia: no long-term cardiac damage in a randomized study of the Dutch Childhood Leukemia Study Group.**
  Author(s): Rammeloo LA, Postma A, Sobotka-Plojhar MA, Bink-Boelkens MT, Berg A, Veerman AJ, Kamps WA.
  Source: Medical and Pediatric Oncology. 2000 July; 35(1): 13-9.
  http://www.ncbi.nlm.nih.gov:80/entrez/query.fcgi?cmd=Retrieve&db=PubMed&list_uids=10881002&dopt=Abstract

- **Lymphomatoid granulomatosis after childhood acute lymphoblastic leukemia: report of effective therapy.**
  Author(s): Moertel CL, Carlson-Green B, Watterson J, Simonton SC.
  Source: Pediatrics. 2001 May; 107(5): E82.
  http://www.ncbi.nlm.nih.gov:80/entrez/query.fcgi?cmd=Retrieve&db=PubMed&list_uids=11331732&dopt=Abstract

- **Male sex and low physical activity are associated with reduced spine bone mineral density in survivors of childhood acute lymphoblastic leukemia.**
  Author(s): Tillmann V, Darlington AS, Eiser C, Bishop NJ, Davies HA.

Source: Journal of Bone and Mineral Research : the Official Journal of the American Society for Bone and Mineral Research. 2002 June; 17(6): 1073-80.
http://www.ncbi.nlm.nih.gov:80/entrez/query.fcgi?cmd=Retrieve&db=PubMed&list_uids=12054163&dopt=Abstract

- **Matched-pair analysis comparing allogeneic PBPCT and BMT from HLA-identical relatives in childhood acute lymphoblastic leukemia.**
  Author(s): Vicent MG, Madero L, Ortega JJ, Martinez A, Gomez P, Verdeguer A, Badell I, Munoz A, Olive T, Maldonado MS, Bureo E, Cubells J, Diaz MA.
  Source: Bone Marrow Transplantation. 2002 July; 30(1): 9-13.
  http://www.ncbi.nlm.nih.gov:80/entrez/query.fcgi?cmd=Retrieve&db=PubMed&list_uids=12105771&dopt=Abstract

- **MDM2 and p53 in childhood acute lymphoblastic leukemia: higher expression in childhood leukemias with poor prognosis compared to long-term survivors.**
  Author(s): Gustafsson B, Axelsson B, Gustafsson B, Christensson B, Winiarski J.
  Source: Pediatric Hematology and Oncology. 2001 December; 18(8): 497-508.
  http://www.ncbi.nlm.nih.gov:80/entrez/query.fcgi?cmd=Retrieve&db=PubMed&list_uids=11764099&dopt=Abstract

- **Messenger RNA analysis of the multidrug resistance related protein (MRP1) and the lung resistance protein (LRP) in de novo and relapsed childhood acute lymphoblastic leukemia.**
  Author(s): Sauerbrey A, Voigt A, Wittig S, Hafer R, Zintl F.
  Source: Leukemia & Lymphoma. 2002 April; 43(4): 875-9.
  http://www.ncbi.nlm.nih.gov:80/entrez/query.fcgi?cmd=Retrieve&db=PubMed&list_uids=12153178&dopt=Abstract

- **Microclustering of TEL-AML1 translocation breakpoints in childhood acute lymphoblastic leukemia.**
  Author(s): Wiemels JL, Alexander FE, Cazzaniga G, Biondi A, Mayer SP, Greaves M.
  Source: Genes, Chromosomes & Cancer. 2000 November; 29(3): 219-28.
  http://www.ncbi.nlm.nih.gov:80/entrez/query.fcgi?cmd=Retrieve&db=PubMed&list_uids=10992297&dopt=Abstract

- **Minimal residual disease quantification in childhood acute lymphoblastic leukemia by real-time polymerase chain reaction using the SYBR green dye.**
  Author(s): Li A, Forestier E, Rosenquist R, Roos G.
  Source: Experimental Hematology. 2002 October; 30(10): 1170.
  http://www.ncbi.nlm.nih.gov:80/entrez/query.fcgi?cmd=Retrieve&db=PubMed&list_uids=12384148&dopt=Abstract

- **Molecular diagnostics in the treatment of childhood acute lymphoblastic leukemia.**
  Author(s): Rubnitz JE.
  Source: J Biol Regul Homeost Agents. 2000 July-September; 14(3): 182-6. Review.
  http://www.ncbi.nlm.nih.gov:80/entrez/query.fcgi?cmd=Retrieve&db=PubMed&list_uids=11037050&dopt=Abstract

- **Motor nervous system impairment persists in long-term survivors of childhood acute lymphoblastic leukemia.**
  Author(s): Lehtinen SS, Huuskonen UE, Harila-Saari AH, Tolonen U, Vainionpaa LK, Lanning BM.
  Source: Cancer. 2002 May 1; 94(9): 2466-73.
  http://www.ncbi.nlm.nih.gov:80/entrez/query.fcgi?cmd=Retrieve&db=PubMed&list_uids=12015772&dopt=Abstract

- **MRD at the end of induction therapy in childhood acute lymphoblastic leukemia: outcome prediction strongly depends on the therapeutic regimen.**
  Author(s): zur Stadt U, Harms DO, Schluter S, Schrappe M, Goebel U, Spaar H, Janka G, Kabisch H.
  Source: Leukemia : Official Journal of the Leukemia Society of America, Leukemia Research Fund, U.K. 2001 February; 15(2): 283-5. No Abstract Available.
  http://www.ncbi.nlm.nih.gov:80/entrez/query.fcgi?cmd=Retrieve&db=PubMed&list_uids=11236947&dopt=Abstract

- **Multicolor spectral karyotyping identifies novel translocations in childhood acute lymphoblastic leukemia.**
  Author(s): Mathew S, Rao PH, Dalton J, Downing JR, Raimondi SC.

Source: Leukemia : Official Journal of the Leukemia Society of America, Leukemia Research Fund, U.K. 2001 March; 15(3): 468-72.
http://www.ncbi.nlm.nih.gov:80/entrez/query.fcgi?cmd=Retrieve&db=PubMed&list_uids=11237073&dopt=Abstract

- **Mutations in the Nijmegen Breakage Syndrome gene (NBS1) in childhood acute lymphoblastic leukemia (ALL).**
  Author(s): Varon R, Reis A, Henze G, von Einsiedel HG, Sperling K, Seeger K.
  Source: Cancer Research. 2001 May 1; 61(9): 3570-2.
  http://www.ncbi.nlm.nih.gov:80/entrez/query.fcgi?cmd=Retrieve&db=PubMed&list_uids=11325820&dopt=Abstract

- **Myelotoxicity, pharmacokinetics, and relapse rate with methotrexate/6-mercaptopurine maintenance therapy of childhood acute lymphoblastic leukemia.**
  Author(s): Schmiegelow K, Ifversen M.
  Source: Pediatric Hematology and Oncology. 1996 September-October; 13(5): 433-41.
  http://www.ncbi.nlm.nih.gov:80/entrez/query.fcgi?cmd=Retrieve&db=PubMed&list_uids=10897815&dopt=Abstract

- **Near haploid childhood acute lymphoblastic leukemia masked by hyperdiploid line: detection by fluorescence in situ hybridization.**
  Author(s): Stark B, Jeison M, Gobuzov R, Krug H, Glaser-Gabay L, Luria D, El-Hasid R, Harush MB, Avrahami G, Fisher S, Stein J, Zaizov R, Yaniv I.
  Source: Cancer Genetics and Cytogenetics. 2001 July 15; 128(2): 108-13.
  http://www.ncbi.nlm.nih.gov:80/entrez/query.fcgi?cmd=Retrieve&db=PubMed&list_uids=11463448&dopt=Abstract

- **Near-haploidy in myeloid antigen positive childhood acute lymphoblastic leukemia.**
  Author(s): Mukherjee S, Das Gupta A, Khodaiji S, Agarwal MB.
  Source: American Journal of Hematology. 2001 August; 67(4): 276-7. No Abstract Available.
  http://www.ncbi.nlm.nih.gov:80/entrez/query.fcgi?cmd=Retrieve&db=PubMed&list_uids=11443648&dopt=Abstract

- **Normal bone mineral density after treatment for childhood acute lymphoblastic leukemia diagnosed between 1991 and 1998.**

Author(s): Kadan-Lottick N, Marshall JA, Baron AE, Krebs NF, Hambidge KM, Albano E.
Source: The Journal of Pediatrics. 2001 June; 138(6): 898-904.
http://www.ncbi.nlm.nih.gov:80/entrez/query.fcgi?cmd=Retrieve&db=PubMed&list_uids=11391336&dopt=Abstract

- **Nutritional and socio-economic status in the prognosis of childhood acute lymphoblastic leukemia.**
  Author(s): Viana MB, Fernandes RA, de Oliveira BM, Murao M, de Andrade Paes C, Duarte AA.
  Source: Haematologica. 2001 February; 86(2): 113-20. Review. No Abstract Available.
  http://www.ncbi.nlm.nih.gov:80/entrez/query.fcgi?cmd=Retrieve&db=PubMed&list_uids=11224478&dopt=Abstract

- **Ocular involvement in childhood acute lymphoblastic leukemia.**
  Author(s): Birinci H, Albayrak D, Oge I, Kaman A.
  Source: J Pediatr Ophthalmol Strabismus. 2001 July-August; 38(4): 242-4. No Abstract Available.
  http://www.ncbi.nlm.nih.gov:80/entrez/query.fcgi?cmd=Retrieve&db=PubMed&list_uids=11495313&dopt=Abstract

- **Origins of "late" relapse in childhood acute lymphoblastic leukemia with TEL-AML1 fusion genes.**
  Author(s): Ford AM, Fasching K, Panzer-Grumayer ER, Koenig M, Haas OA, Greaves MF.
  Source: Blood. 2001 August 1; 98(3): 558-64.
  http://www.ncbi.nlm.nih.gov:80/entrez/query.fcgi?cmd=Retrieve&db=PubMed&list_uids=11468150&dopt=Abstract

- **Outcome after relapse in childhood acute lymphoblastic leukemia.**
  Author(s): Yumura-Yagi K, Hara J, Horibe K, Tawa A, Komada Y, Oda M, Nishimura S, Yoshida M, Kudo T, Ueda K.
  Source: International Journal of Hematology. 2002 July; 76(1): 61-8.
  http://www.ncbi.nlm.nih.gov:80/entrez/query.fcgi?cmd=Retrieve&db=PubMed&list_uids=12138898&dopt=Abstract

- **Outcomes of growth hormone replacement therapy in survivors of childhood acute lymphoblastic leukemia.**
  Author(s): Leung W, Rose SR, Zhou Y, Hancock ML, Burstein S, Schriock EA, Lustig R, Danish RK, Evans WE, Hudson MM, Pui CH.

Source: Journal of Clinical Oncology : Official Journal of the American Society of Clinical Oncology. 2002 July 1; 20(13): 2959-64.
http://www.ncbi.nlm.nih.gov:80/entrez/query.fcgi?cmd=Retrieve&db=PubMed&list_uids=12089225&dopt=Abstract

- **#14-S breast-feeding and risk of childhood acute lymphoblastic leukemia. Results and commentary from a case-control study.**
  Author(s): Kwan M, Buffler P.
  Source: Annals of Epidemiology. 2002 October; 12(7): 495.
  http://www.ncbi.nlm.nih.gov:80/entrez/query.fcgi?cmd=Retrieve&db=PubMed&list_uids=12377440&dopt=Abstract

- **6-mercaptopurine: efficacy and bone marrow toxicity in childhood acute lymphoblastic leukemia. Association with low (thio)purine enzyme activity.**
  Author(s): De Abreu RA, Lambooy LH, Ahment K, Brouwer C, Keizer-Garritsen JJ, Bokkerink JP, Trijbels FJ.
  Source: Advances in Experimental Medicine and Biology. 2000; 486: 271-5. Review. No Abstract Available.
  http://www.ncbi.nlm.nih.gov:80/entrez/query.fcgi?cmd=Retrieve&db=PubMed&list_uids=11783498&dopt=Abstract

- **Abnormalities of chromosome bands 13q12 to 13q14 in childhood acute lymphoblastic leukemia.**
  Author(s): Heerema NA, Sather HN, Sensel MG, Lee MK, Hutchinson RJ, Nachman JB, Reaman GH, Lange BJ, Steinherz PG, Bostrom BC, Gaynon PS, Uckun FM.
  Source: Journal of Clinical Oncology : Official Journal of the American Society of Clinical Oncology. 2000 November 15; 18(22): 3837-44.
  http://www.ncbi.nlm.nih.gov:80/entrez/query.fcgi?cmd=Retrieve&db=PubMed&list_uids=11078497&dopt=Abstract

- **Abnormalities of chromosome bands 15q13-15 in childhood acute lymphoblastic leukemia.**
  Author(s): Heerema NA, Sather HN, Sensel MG, La MK, Hutchinson RJ, Nachman JB, Reaman GH, Lange BJ, Steinherz PG, Bostrom BC, Gaynon PS, Uckun FM.
  Source: Cancer. 2002 February 15; 94(4): 1102-10.
  http://www.ncbi.nlm.nih.gov:80/entrez/query.fcgi?cmd=Retrieve&db=PubMed&list_uids=11920481&dopt=Abstract

- **Absence of mutations in the CDKN2 binding site of CDK4 in childhood acute lymphoblastic leukemia.**
  Author(s): Einsiedel HG, Taube T, Beyermann B, Dragon S, Moricke A, Kebelmann-Betzig C, Kochling J, Henze G, Seeger K.
  Source: Leukemia & Lymphoma. 2001 January; 40(3-4): 413-7.
  http://www.ncbi.nlm.nih.gov:80/entrez/query.fcgi?cmd=Retrieve&db=PubMed&list_uids=11426564&dopt=Abstract

- **Adhesion molecule expression, clinical features and therapy outcome in childhood acute lymphoblastic leukemia.**
  Author(s): Mengarelli A, Zarcone D, Caruso R, Tenca C, Rana I, Pinto RM, Grossi CE, De Rossi G.
  Source: Leukemia & Lymphoma. 2001 February; 40(5-6): 625-30.
  http://www.ncbi.nlm.nih.gov:80/entrez/query.fcgi?cmd=Retrieve&db=PubMed&list_uids=11426534&dopt=Abstract

- **Altered bone mineral density and body composition, and increased fracture risk in childhood acute lymphoblastic leukemia.**
  Author(s): van der Sluis IM, van den Heuvel-Eibrink MM, Hahlen K, Krenning EP, de Muinck Keizer-Schrama SM.
  Source: The Journal of Pediatrics. 2002 August; 141(2): 204-10.
  http://www.ncbi.nlm.nih.gov:80/entrez/query.fcgi?cmd=Retrieve&db=PubMed&list_uids=12183715&dopt=Abstract

- **AML1 amplification in a case of childhood acute lymphoblastic leukemia.**
  Author(s): Morel F, Herry A, Le Bris MJ, Douet-Guilbert N, Le Calvez G, Marion V, Berthou C, De Braekeeler M.
  Source: Cancer Genetics and Cytogenetics. 2002 September; 137(2): 142.
  http://www.ncbi.nlm.nih.gov:80/entrez/query.fcgi?cmd=Retrieve&db=PubMed&list_uids=12393286&dopt=Abstract

- **AML1 gene over-expression in childhood acute lymphoblastic leukemia.**
  Author(s): Mikhail FM, Serry KA, Hatem N, Mourad ZI, Farawela HM, El Kaffash DM, Coignet L, Nucifora G.
  Source: Leukemia : Official Journal of the Leukemia Society of America, Leukemia Research Fund, U.K. 2002 April; 16(4): 658-68.
  http://www.ncbi.nlm.nih.gov:80/entrez/query.fcgi?cmd=Retrieve&db=PubMed&list_uids=11960347&dopt=Abstract

- **Amplification of AML1 gene is present in childhood acute lymphoblastic leukemia but not in adult, and is not associated with AML1 gene mutation.**
  Author(s): Penther D, Preudhomme C, Talmant P, Roumier C, Godon A, Mechinaud F, Milpied N, Bataille R, Avet-Loiseau H.
  Source: Leukemia : Official Journal of the Leukemia Society of America, Leukemia Research Fund, U.K. 2002 June; 16(6): 1131-4.
  http://www.ncbi.nlm.nih.gov:80/entrez/query.fcgi?cmd=Retrieve&db=PubMed&list_uids=12040444&dopt=Abstract

- **Amplification of AML1 in childhood acute lymphoblastic leukemias.**
  Author(s): Dal Cin P, Atkins L, Ford C, Ariyanayagam S, Armstrong SA, George R, Cleary A, Morton CC.
  Source: Genes, Chromosomes & Cancer. 2001 April; 30(4): 407-9.
  http://www.ncbi.nlm.nih.gov:80/entrez/query.fcgi?cmd=Retrieve&db=PubMed&list_uids=11241794&dopt=Abstract

- **Analysis of TP53 mutations in relapsed childhood acute lymphoblastic leukemia.**
  Author(s): Gump J, McGavran L, Wei Q, Hunger SP.
  Source: Journal of Pediatric Hematology/Oncology : Official Journal of the American Society of Pediatric Hematology/Oncology. 2001 October; 23(7): 416-9.
  http://www.ncbi.nlm.nih.gov:80/entrez/query.fcgi?cmd=Retrieve&db=PubMed&list_uids=11878574&dopt=Abstract

- **Anti-Erwinia asparaginase antibodies during treatment of childhood acute lymphoblastic leukemia and their relationship to outcome: a case-control study.**
  Author(s): Klug Albertsen B, Schmiegelow K, Schroder H, Carlsen NT, Rosthoj S, Avramis VI, Jakobsen P.
  Source: Cancer Chemotherapy and Pharmacology. 2002 August; 50(2): 117-20.
  http://www.ncbi.nlm.nih.gov:80/entrez/query.fcgi?cmd=Retrieve&db=PubMed&list_uids=12172975&dopt=Abstract

- **Application of a chemiluminescent methodology for detection of minimal residual disease in childhood acute lymphoblastic leukemia.**
  Author(s): Lo Nigro L, Poli A, Mirabile E, Costantino F, Schiliro G.

Source: Haematologica. 2001 December; 86(12): 1314-6. No Abstract Available.
http://www.ncbi.nlm.nih.gov:80/entrez/query.fcgi?cmd=Retrieve&db=PubMed&list_uids=11726326&dopt=Abstract

- **Autologous bone marrow transplantation for childhood acute lymphoblastic leukemia in second remission.**
  Author(s): Maldonado MS, Munoz A.
  Source: Bone Marrow Transplantation. 2000 November; 26(10): 1136-7. No Abstract Available.
  http://www.ncbi.nlm.nih.gov:80/entrez/query.fcgi?cmd=Retrieve&db=PubMed&list_uids=11108320&dopt=Abstract

- **Autologous bone marrow transplantation for childhood acute lymphoblastic leukemia: a novel combined approach consisting of ex vivo marrow purging, modulation of multi-drug resistance, induction of autograft vs leukemia effect, and post-transplant immuno- and chemotherapy (PTIC).**
  Author(s): Houtenbos I, Bracho F, Davenport V, Slack R, van de Ven C, Suen Y, Killen R, Shen V, Cairo MS.
  Source: Bone Marrow Transplantation. 2001 January; 27(2): 145-53.
  http://www.ncbi.nlm.nih.gov:80/entrez/query.fcgi?cmd=Retrieve&db=PubMed&list_uids=11281383&dopt=Abstract

- **Beginning treatment for childhood acute lymphoblastic leukemia: insights from the parents' perspective.**
  Author(s): McGrath P.
  Source: Oncology Nursing Forum. 2002 July; 29(6): 988-96.
  http://www.ncbi.nlm.nih.gov:80/entrez/query.fcgi?cmd=Retrieve&db=PubMed&list_uids=12096296&dopt=Abstract

- **Bone marrow transplantation versus chemotherapy in the treatment of very high-risk childhood acute lymphoblastic leukemia in first remission: results from Medical Research Council UKALL X and XI.**
  Author(s): Wheeler KA, Richards SM, Bailey CC, Gibson B, Hann IM, Hill FG, Chessells JM.
  Source: Blood. 2000 October 1; 96(7): 2412-8.
  http://www.ncbi.nlm.nih.gov:80/entrez/query.fcgi?cmd=Retrieve&db=PubMed&list_uids=11001892&dopt=Abstract

- **Bone mineral decrements in survivors of childhood acute lymphoblastic leukemia: frequency of occurrence and risk factors for**

their development.
Author(s): Kaste SC, Jones-Wallace D, Rose SR, Boyett JM, Lustig RH, Rivera GK, Pui CH, Hudson MM.
Source: Leukemia : Official Journal of the Leukemia Society of America, Leukemia Research Fund, U.K. 2001 May; 15(5): 728-34.
http://www.ncbi.nlm.nih.gov:80/entrez/query.fcgi?cmd=Retrieve&db=PubMed&list_uids=11368432&dopt=Abstract

- **Cardiovascular risk factors in young adult survivors of childhood acute lymphoblastic leukemia.**
  Author(s): Oeffinger KC, Buchanan GR, Eshelman DA, Denke MA, Andrews TC, Germak JA, Tomlinson GE, Snell LE, Foster BM.
  Source: Journal of Pediatric Hematology/Oncology : Official Journal of the American Society of Pediatric Hematology/Oncology. 2001 October; 23(7): 424-30.
  http://www.ncbi.nlm.nih.gov:80/entrez/query.fcgi?cmd=Retrieve&db=PubMed&list_uids=11878576&dopt=Abstract

- **CD40 ligand-stimulated B cell precursor leukemic cells elicit interferon-gamma production by autologous bone marrow T cells in childhood acute lymphoblastic leukemia.**
  Author(s): Todisco E, Gaipa G, Biagi E, Bonamino M, Gramigna R, Introna M, Biondi A.
  Source: Leukemia : Official Journal of the Leukemia Society of America, Leukemia Research Fund, U.K. 2002 October; 16(10): 2046-54.
  http://www.ncbi.nlm.nih.gov:80/entrez/query.fcgi?cmd=Retrieve&db=PubMed&list_uids=12357356&dopt=Abstract

- **Central nervous system-directed therapy in the treatment of childhood acute lymphoblastic leukemia and studies of neurobehavioral outcome: Children's Cancer Group trials.**
  Author(s): Kaleita TA.
  Source: Current Oncology Reports. 2002 March; 4(2): 131-41. Review.
  http://www.ncbi.nlm.nih.gov:80/entrez/query.fcgi?cmd=Retrieve&db=PubMed&list_uids=11822985&dopt=Abstract

- **Changes in body mass index and prevalence of overweight in survivors of childhood acute lymphoblastic leukemia: role of cranial irradiation.**
  Author(s): Sklar CA, Mertens AC, Walter A, Mitchell D, Nesbit ME, O'Leary M, Hutchinson R, Meadows AT, Robison LL.

Source: Medical and Pediatric Oncology. 2000 August; 35(2): 91-5.
http://www.ncbi.nlm.nih.gov:80/entrez/query.fcgi?cmd=Retrieve&db=PubMed&list_uids=10918229&dopt=Abstract

- **Characterization of additional genetic events in childhood acute lymphoblastic leukemia with TEL/AML1 gene fusion: a molecular cytogenetics study.**
  Author(s): Ma SK, Wan TS, Cheuk AT, Fung LF, Chan GC, Chan SY, Ha SY, Chan LC.
  Source: Leukemia : Official Journal of the Leukemia Society of America, Leukemia Research Fund, U.K. 2001 September; 15(9): 1442-7.
  http://www.ncbi.nlm.nih.gov:80/entrez/query.fcgi?cmd=Retrieve&db=PubMed&list_uids=11516105&dopt=Abstract

- **Childhood acute lymphoblastic leukemia associated with parental alcohol consumption and polymorphisms of carcinogen-metabolizing genes.**
  Author(s): Infante-Rivard C, Krajinovic M, Labuda D, Sinnett D.
  Source: Epidemiology (Cambridge, Mass.). 2002 May; 13(3): 277-81.
  http://www.ncbi.nlm.nih.gov:80/entrez/query.fcgi?cmd=Retrieve&db=PubMed&list_uids=11964928&dopt=Abstract

- **Childhood acute lymphoblastic leukemia presenting with severe hepatic dysfunction.**
  Author(s): Belgaumi AF, Hudson MM.
  Source: Medical and Pediatric Oncology. 2001 August; 37(2): 142-4. No Abstract Available.
  http://www.ncbi.nlm.nih.gov:80/entrez/query.fcgi?cmd=Retrieve&db=PubMed&list_uids=11496355&dopt=Abstract

- **Childhood acute lymphoblastic leukemia with a novel der(10)t(7;10)(q11;q26).**
  Author(s): So CC, Wong KF.
  Source: Cancer Genetics and Cytogenetics. 2001 July 15; 128(2): 175-7. No Abstract Available.
  http://www.ncbi.nlm.nih.gov:80/entrez/query.fcgi?cmd=Retrieve&db=PubMed&list_uids=11478301&dopt=Abstract

- **Childhood acute lymphoblastic leukemia.**
  Author(s): Pui CH, Relling MV, Campana D, Evans WE.

Source: Reviews in Clinical and Experimental Hematology. 2002 June; 6(2): 161-80.
http://www.ncbi.nlm.nih.gov:80/entrez/query.fcgi?cmd=Retrieve&db=PubMed&list_uids=12196214&dopt=Abstract

- **Childhood acute lymphoblastic leukemia: current perspectives.**
  Author(s): Landier W.
  Source: Oncology Nursing Forum. 2001 June; 28(5): 823-33; Quiz 834-5. Review.
  http://www.ncbi.nlm.nih.gov:80/entrez/query.fcgi?cmd=Retrieve&db=PubMed&list_uids=11421142&dopt=Abstract

- **Childhood acute lymphoblastic leukemia: genetic determinants of susceptibility and disease outcome.**
  Author(s): Krajinovic M, Labuda D, Sinnett D.
  Source: Rev Environ Health. 2001 July-September; 16(4): 263-79. Review.
  http://www.ncbi.nlm.nih.gov:80/entrez/query.fcgi?cmd=Retrieve&db=PubMed&list_uids=12041882&dopt=Abstract

- **Childhood acute lymphoblastic leukemia: prognostic value of initial peripheral blast count in good responders to prednisone.**
  Author(s): Felice MS, Zubizarreta PA, Alfaro EM, Sackmann-Muriel F.
  Source: Journal of Pediatric Hematology/Oncology : Official Journal of the American Society of Pediatric Hematology/Oncology. 2001 October; 23(7): 411-5.
  http://www.ncbi.nlm.nih.gov:80/entrez/query.fcgi?cmd=Retrieve&db=PubMed&list_uids=11878573&dopt=Abstract

- **Children's Cancer Group trials in childhood acute lymphoblastic leukemia: 1983-1995.**
  Author(s): Gaynon PS, Trigg ME, Heerema NA, Sensel MG, Sather HN, Hammond GD, Bleyer WA.
  Source: Leukemia : Official Journal of the Leukemia Society of America, Leukemia Research Fund, U.K. 2000 December; 14(12): 2223-33.
  http://www.ncbi.nlm.nih.gov:80/entrez/query.fcgi?cmd=Retrieve&db=PubMed&list_uids=11187913&dopt=Abstract

- **Clinical trials in childhood acute lymphoblastic leukemia: a common prognostic classification and a common induction therapy are now warranted.**
  Author(s): Donadieu J, Hill C.

Source: Journal of Pediatric Hematology/Oncology : Official Journal of the American Society of Pediatric Hematology/Oncology. 2002 August-September; 24(6): 424-5. No Abstract Available.
http://www.ncbi.nlm.nih.gov:80/entrez/query.fcgi?cmd=Retrieve&db=PubMed&list_uids=12218586&dopt=Abstract

- **Comparative genomic hybridization in childhood acute lymphoblastic leukemia: correlation with interphase cytogenetics and loss of heterozygosity analysis.**
  Author(s): Scholz I, Popp S, Granzow M, Schoell B, Holtgreve-Grez H, Takeuchi S, Schrappe M, Harbott J, Teigler-Schlegel A, Zimmermann M, Fischer C, Koeffler HP, Bartram CR, Jauch A.
  Source: Cancer Genetics and Cytogenetics. 2001 January 15; 124(2): 89-97.
  http://www.ncbi.nlm.nih.gov:80/entrez/query.fcgi?cmd=Retrieve&db=PubMed&list_uids=11172898&dopt=Abstract

- **Concordant childhood acute lymphoblastic leukemia in monozygotic twins.**
  Author(s): Chin YM, Wan Ariffin A, Lin HP, Chan YS.
  Source: Med J Malaysia. 1996 March; 51(1): 145-8.
  http://www.ncbi.nlm.nih.gov:80/entrez/query.fcgi?cmd=Retrieve&db=PubMed&list_uids=10967997&dopt=Abstract

- **Co-operative study group for childhood acute lymphoblastic leukemia (COALL): long-term follow-up of trials 82, 85, 89 and 92.**
  Author(s): Harms DO, Janka-Schaub GE.
  Source: Leukemia : Official Journal of the Leukemia Society of America, Leukemia Research Fund, U.K. 2000 December; 14(12): 2234-9.
  http://www.ncbi.nlm.nih.gov:80/entrez/query.fcgi?cmd=Retrieve&db=PubMed&list_uids=11187914&dopt=Abstract

- **Cotrimoxazole prophylaxis of Pneumocystis carinii infection during the treatment of childhood acute lymphoblastic leukemia--beware non compliance in older children and adolescents.**
  Author(s): Castagnola E, Zarri D, Caprino D, Losurdo G, Micalizzi C.
  Source: Supportive Care in Cancer : Official Journal of the Multinational Association of Supportive Care in Cancer. 2001 October; 9(7): 552-3. No Abstract Available.
  http://www.ncbi.nlm.nih.gov:80/entrez/query.fcgi?cmd=Retrieve&db=PubMed&list_uids=11680836&dopt=Abstract

- **Current chemotherapy protocols for childhood acute lymphoblastic leukemia induce loss of humoral immunity to viral vaccination antigens.**
  Author(s): Nilsson A, De Milito A, Engstrom P, Nordin M, Narita M, Grillner L, Chiodi F, Bjork O.
  Source: Pediatrics. 2002 June; 109(6): E91.
  http://www.ncbi.nlm.nih.gov:80/entrez/query.fcgi?cmd=Retrieve&db=PubMed&list_uids=12042585&dopt=Abstract

- **Cytogenetic and FISH studies of a single center consecutive series of 152 childhood acute lymphoblastic leukemias.**
  Author(s): Andreasson P, Hoglund M, Bekassy AN, Garwicz S, Heldrup J, Mitelman F, Johansson B.
  Source: European Journal of Haematology. 2000 July; 65(1): 40-51.
  http://www.ncbi.nlm.nih.gov:80/entrez/query.fcgi?cmd=Retrieve&db=PubMed&list_uids=10914938&dopt=Abstract

- **Deletion analysis of p16(INKa) and p15(INKb) in relapsed childhood acute lymphoblastic leukemia.**
  Author(s): Graf Einsiedel H, Taube T, Hartmann R, Wellmann S, Seifert G, Henze G, Seeger K.
  Source: Blood. 2002 June 15; 99(12): 4629-31.
  http://www.ncbi.nlm.nih.gov:80/entrez/query.fcgi?cmd=Retrieve&db=PubMed&list_uids=12036898&dopt=Abstract

- **p16(INK4a) immunocytochemical analysis is an independent prognostic factor in childhood acute lymphoblastic leukemia.**
  Author(s): Dalle JH, Fournier M, Nelken B, Mazingue F, Lai JL, Bauters F, Fenaux P, Quesnel B.
  Source: Blood. 2002 April 1; 99(7): 2620-3.
  http://www.ncbi.nlm.nih.gov:80/entrez/query.fcgi?cmd=Retrieve&db=PubMed&list_uids=11895806&dopt=Abstract

Vocabulary Builder

Abscess: A localized collection of pus caused by suppuration buried in tissues, organs, or confined spaces. [EU]

Alleles: Mutually exclusive forms of the same gene, occupying the same locus on homologous chromosomes, and governing the same biochemical and developmental process. [NIH]

Antigens: Substances that cause the immune system to make a specific immune response. [NIH]

Apoptosis: A normal series of events in a cell that leads to its death. [NIH]

Asparaginase: An anticancer drug that is an enzyme. [NIH]

Aspiration: Removal of fluid from a lump, often a cyst, with a needle and a syringe. [NIH]

Assay: Determination of the amount of a particular constituent of a mixture, or of the biological or pharmacological potency of a drug. [EU]

Biomarkers: Substances sometimes found in an increased amount in the blood, other body fluids, or tissues and that may suggest the presence of some types of cancer. Biomarkers include CA 125 (ovarian cancer), CA 15-3 (breast cancer), CEA (ovarian, lung, breast, pancreas, and GI tract cancers), and PSA (prostate cancer). Also called tumor markers. [NIH]

Carcinogen: Any substance that causes cancer. [NIH]

Cardiac: Having to do with the heart. [NIH]

Cardiomyopathy: A general diagnostic term designating primary myocardial disease, often of obscure or unknown etiology. [EU]

Carnitine: Constituent of striated muscle and liver. It is used therapeutically to stimulate gastric and pancreatic secretions and in the treatment of hyperlipoproteinemias. [NIH]

Catechol: A chemical originally isolated from a type of mimosa tree. Catechol is used as an astringent, an antiseptic, and in photography, electroplating, and making other chemicals. It can also be man-made. [NIH]

Chromosomal: Pertaining to chromosomes. [EU]

Cisplatin: An anticancer drug that belongs to the family of drugs called platinum compounds. [NIH]

Cranial: Pertaining to the cranium, or to the anterior (in animals) or superior (in humans) end of the body. [EU]

Cytogenetics: A branch of genetics which deals with the cytological and molecular behavior of genes and chromosomes during cell division. [NIH]

Daunorubicin: An anticancer drug that belongs to the family of drugs called antitumor antibiotics. [NIH]

Dexrazoxane: A drug used to protect the heart from the toxic effects of anthracycline drugs such as doxorubicin. It belongs to the family of drugs called chemoprotective agents. [NIH]

Disposition: A tendency either physical or mental toward certain diseases. [EU]

Doxorubicin: An anticancer drug that belongs to the family of drugs called antitumor antibiotics. It is an anthracycline. [NIH]

Encephalopathy: A disorder of the brain that can be caused by disease, injury, drugs, or chemicals. [NIH]

Endogenous: Produced inside an organism or cell. The opposite is external (exogenous) production. [NIH]

Erwinia: A genus of gram-negative, facultatively anaerobic, rod-shaped bacteria whose organisms are associated with plants as pathogens, saprophytes, or as constituents of the epiphytic flora. [NIH]

Etoposide: An anticancer drug that is a podophyllotoxin derivative and belongs to the family of drugs called mitotic inhibitors. [NIH]

Exogenous: Developed or originating outside the organism, as exogenous disease. [EU]

Fluorescence: The property of emitting radiation while being irradiated. The radiation emitted is usually of longer wavelength than that incident or absorbed, e.g., a substance can be irradiated with invisible radiation and emit visible light. X-ray fluorescence is used in diagnosis. [NIH]

Genotype: The genetic constitution of the individual; the characterization of the genes. [NIH]

Glucocorticoid: A compound that belongs to the family of compounds called corticosteroids (steroids). Glucocorticoids affect metabolism and have anti-inflammatory and immunosuppressive effects. They may be naturally produced (hormones) or synthetic (drugs). [NIH]

Glycoprotein: A protein that has sugar molecules attached to it. [NIH]

Haploidy: The number of chromosomes in the gametes, which is half the number normally found in somatic cells. Symbol: N. [NIH]

Hepatic: Refers to the liver. [NIH]

Histiocytosis: General term for the abnormal appearance of histiocytes in the blood. Based on the pathological features of the cells involved rather than on clinical findings, the histiocytic diseases are subdivided into three groups: histiocytosis, langerhans cell; histiocytosis, non-langerhans cell; and histiocytic disorders, malignant. [NIH]

Humoral: Of, relating to, proceeding from, or involving a bodily humour - now often used of endocrine factors as opposed to neural or somatic. [EU]

Hunger: The desire for food generated by a sensation arising from the lack of food in the stomach. [NIH]

Hybridization: The genetic process of crossbreeding to produce a hybrid. Hybrid nucleic acids can be formed by nucleic acid hybridization of DNA and RNA molecules. Protein hybridization allows for hybrid proteins to be formed from polypeptide chains. [NIH]

Hypoglycemia: Abnormally low blood sugar [NIH]

Immunity: The condition of being immune; the protection against infectious disease conferred either by the immune response generated by immunization or previous infection or by other nonimmunologic factors (innate i.). [EU]

Immunocompromised: Having a weakened immune system caused by certain diseases or treatments. [NIH]

Infusion: A method of putting fluids, including drugs, into the bloodstream. Also called intravenous infusion. [NIH]

Interferon: A biological response modifier (a substance that can improve the body's natural response to disease). Interferons interfere with the division of cancer cells and can slow tumor growth. There are several types of interferons, including interferon-alpha, -beta, and -gamma. These substances are normally produced by the body. They are also made in the laboratory for use in treating cancer and other diseases. [NIH]

Interphase: The interval between two successive cell divisions during which the chromosomes are not individually distinguishable and DNA replication occurs. [NIH]

Invasive: 1. having the quality of invasiveness. 2. involving puncture or incision of the skin or insertion of an instrument or foreign material into the body; said of diagnostic techniques. [EU]

LH: A small glycoprotein hormone secreted by the anterior pituitary. LH plays an important role in controlling ovulation and in controlling secretion of hormones by the ovaries and testes. [NIH]

Malignancy: A cancerous tumor that can invade and destroy nearby tissue and spread to other parts of the body. [NIH]

Membrane: A very thin layer of tissue that covers a surface. [NIH]

Mercaptopurine: An anticancer drug that belongs to the family of drugs called antimetabolites. [NIH]

Metabolite: Any substance produced by metabolism or by a metabolic process. [EU]

Methotrexate: An anticancer drug that belongs to the family of drugs called antimetabolites. [NIH]

Molecular: Of, pertaining to, or composed of molecules : a very small mass of matter. [EU]

Molecule: A chemical made up of two or more atoms. The atoms in a molecule can be the same (an oxygen molecule has two oxygen atoms) or different (a water molecule has two hydrogen atoms and one oxygen atom). Biological molecules, such as proteins and DNA, can be made up of many thousands of atoms. [NIH]

Mutagenic: Inducing genetic mutation. [EU]

Necrosis: Refers to the death of living tissues. [NIH]

Oncogene: A gene that normally directs cell growth. If altered, an oncogene can promote or allow the uncontrolled growth of cancer. Alterations can be inherited or caused by an environmental exposure to carcinogens. [NIH]

Paradoxical: Occurring at variance with the normal rule. [EU]

Pharmacodynamics: The study of the biochemical and physiological effects of drugs and the mechanisms of their actions, including the correlation of actions and effects of drugs with their chemical structure; also, such effects on the actions of a particular drug or drugs. [EU]

Pharmacokinetics: The activity of drugs in the body over a period of time, including the processes by which drugs are absorbed, distributed in the body, localized in the tissues, and excreted. [NIH]

Phenotype: The outward appearance of the individual. It is the product of interactions between genes and between the genotype and the environment. This includes the killer phenotype, characteristic of yeasts. [NIH]

Plasma: The clear, yellowish, fluid part of the blood that carries the blood cells. The proteins that form blood clots are in plasma. [NIH]

Ploidy: The number of sets of chromosomes in a cell or an organism. For example, haploid means one set and diploid means two sets. [NIH]

Postnatal: Occurring after birth, with reference to the newborn. [EU]

Precursor: Something that precedes. In biological processes, a substance from which another, usually more active or mature substance is formed. In clinical medicine, a sign or symptom that heralds another. [EU]

Prednisone: Belongs to the family of drugs called steroids and is used to treat several types of cancer and other disorders. Prednisone also inhibits the body's immune response. [NIH]

Prenatal: Existing or occurring before birth, with reference to the fetus. [EU]

Prevalence: The total number of cases of a given disease in a specified population at a designated time. It is differentiated from incidence, which refers to the number of new cases in the population at a given time. [NIH]

Proteins: Polymers of amino acids linked by peptide bonds. The specific sequence of amino acids determines the shape and function of the protein. [NIH]

Pseudomonas: A genus of gram-negative, aerobic, rod-shaped bacteria widely distributed in nature. Some species are pathogenic for humans, animals, and plants. [NIH]

Receptor: A molecule inside or on the surface of a cell that binds to a specific substance and causes a specific physiologic effect in the cell. [NIH]

Recombinant: 1. a cell or an individual with a new combination of genes not found together in either parent; usually applied to linked genes. [EU]

Recurrence: The return of cancer, at the same site as the original (primary) tumor or in another location, after the tumor had disappeared. [NIH]

Solvent: 1. dissolving; effecting a solution. 2. a liquid that dissolves or that is capable of dissolving; the component of a solution that is present in greater amount. [EU]

Somatic: 1. pertaining to or characteristic of the soma or body. 2. pertaining to the body wall in contrast to the viscera. [EU]

Strabismus: Deviation of the eye which the patient cannot overcome. The visual axes assume a position relative to each other different from that required by the physiological conditions. The various forms of strabismus are spoken of as tropias, their direction being indicated by the appropriate prefix, as cyclo tropia, esotropia, exotropia, hypertropia, and hypotropia. Called also cast, heterotropia, manifest deviation, and squint. [EU]

Teniposide: An anticancer drug that is a podophyllotoxin derivative and belongs to the family of drugs called mitotic inhibitors. [NIH]

Toxicity: The quality of being poisonous, especially the degree of virulence of a toxic microbe or of a poison. [EU]

Vaccination: Treatment with a vaccine. [NIH]

Viral: Pertaining to, caused by, or of the nature of virus. [EU]

CHAPTER 5. BOOKS ON CHILDHOOD ACUTE LYMPHOBLASTIC LEUKEMIA

Overview

This chapter provides bibliographic book references relating to childhood acute lymphoblastic leukemia. You have many options to locate books on childhood acute lymphoblastic leukemia. The simplest method is to go to your local bookseller and inquire about titles that they have in stock or can special order for you. Some parents, however, prefer online sources (e.g. **www.amazon.com** and **www.bn.com**). In addition to online booksellers, excellent sources for book titles on childhood acute lymphoblastic leukemia include the Combined Health Information Database and the National Library of Medicine. Once you have found a title that interests you, visit your local public or medical library to see if it is available for loan.

The National Library of Medicine Book Index

The National Library of Medicine at the National Institutes of Health has a massive database of books published on healthcare and biomedicine. Go to the following Internet site, **http://locatorplus.gov/**, and then select "Search LOCATORplus." Once you are in the search area, simply type "childhood acute lymphoblastic leukemia" (or synonyms) into the search box, and select "books only." From there, results can be sorted by publication date, author, or relevance. The following was recently catalogued by the National Library of Medicine:[31]

---

[31] In addition to LOCATORPlus, in collaboration with authors and publishers, the National Center for Biotechnology Information (NCBI) is adapting biomedical books for the Web. The

- **Acute lymphatic leukemia in childhood.** Author: Mills, Stephen Dow, 1906-; Year: 1933; [Minneapolis, 1933?]
- **Acute lymphoblastic leukemia: proceedings of a Wyeth-Ayerst-UCLA Western Workshop on Acute Lymphoblastic Leukemia, held at Tapatio Springs, Texas, November 29-December 2, 1988.** Author: editors, Robert Peter Gale, Dieter Hoelzer; Year: 1990; New York: Wiley-Liss, c1990; ISBN: 0471567191
http://www.amazon.com/exec/obidos/ASIN/0471567191/icongroupinterna
- **Acute myelogenous leukemia: progress and controversies: proceedings of a Wyeth-Ayerst-UCLA Symposia Western Workshop held at Lake Lanier, Georgia, November 28-December 1, 1989.** Author: editor, Robert Peter Gale; Year: 1990; New York: Wiley-Liss, c1990; ISBN: 0471568724
http://www.amazon.com/exec/obidos/ASIN/0471568724/icongroupinterna
- **Acute myelogenous leukemia in childhood: implications of therapy studies for future risk-adapted treatment strategies.** Author: U. Creutzig, J. Ritter, G. Schellong (eds.); Year: 1990; Berlin; New York: Springer-Verlag, c1990; ISBN: 3540520708 (alk. paper)
http://www.amazon.com/exec/obidos/ASIN/3540520708/icongroupinterna
- **Biology of acute lymphoblastic leukemia: sixteenth annual guest lecture delivered at the Institute of Education, University of London, on 29th October 1980.** Author: by Melvyn F. Greaves; Year: 1981; London, England: Leukemia Research Fund, 1981
- **Cell proliferation patterns in acute leukemia monitored by pulse-cytophotometry.** Author: H. F. P. Hillen, J. M. C. Wessels, C. A. M. Haanen; Year: 1975; Ghent, Belgium: European Press Medikon, c1975
- **Childhood leukemia: the facts.** Author: John S. Lilleyman; Year: 1994; Oxford; New York: Oxford University Press, 1994; ISBN: 0192624512 (pbk.)
http://www.amazon.com/exec/obidos/ASIN/0192624512/icongroupinterna

---

books may be accessed in two ways: (1) by searching directly using any search term or phrase (in the same way as the bibliographic database PubMed), or (2) by following the links to PubMed abstracts. Each PubMed abstract has a "Books" button that displays a facsimile of the abstract in which some phrases are hypertext links. These phrases are also found in the books available at NCBI. Click on hyperlinked results in the list of books in which the phrase is found. Currently, the majority of the links are between the books and PubMed. In the future, more links will be created between the books and other types of information, such as gene and protein sequences and macromolecular structures. See **http://www.ncbi.nlm.nih.gov/entrez/query.fcgi?db=Books.**

- **Childhood lymphoblastic leukemia.** Author: edited by Carl Pochedly; foreword by Emil Frei III; Year: 1985; New York: Praeger, 1985; ISBN: 003717388 (alk. paper)
- **Chromosome changes in acute myelomonocytic leukemia.** Author: Hoagland, Howard Clark, 1936-; Year: 1971; [Minneapolis] 1971
- **Chromosomes and genes in acute lymphoblastic leukemia.** Author: Lorna M. Secker-Walker; Year: 1997; Austin,: R.G. Landes Co.; New York: Chapman ; Hall, 1997; ISBN: 1570594112 (alk. paper)
  http://www.amazon.com/exec/obidos/ASIN/1570594112/icongroupinterna
- **Chronic myeloid leukemia and blastic crisis.** Author: guest editor, Michele Baccarani; Year: 1975; Copenhagen: Munksgaard, 1975; ISBN: 8716023870
- **Clinical and pharmacological studies on cytosine arabinoside in acute leukemia.** Author: door Aleida Maria Schonk; Year: 1982; Meppel: Krips Repro, [1982?]
- **Cure of childhood leukemia: into the age of miracles.** Author: John Laszlo; Year: 1995; New Brunswick, N.J.: Rutgers University Press, c1995; ISBN: 0813521866
  http://www.amazon.com/exec/obidos/ASIN/0813521866/icongroupinterna
- **Current management of childhood leukemia.** Author: Alvin M. Mauer, consulting reviewer; Year: 1991; Bethesda, MD: U.S. Dept. of Health and Human Services, Public Health Service, National Institutes of Health, National Cancer Institute, International Cancer Research Data Bank; Washington, D.C.: For sale by the Supt. of Docs., U.S. G.P.O., [1991]
- **Effect of granulocyte chalone on acute and chronic granulocytic leukaemia in man: report of seven cases.** Author: T. Rytömaa ... [et al.]; Year: 1976; Copenhagen: Munksgaard, 1976; ISBN: 8716022513
  http://www.amazon.com/exec/obidos/ASIN/8716022513/icongroupinterna
- **Glucocorticoid receptor structure and leukemic cell responses.** Author: [edited by] Bahiru Gametchu; Year: 1995; New York: Springer-Verlag; Austin: R.G. Landes, 1995; ISBN: 1570592527 (hard cover: alk. paper)
  http://www.amazon.com/exec/obidos/ASIN/1570592527/icongroupinterna
- **Life after leukemia.** Author: [Wayne Reed]; Year: 1989; Carlton, Victoria: W. Reed, c1989
- **Lymphosarcoma and acute lymphatic leukemia in childhood; a comparative study with particular reference to bone marrow and blood**

smear morphology. Author: Shea, Daniel W. (Daniel Wright), 1928-; Year: 1957; [Minneapolis] 1957

- **Methotrexate in the central nervous system prophylaxis of children with acute lymphoblastic leukemia.** Author: door Robert Jozef Joost Lippens; Year: 1981; Beetsterzwaag [Netherlands]: Mefar, 1981
- **Monetary costs of childhood cancer to the families of patients.** Author: J. Horsman ... [et al.]; Year: 1994; Ontario: CHEPA, 1994
- **Myelodysplastic syndromes & secondary acute myelogenous leukemia: directions for the new millennium.** Author: edited by Azra Raza, Suneel D. Mundle; Year: 2001; Boston: Kluwer Academic Publishers, c2001; ISBN: 0792373960 (alk. paper)
http://www.amazon.com/exec/obidos/ASIN/0792373960/icongroupinterna
- **Neurological survey of children with acute lymphoblastic leukaemia at diagnosis and during treatment.** Author: Leena Vainionpää; Year: 1991; Oulu: University of Oulu, 1991; ISBN: 9514232348
- **Preleukemic disorders.** Author: by Lawrence Kass; Year: 1979; Springfield, Ill.: Thomas, c1979; ISBN: 0398037965
http://www.amazon.com/exec/obidos/ASIN/0398037965/icongroupinterna
- **Prestorage filtration of blood components for patients who are chronically transfusion dependent.** Author: S. Beck, A. Stevens; Year: 1996; Bristol, England: U.K. National Health Service, South and West Regional Health Authority, 1996
- **Rapid structured review of studies on health-related quality of life and economic evaluation in pediatric acute lymphoblastic leukemia.** Author: A. Simon Pickard, Leigh-Ann Topfer, and David H. Feeny; Year: 2000; Edmonton, Alta.: Institute of Health Economics, [2000]
- **Therapy of acute leukemias: proceedings of international meeting, Rome, December 6-8, 1973.** Author: edited by F. Mandelli, S. Amadori, G. Mariani; Year: 1975; [Torino]: Minerva medica, 1975

Chapters on Childhood Acute Lymphoblastic Leukemia

Frequently, childhood acute lymphoblastic leukemia will be discussed within a book, perhaps within a specific chapter. In order to find chapters that are specifically dealing with childhood acute lymphoblastic leukemia, an excellent source of abstracts is the Combined Health Information Database. You will need to limit your search to book chapters and childhood acute lymphoblastic leukemia using the "Detailed Search" option. Go directly to the following hyperlink: **http://chid.nih.gov/detail/detail.html**. To find book chapters, use the drop boxes at the bottom of the search page where "You may refine your search by." Select the dates and language you prefer, and the format option "Book Chapter." By making these selections and typing in "childhood acute lymphoblastic leukemia" (or synonyms) into the "For these words:" box, you will only receive results on chapters in books.

General Home References

In addition to references for childhood acute lymphoblastic leukemia, you may want a general home medical guide that spans all aspects of home healthcare. The following list is a recent sample of such guides (sorted alphabetically by title; hyperlinks provide rankings, information, and reviews at Amazon.com):

- **American Academy of Pediatrics Guide to Your Child's Symptoms: The Official, Complete Home Reference, Birth Through Adolescence** by Donald Schiff (Editor), et al; Paperback - 256 pages (January 1997), Villard Books; ISBN: 0375752579;
  http://www.amazon.com/exec/obidos/ASIN/0375752579/icongroupinterna

- **Cancer: 50 Essential Things to Do** by Greg Anderson, O. Carl Simonton; Paperback - 184 pages; Revised & Updated edition (August 1999), Plume; ISBN: 0452280745;
  http://www.amazon.com/exec/obidos/ASIN/0452280745/icongroupinterna

- **Cancer Encyclopedia -- Collections of Anti-Cancer & Anti-Carcinogenic Agents, Chemicals, Drugs and Substances** by John C. Bartone; Paperback (January 2002), ABBE Publishers Association of Washington, DC; ISBN: 0788326791;
  http://www.amazon.com/exec/obidos/ASIN/0788326791/icongroupinterna

- **Cancer Sourcebook: Basic Consumer Health Information About Major Forms and Stages of Cancer** by Edward J. Prucha (Editor); Library Binding - 1100 pages, 3rd edition (August 1, 2000), Omnigraphics, Inc.; ISBN: 0780802276;
  http://www.amazon.com/exec/obidos/ASIN/0780802276/icongroupinterna

- **Cancer Supportive Care: A Comprehensive Guide for Patients and Their Families** by Ernest H. Rosenbaum, M.D., Isadora Rosenbaum, M.A.; Paperback - 472 pages (November 5, 1998), Somerville House Books Limited; ISBN: 1894042115;
  http://www.amazon.com/exec/obidos/ASIN/1894042115/icongroupinterna

- **Cancer Symptom Management: Patient Self-Care Guides (Book with CD-ROM for Windows & Macintosh)** by Connie Henke Yarbro (Editor), et al; CD-ROM - 264 pages, 2nd Book & CD-Rom edition (January 15, 2000), Jones & Bartlett Publishing; ISBN: 0763711675;
  http://www.amazon.com/exec/obidos/ASIN/0763711675/icongroupinterna

- **Children with Cancer: A Comprehensive Reference Guide for Parents** by Jeanne Munn Bracken; Hardcover (May 2001), Replica Books; ISBN: 0735104123;
  http://www.amazon.com/exec/obidos/ASIN/0735104123/icongroupinterna

- **The Children's Hospital Guide to Your Child's Health and Development** by Alan D. Woolf (Editor), et al; Hardcover - 796 pages, 1st edition (January 15, 2001), Perseus Books; ISBN: 073820241X;
  http://www.amazon.com/exec/obidos/ASIN/073820241X/icongroupinterna

- **Diagnosis Cancer: Your Guide Through the First Few Months** by Wendy Schlessel Harpham, Ann Bliss Pilcher (Illustrator); Paperback: 230 pages; Revised & Updated edition (November 1997), .W. Norton & Company; ISBN: 0393316912;
  http://www.amazon.com/exec/obidos/ASIN/0393316912/icongroupinterna

- **Helping Your Child in the Hospital: A Practical Guide for Parents** by Nancy Keene, Rachel Prentice; Paperback - 176 pages, 3rd edition (April 15, 2002), O'Reilly & Associates; ISBN: 0596500114;
  http://www.amazon.com/exec/obidos/ASIN/0596500114/icongroupinterna

- **The Human Side of Cancer: Living with Hope, Coping with Uncertainty** by Jimmie C. Holland, M.D., Sheldon Lewis; Paperback - 368 pages (October 2, 2001), Quill; ISBN: 006093042X;
  http://www.amazon.com/exec/obidos/ASIN/006093042X/icongroupinterna

- **Medical Emergencies & Childhood Illnesses: Includes Your Child's Personal Health Journal (Parent Smart)** by Penny A. Shore, William Sears (Contributor); Paperback - 115 pages (February 2002), Parent Kit Corporation; ISBN: 1896833187;
  http://www.amazon.com/exec/obidos/ASIN/1896833187/icongroupinterna

- **Taking Care of Your Child: A Parent's Guide to Complete Medical Care** by Robert H. Pantell, M.D., et al; Paperback - 524 pages, 6th edition (March 5, 2002), Perseus Press; ISBN: 0738206016;
  http://www.amazon.com/exec/obidos/ASIN/0738206016/icongroupinterna

- **You and Your Cancer: A Child's Guide** by Lynda Cranston, et al; Paperback - 56 pages, 1st edition (July 15, 2001), B C Decker; ISBN: 1550091476;
  http://www.amazon.com/exec/obidos/ASIN/1550091476/icongroupinterna

Vocabulary Builder

Aclarubicin: An anthracycline antibiotic produced by Streptomyces galilaeus. It has potent antineoplastic activity, especially in the treatment of leukemias, with reduced cardiac toxicity in comparison to daunorubicin or doxorubicin. [NIH]

Carcinogenic: Producing carcinoma. [EU]

Cytophotometry: A method for the study of certain organic compounds within cells, in situ, by measuring the light intensities of the selectively stained areas of cytoplasm. The compounds studied and their locations in the cells are made to fluoresce and are observed under a microscope. [NIH]

Cytosine: A pyrimidine base that is a fundamental unit of nucleic acids. [NIH]

Filtration: The passage of a liquid through a filter, accomplished by gravity, pressure, or vacuum (suction). [EU]

Granulocyte: A type of white blood cell that fights bacterial infection. Neutrophils, eosinophils, and basophils are granulocytes. [NIH]

Herbicide: A chemical that kills plants. [NIH]

Morphology: The science of the form and structure of organisms (plants, animals, and other forms of life). [NIH]

Pulse: The rhythmical expansion and contraction of an artery produced by waves of pressure caused by the ejection of blood from the left ventricle of the heart as it contracts. [NIH]

CHAPTER 6. MULTIMEDIA ON CHILDHOOD ACUTE LYMPHOBLASTIC LEUKEMIA

Overview

Information on childhood acute lymphoblastic leukemia can come in a variety of formats. Among multimedia sources, video productions, slides, audiotapes, and computer databases are often available. In this chapter, we show you how to keep current on multimedia sources of information on childhood acute lymphoblastic leukemia. We start with sources that have been summarized by federal agencies, and then show you how to find bibliographic information catalogued by the National Library of Medicine. If you see an interesting item, visit your local medical library to check on the availability of the title.

Bibliography: Multimedia on Childhood Acute Lymphoblastic Leukemia

The National Library of Medicine is a rich source of information on healthcare-related multimedia productions including slides, computer software, and databases. To access the multimedia database, go to the following Web site: **http://locatorplus.gov/**. Select "Search LOCATORplus." Once in the search area, simply type in childhood acute lymphoblastic leukemia (or synonyms). Then, in the option box provided below the search box, select "Audiovisuals and Computer Files." From there, you can choose to sort results by publication date, author, or relevance. The following multimedia has been indexed on childhood acute lymphoblastic leukemia. For more information, follow the hyperlink indicated:

- **Acute and chronic leukemias.** Source: [produced and published by Gower Medical Publishing]; Year: 1991; Format: Slide; New York, NY: Gower Medical Pub., c1991
- **Acute leukemia: the nursing approach.** Source: Roswell Park Memorial Institute, in cooperation with the Lakes Area Regional Medical Program; Year: 1975; Format: Slide; [Buffalo]: Communications in Learning, 1975
- **Acute leukemia morphology II.** Source: a collaborative effort of the following University of Washington departments and facilities, Department of Laboratory Medicine ... [et al.], with the collaboration of the American Society ofHematology; Heal; Year: 1984; Format: Videorecording; Seattle, WA: University of Washington, c1984
- **Acute leukemia.** Source: [American Society of Hematology]; Year: 1974; Format: Slide; [Seattle: The Society: for sale by University of Washington Health Sciences Center for Educational Resources, 1974]
- **Acute myelomonocytic leukemia, monocytic leukemia, and erythroleukemia.** Source: Virginia Minnich; Year: 1982; Format: Slide; Chicago: American Society of Clinical Pathologists, c1982
- **Adults with acute leukemia.** Source: University of Texas System Cancer Center; Year: 1976; Format: Videorecording; Houston: The Center, 1976
- **Advances in acute promyelocytic leukemia.** Source: Raymond P. Warrell, Jr; Year: 1994; Format: Videorecording; Secaucus, N.J.: Network for Continuing Medical Education, 1994
- **Basic hematology.** Source: Trainex Corporation; Year: 1972; Format: Filmstrip; [Garden Grove, Calif.]: Trainex, c1972
- **Bone marrow transplantation for treatment of leukemia.** Source: a production of the UCLA Public Information Office, in association with

UCLA Media Center; Year: 1976; Format: Videorecording; Berkeley, Calif.: Regents of the University of California, c1976

- **Bone marrow transplantation in acute leukemia.** Source: produced by Biomedical Communications, University of Arizona, Health Sciences Center; Year: 1983; Format: Videorecording; Tucson, AZ: The University, c1983
- **Children with acute lymphocytic leukemia.** Source: University of Texas System Cancer Center M. D. Anderson Hospital and Tumor Institute; Year: 1976; Format: Videorecording; Houston: The Institute, 1976
- **Classification and management of the leukemias.** Source: John M. Bennett, Claude Sultan; Year: 9999; Format: Slide; [New York]: Medcom, c1982-
- **Hematuria: don't stop the workup too soon.** Source: Vincent J. 0'Conor, Jr. Acute myelogenous leukemia: the diagnosis; Acute myelogenous leukemia: the treatment / Monroe Dowling; Year: 1975; Format: Videorecording; New York: Network for Continuing Medical Education, 1975
- **Leukemia: ASCO fall conference.** Year: 1990; Format: Sound recording; Chicago, IL: Teach'em, [1990]
- **Leukocytes in health and disease.** Source: Center for Disease Control, Bureau of Laboratories, Laboratory Training and Consultation Division; Year: 1977; Format: Slide; Atlanta: The Center; [Buffalo, N. Y.: for sale by Communications in Learning, 1977]
- **Management of acute leukemia.** Source: University of Texas System Cancer Center M. D. Anderson Hospital and Tumor Institute; Year: 1976; Format: Videorecording; Houston: The Institute, 1976
- **Medical applications videodisc: hematology.** Source: a collaborative effort of the following University of Washington departments and facilities, Department of Laboratory Medicine ... [et al.], with the collaboration of the American Society of H; Year: 1984; Format: Videorecording; [Seattle, Wash.]: University of Washington, c1984
- **Morphology of white blood cells.** Source: Cleveland Clinic Educational Foundation; Year: 1975; Format: Videorecording; Cleveland, Ohio: The Foundation; [for sale by Cleveland Clinic Educational Foundation, Audiovisual Dept.], 1975
- **Most common childhood malignancy.** Source: with Eva Radel; Year: 1987; Format: Videorecording; Secaucus, N.J.: Network for Continuing Medical Education, 1987
- **Musculoskeletal manifestations of leukemia in childhood.** Source: [presented by] the Emory Medical Television Network, Emory University

School of Medicine of the Robert Woodruff Health Sciences Center; Year: 1992; Format: Videorecording; Atlanta, Ga.: The University, c1992

- **New insights into the pathogenesis, manifestations and treatment of acute promyelocytic leukemia.** Source: [presented by] Marshfield Clinic, Saint Joseph's Hospital, [and] Marshfield Medical Research Foundation; Year: 1993; Format: Videorecording; Marshfield, WI: The Clinic, [1993]
- **Oral manifestations and management of leukemia in children: a self-instructional program.** Source: Frank H. Farrington, in cooperation with the Office of Educational Services, Medical University of South Carolina; Year: 1979; Format: Slide; Chapel Hill, N. C.: Health Sciences Consortium, c1979
- **Pediatric hematology.** Source: Sergio Piomelli, Laurence M. Corash; Year: 1971; Format: Slide; New York: Medcom, c1971
- **Radiation therapy in the management of childhood cancer.** Source: the Radiological Society of North America; Year: 1988; Format: Slide; [Oak Brook, Ill.]: RSNA, [1988]
- **T-cell acute lymphoblastic leukemia: pathogenesis and therapy.** Source: the University of Texas Medical School at Houston; produced by UT-TV, Houston; Year: 1991; Format: Videorecording; [Houston, Tex.: UT-TV], c1991
- **Technique of platelet transfusion.** Source: Acute Leukemia Task Force, with assistance from American Red Cross ... [et al.]; produced by Medical Arts and Photography Branch, National Institutes of Health; Year: 1966; Format: Motion picture; [Bethesda, Md.]: National Cancer Institute; [Atlanta: for loan by National Medical Audiovisual Center, 1966]
- **Treatment of acute leukemia.** Source: Roswell Park Memorial Institute, in cooperation with the Lakes Area Regional Medical Program; Year: 1975; Format: Slide; [Buffalo]: Communications in Learning, 1975
- **Update on the treatment of acute leukemia.** Source: [presented by] Marshfield Clinic ... [et al.]; Year: 1993; Format: Videorecording; Marshfield, WI: The Clinic, [1993?]

Vocabulary Builder

Dermatology: A medical specialty concerned with the skin, its structure, functions, diseases, and treatment. [NIH]

Erythroleukemia: Cancer of the blood-forming tissues in which large numbers of immature, abnormal red blood cells are found in the blood and bone marrow. [NIH]

CHAPTER 7. PHYSICIAN GUIDELINES AND DATABASES

Overview

Doctors and medical researchers rely on a number of information sources to help children with childhood acute lymphoblastic leukemia. Many will subscribe to journals or newsletters published by their professional associations or refer to specialized textbooks or clinical guides published for the medical profession. In this chapter, we focus on databases and Internet-based guidelines created or written for this professional audience.

NIH Guidelines

For the more common medical conditions, the National Institutes of Health publish guidelines that are frequently consulted by physicians. Publications are typically written by one or more of the various NIH Institutes. For physician guidelines, commonly referred to as "clinical" or "professional" guidelines, you can visit the following Institutes:

- Office of the Director (OD); guidelines consolidated across agencies available at **http://www.nih.gov/health/consumer/conkey.htm**

- National Institute of General Medical Sciences (NIGMS); fact sheets available at **http://www.nigms.nih.gov/news/facts/**

- National Library of Medicine (NLM); extensive encyclopedia (A.D.A.M., Inc.) with guidelines:
  http://www.nlm.nih.gov/medlineplus/healthtopics.html

- National Cancer Institute (NCI); guidelines available at
  http://cancernet.nci.nih.gov/pdq/pdq_treatment.shtml

In this chapter, we begin by reproducing one such guideline for childhood acute lymphoblastic leukemia:

What Is Childhood Acute Lymphoblastic Leukemia?[32]

This treatment information summary on childhood acute lymphoblastic leukemia (ALL) is an overview of prognosis, diagnosis, classification, and patient treatment. The National Cancer Institute (NCI) created the PDQ database to increase the availability of new treatment information and its use in treating patients. Information and references from the most recently published literature are included after review by pediatric oncology specialists.

Cancer in children and adolescents is rare. Children and adolescents with cancer should be referred to medical centers that have a multidisciplinary team of cancer specialists with experience treating the cancers that occur during childhood and adolescence. This multidisciplinary team incorporates the skills of the primary care physician, pediatric surgical subspecialists, radiation oncologists, pediatric medical oncologists/hematologists, rehabilitation specialists, pediatric nurse specialists, social workers, and others in order to ensure that children receive treatment, supportive care, and rehabilitation that will achieve optimal survival and quality of life. Guidelines for pediatric cancer centers and their role in the treatment of pediatric patients with cancer have been outlined by the American Academy of Pediatrics.[33] Since treatment of children with ALL entails many potential complications and requires aggressive supportive care (transfusions; management of infectious complications; and emotional, financial, and developmental support), this treatment is best coordinated by pediatric oncologists and performed in cancer centers or hospitals with all of the necessary pediatric supportive care facilities. Specialized care is essential for all children with ALL, including those in whom specific clinical and laboratory features might confer a favorable prognosis. At the same time, it is equally important that the clinical centers and the specialists directing the patient's care maintain contact with the referring physician in the community. Strong lines of communication optimize any urgent or interim care required when the child is at home.

---

[32] The following guidelines appeared on the NCI website on Aug 26, 2002. The text was last modified May, 2002. The text has been adapted for this sourcebook.
[33] Sanders J, Glader B, Cairo M, et al.: Guidelines for the pediatric cancer center and role of such centers in diagnosis and treatment. American Academy of Pediatrics Section Statement Section on Hematology/Oncology. Pediatrics 99(1): 139-141, 1997.

ALL is the most common cancer occurring in children, representing 23% of cancer diagnoses among children younger than 15 years of age and occurring at an annual rate of approximately 31 per million.[34] There are approximately 2,400 children and adolescents younger than 20 years of age diagnosed with ALL each year in the United States.[35] There is a sharp peak in ALL incidence among children ages 2 to 3 years (> 80 per million per year), with rates decreasing to 20 per million for ages 8 to 10 years. The incidence of ALL among children ages 2 to 3 years is approximately fourfold greater than that for infants and is nearly 10-fold greater than that for children who are 19 years old. For unexplained reasons, the incidence of ALL is substantially higher for white children than for black children, with a nearly threefold higher incidence at 2 to 3 years of age for white children compared to black children.[36]

Risk Factors

There are few identified factors associated with increased risk of ALL.[37] The primary accepted nongenetic risk factors for ALL are prenatal exposure to x-rays and postnatal exposure to high doses of radiation (e.g., therapeutic radiation as previously used for conditions such as tinea capitis and thymus enlargement).[38] Children with Down syndrome have increased risk for developing both ALL and acute myeloid leukemia,[39] with a cumulative risk for developing leukemia of approximately 2.1% by aged 5 years and 2.7% by aged 30 years.[40] Approximately two-thirds of the cases of acute leukemia in

---

[34] Ries LA, Kosary CL, Hankey BF, et al., eds.: SEER Cancer Statistics Review, 1973-1996. Available at: **http://www-seer.ims.nci.nih.gov/Publications/CSR1973_1996**

[35] Smith MA, Ries LA, Gurney JG, et al.: Leukemia. In: Ries LA, Smith MA, Gurney JG, et al., eds.: Cancer Incidence and Survival Among Children and Adolescents: United States SEER Program 1975-1995. Bethesda, Md: National Cancer Institute, SEER Program, NIH Pub.No. 99-4649, 1999, pp 17-34.

[36] Smith MA, Ries LA, Gurney JG, et al.: Leukemia. In: Ries LA, Smith MA, Gurney JG, et al., eds.: Cancer Incidence and Survival Among Children and Adolescents: United States SEER Program 1975-1995. Bethesda, Md: National Cancer Institute, SEER Program, NIH Pub.No. 99-4649, 1999, pp 17-34.

[37] Smith MA, Ries LA, Gurney JG, et al.: Leukemia. In: Ries LA, Smith MA, Gurney JG, et al., eds.: Cancer Incidence and Survival Among Children and Adolescents: United States SEER Program 1975-1995. Bethesda, Md: National Cancer Institute, SEER Program, NIH Pub.No. 99-4649, 1999, pp 17-34.

[38] Ross JA, Davies SM, Potter JD, et al.: Epidemiology of childhood leukemia, with a focus on infants. Epidemiologic Reviews 16(2): 243-272, 1994.

[39] Avet-Loiseau H, Mechinaud F, Harousseau L: Clonal hematologic disorders in Down syndrome. Journal of Pediatric Hematology/Oncology 17(1): 19-24, 1995.

[40] Hasle H, Clemmensen H, Mikkelsen M: Risks of leukaemia and solid tumours in individuals with Down's syndrome. Lancet 355(9199): 165-169, 2000.

children with Down syndrome are ALL.[41] Increased occurrence of ALL is also associated with certain genetic conditions, including neurofibromatosis,[42] Shwachman syndrome,[43] Bloom syndrome,[44] and ataxia telangiectasia.[45]

Prognosis

Seventy-five percent to 80% of children with ALL survive at least 5 years from diagnosis with current treatments that incorporate systemic therapy (e.g., combination chemotherapy) and specific central nervous system (CNS) preventive therapy (i.e., intrathecal chemotherapy with or without cranial irradiation).[46] Ten-year event-free survival of multiple large prospective trials conducted in different countries for children treated primarily in the 1980s is approximately 70%.[47] Since nearly all children with ALL achieve an initial

---

[41] Hasle H, Clemmensen H, Mikkelsen M: Risks of leukaemia and solid tumours in individuals with Down's syndrome. Lancet 355(9199): 165-169, 2000.

[42] Stiller CA, Chessells JM, Fitchett M: Neurofibromatosis and childhood leukaemia/lymphoma: a population-based UKCCSG study. British Journal of Cancer 70(5): 969-972, 1994.

[43] Strevens MJ, Lilleyman JS, Williams RB: Shwachman's syndrome and acute lymphoblastic leukaemia. British Medical Journal 2(6129): 18, 1978.

Woods WG, Roloff JS, Lukens JN, et al.: The occurrence of leukemia in patients with the Shwachman syndrome. The Journal of Pediatrics 99(3): 425-428, 1981.

[44] Passarge E: Bloom's syndrome: the German experience. Annales de Genetique 34(3-4): 179-197, 1991.

[45] Taylor AM, Metcalfe JA, Thick J, et al.: Leukemia and lymphoma in ataxia telangiectasia. Blood 87(2): 423-438, 1996.

[46] Ries LA, Kosary CL, Hankey BF, et al., eds.: SEER Cancer Statistics Review, 1973-1996. Available at: **http://www-seer.ims.nci.nih.gov/Publications/CSR1973_1996**

Smith MA, Ries LA, Gurney JG, et al.: Leukemia. In: Ries LA, Smith MA, Gurney JG, et al., eds.: Cancer Incidence and Survival Among Children and Adolescents: United States SEER Program 1975-1995. Bethesda, Md: National Cancer Institute, SEER Program, NIH Pub.No. 99-4649, 1999, pp 17-34.

Pui CH, Evans WE: Acute lymphoblastic leukemia. New England Journal of Medicine 339(9): 605-615, 1998.

Pui CH: Acute lymphoblastic leukemia in children. Current Opinion in Oncology 12(1): 3-12, 2000.

[47] Gaynon PS, Trigg ME, Heerema NA, et al.: Children's Cancer Group trials in childhood acute lymphoblastic leukemia: 1983-1995. Leukemia 14(12): 2223-2233, 2000.

Schrappe M, Reiter A, Zimmermann M, et al.: Long-term results of four consecutive trials in childhood ALL performed by the ALL-BFM study group from 1981 to 1995. Leukemia 14(12): 2205-2222, 2000.

Harms DO, Janka-Schaub GE: Co-operative study group for childhood acute lymphoblastic leukemia (COALL): long-term follow-up of trials 82, 85, 89 and 92 on behalf of the COALL study group. Leukemia 14(12): 2234-2239, 2000.

remission, the major obstacle to cure is bone marrow and/or extramedullary (e.g., CNS, testicular) relapse. Relapse from remission can occur during therapy or after completion of treatment. While the majority of children with recurrent ALL attain a second remission, the likelihood of cure is generally poor, particularly for those with bone marrow relapse following a short initial remission duration.[48]

Lymphoblasts from a particular patient carry antigen receptors unique to that patient. There is evidence to suggest that the specific antigen receptor may be present at birth in some patients with ALL, suggesting a prenatal origin for the leukemic clone. Similarly, some patients with ALL characterized by specific translocations have been shown to have cells showing the translocation at the time of birth.[49]

Despite the treatment advances noted in childhood ALL, numerous important biologic and therapeutic questions remain to be answered in order to achieve the goal of curing every child with ALL. The systematic investigation of these issues requires large clinical trials, and the opportunity to participate in these trials is offered to most patients/families. Clinical trials for children and adolescents with ALL are generally designed to compare potentially better therapy with therapy that is currently accepted as standard. Much of the progress made in identifying curative therapies for childhood ALL and other childhood cancers has been achieved through

---

Silverman LB, Declerck L, Gelber RD, et al.: Results of Dana-Farber Cancer Institute consortium protocols for children with newly diagnosed acute lymphoblastic leukemia (1981-1995). Leukemia 14(12): 2247-2256, 2000.

Maloney KW, Shuster JJ, Murphy S, et al.: Long-term results of treatment studies for childhood acute lymphoblastic leukemia: Pediatric Oncology Group studies from 1986-1994. Leukemia 14(12): 2276-2285, 2000.

Pui C-H, Boyett JM, Rivera GK, et al.: Long-term results of Total Therapy studies 11, 12 and 13A for childhood acute lymphoblastic leukemia at St Jude Children's Research Hospital. Leukemia 14(12): 2286-2294, 2000.

Eden OB, Harrison G, Richards S, et al.: Long-term follow-up of the United Kingdom Medical Research Council protocols for childhood acute lymphoblastic leukaemia, 1980-1997. Leukemia 14(12): 2307-2320, 2000.

[48] Gaynon PS, Qu RP, Chappell RJ, et al.: Survival after relapse in childhood acute lymphoblastic leukemia: impact of site and time to first relapse--the Children's Cancer Group Experience. Cancer 82(7): 1387-1395, 1998.

[49] Yagi T, Hibi S, Tabata Y, et al.: Detection of clonotypic IGH and TCR rearrangements in the neonatal blood spots of infants and children with B-cell precursor acute lymphoblastic leukemia. Blood 96(1): 264-268, 2000.

Fasching K, Panzer S, Haas OA, et al.: Presence of clone-specific antigen receptor gene rearrangements at birth indicates an in utero origin of diverse types of early childhood acute lymphoblastic leukemia. Blood 95(8): 2722-2724, 2000.

clinical trials.[50] Information about ongoing clinical trials is available from the NCI (**http://cancer.gov/clinical_trials/**).

Cellular Classification

Children with acute lymphoblastic leukemia (ALL) are usually treated according to risk groups defined by both clinical and laboratory features. The intensity of treatment required for favorable outcome varies substantially among subsets of children with ALL. Risk-based treatment assignment is utilized for children with ALL so that those children who have a very good outcome with modest therapy can be spared more intensive and toxic treatment, while a more aggressive (and thus more toxic) therapeutic approach can be provided for patients who have a lower probability of long-term survival.[51]

Risk-based treatment assignment requires the availability of prognostic factors that reliably predict outcome. For children with ALL, a number of clinical and laboratory features have demonstrated prognostic value, some of which are described below. The factors described are grouped into the following categories: clinical and laboratory features at diagnosis; molecular characteristics of leukemia cells at diagnosis; and response to initial treatment. As in any discussion of prognostic factors, it is critical to remember that the relative order of significance and the interrelationship of the variables are often treatment dependent and require multivariate analysis to determine which factors operate independently as prognostic variables.[52] Because prognostic factors are treatment dependent, improvements in therapy may diminish the importance of or abrogate any of these presumed prognostic factors. For example, a report from the Children's Cancer Group (CCG) showed that the adverse prognostic significance of

---

[50] Vietti TJ, Land V, et al, for the Pediatric Oncology Group: Progress against childhood cancer: the Pediatric Oncology Group experience. Pediatrics 89(4 pt 1): 597-600, 1992.
Bleyer WA: The U.S. pediatric cancer clinical trials programmes: international implications and the way forward. European Journal of Cancer 33(9): 1439-1447, 1997.
[51] Smith M, Arthur D, Camitta B, et al.: Uniform approach to risk classification and treatment assignment for children with acute lymphoblastic leukemia. Journal of Clinical Oncology 14(1): 18-24, 1996.
[52] Uckun FM, Sensel MG, Sun L, et al.: Biology and treatment of childhood T-lineage acute lymphoblastic leukemia. Blood 91(3): 735-746, 1998.
Pullen J, Shuster JJ, Link M, et al.: Significance of commonly used prognostic factors differs for children with T-cell acute lymphocytic leukemia (ALL), as compared to those with B-precursor ALL. A Pediatric Oncology Group study. Leukemia 13(11): 1696-1707, 1999.

slow early response disappears when these patients receive intensified post induction chemotherapy.[53]

A subset of the prognostic factors discussed below is used for the initial stratification of children with ALL for treatment assignment, and at the end of this section there are brief descriptions of the prognostic groupings currently applied for clinical trials in the United States.

Clinical and Laboratory Features at Diagnosis

Clinical and laboratory features at diagnosis which are associated with outcome include the following:

Age at Diagnosis

Age at diagnosis has strong prognostic significance, reflecting the different underlying biology of ALL in different age groups.

Infants with ALL have a particularly high risk of treatment failure, with the risk of treatment failure being greatest for young infants (< 6 months) compared to older infants (>/= 6-9 months).[54] Rearrangement of the MLL gene at chromosome band 11q23 can be detected in the leukemia cells of a large percentage of infants with ALL,[55] and the poor outcome for infants with ALL is strongly associated with the presence of the t(4;11) translocation involving the MLL gene.[56] ALL in infants is also associated with a

---

[53] Nachman JB, Sather HN, Sensel MG, et al.: Augmented post-induction therapy for children with high-risk acute lymphoblastic leukemia and a slow response to initial therapy. New England Journal of Medicine 338(23): 1663-1671, 1998.

[54] Reaman GH, Sposto R, Sensel MG, et al.: Treatment outcome and prognostic factors for infants with acute lymphoblastic leukemia treated on two consecutive trials of the Children's Cancer Group. Journal of Clinical Oncology 17(2): 445-455, 1999.
Frankel LS, Ochs J, Shuster JJ, et al.: Therapeutic trial for infant acute lymphoblastic leukemia: the Pediatric Oncology Group experience (POG 8493). Journal of Pediatric Hematology/Oncology 19(1): 35-42, 1997.
Dordelmann M, Reiter A, et al, for the ALL-BFM Group: Prednisone response is the strongest predictor of treatment outcome in infant acute lymphoblastic leukemia. Blood 94(4): 1209-1217, 1999.
Biondi A, Cimino G, Pieters R, et al.: Biological and therapeutic aspects of infant leukemia. Blood 96(1): 24-33, 2000.

[55] Rubnitz JE, Link MP, Shuster JJ, et al.: Frequency and prognostic significance of HRX rearrangements in infant acute lymphoblastic leukemia: a Pediatric Oncology Group study. Blood 84(2): 570-573, 1994.

[56] Felix CA, Lange BJ: Leukemia in infants. Oncologist 4(3): 225-240, 1999.

constellation of other characteristics associated with poor outcome, including elevated white blood cell (WBC) count, central nervous system leukemia, lack of CD10 (cALLa antigen) expression, and poor response to initial treatment.[57]

Young children (1-9 years) have a favorable outcome in comparison to either older children and adolescents or in comparison to infants.[58]

Older children and adolescents (>/= 10 years) have a less favorable outcome than young children, and more aggressive treatments are generally employed in order to improve outcome for these patients.

WBC Count at Diagnosis

Patients with higher WBC counts at diagnosis have a higher risk for treatment failure than do patients with lower WBC counts. A WBC count of 50,000/mm3 is generally used as an operational cut point between better and poorer prognosis,[59] although the relationship between WBC count and prognosis is a continuous rather than a step function.[60] Elevated WBC count

---

Heerema NA, Sather HN, Ge J, et al.: Cytogenetic studies of infant acute lymphoblastic leukemia: poor prognosis of infants with t(4;11) - a report of the Children's Cancer Group. Leukemia 13(5): 679-686, 1999.

[57] Reaman GH, Sposto R, Sensel MG, et al.: Treatment outcome and prognostic factors for infants with acute lymphoblastic leukemia treated on two consecutive trials of the Children's Cancer Group. Journal of Clinical Oncology 17(2): 445-455, 1999.

Dordelmann M, Reiter A, et al, for the ALL-BFM Group: Prednisone response is the strongest predictor of treatment outcome in infant acute lymphoblastic leukemia. Blood 94(4): 1209-1217, 1999.

[58] Smith M, Arthur D, Camitta B, et al.: Uniform approach to risk classification and treatment assignment for children with acute lymphoblastic leukemia. Journal of Clinical Oncology 14(1): 18-24, 1996.

Trueworthy R, Shuster J, Look T, et al.: Ploidy of lymphoblasts is the strongest predictor of treatment outcome in B-progenitor cell acute lymphoblastic leukemia of childhood: a Pediatric Oncology Group study. Journal of Clinical Oncology 10(4): 606-613, 1992.

Reiter A, Schrappe M, Ludwig W, et al.: Chemotherapy in 998 unselected childhood acute lymphoblastic leukemia patients: results and conclusions of the multicenter trial ALL-BFM 86. Blood 84(9): 3122-3133, 1994.

[59] Smith M, Arthur D, Camitta B, et al.: Uniform approach to risk classification and treatment assignment for children with acute lymphoblastic leukemia. Journal of Clinical Oncology 14(1): 18-24, 1996.

[60] Reiter A, Schrappe M, Ludwig W, et al.: Chemotherapy in 998 unselected childhood acute lymphoblastic leukemia patients: results and conclusions of the multicenter trial ALL-BFM 86. Blood 84(9): 3122-3133, 1994.

Chessells JM, Bailey C, Richards SM, et al.: Intensification of treatment and survival in all children with lymphoblastic leukaemia: results of UK Medical Research Council trial

is associated with other high-risk prognostic factors, including unfavorable chromosomal translocations such as t(4;11) and t(9;22) (see below).

Gender

The prognosis for girls with ALL is slightly better than that for boys with ALL.[61] One reason for the superior prognosis for girls is the occurrence of testicular relapses among boys, but boys also appear to be at increased risk for bone marrow relapse for reasons that are not well understood.[62]

Race

Survival rates for black children with ALL are somewhat lower than those for white children with ALL.[63] The reason for the better outcome for white children compared to black children is not known, but it can not be completely explained based on known prognostic factors.[64]

UKALL X. Medical Research Council Working Party on Childhood Leukaemia. Lancet 345(8943): 143-148, 1995.

[61] Pui CH, Boyett JM, Relling MV, et al.: Sex differences in prognosis for children with acute lymphoblastic leukemia. Journal of Clinical Oncology 17(3): 818-824, 1999.

Shuster JJ, Wacker P, Pullen J, et al.: Prognostic significance of sex in childhood B-precursor acute lymphoblastic leukemia: a Pediatric Oncology Group study. Journal of Clinical Oncology 16(8): 2854-2863, 1998.

Chessells JM, Richards SM, Bailey CC, et al.: Gender and treatment outcome in childhood lymphoblastic leukaemia: report from the MRC UKALL trials. British Journal of Haematology 89(2): 364-372, 1995.

[62] Chessells JM, Richards SM, Bailey CC, et al.: Gender and treatment outcome in childhood lymphoblastic leukaemia: report from the MRC UKALL trials. British Journal of Haematology 89(2): 364-372, 1995.

[63] Trueworthy R, Shuster J, Look T, et al.: Ploidy of lymphoblasts is the strongest predictor of treatment outcome in B-progenitor cell acute lymphoblastic leukemia of childhood: a Pediatric Oncology Group study. Journal of Clinical Oncology 10(4): 606-613, 1992.

Pui CH, Boyett JM, Hancock ML, et al.: Outcome of treatment for childhood cancer in black as compared with white children: the St Jude Children's Research Hospital experience, 1962 through 1992. JAMA: Journal of the American Medical Association 273(8): 633-637, 1995.

Bhatia S, Sather H, Zhang J, et al.: Ethnicity and survival following childhood acute lymphoblastic leukemia (ALL): follow-up of the Children's Cancer Group (CCG) cohort. Proceedings of the American Society of Clinical Oncology 18: A2190, 568a, 1999.

Pollock BH, DeBaun MR, Camitta BM, et al.: Racial differences in the survival of childhood B-precursor acute lymphoblastic leukemia: a pediatric oncology group study. Journal of Clinical Oncology 18(4): 813-823, 2000.

[64] Bhatia S, Sather H, Zhang J, et al.: Ethnicity and survival following childhood acute lymphoblastic leukemia (ALL): follow-up of the Children's Cancer Group (CCG) cohort. Proceedings of the American Society of Clinical Oncology 18: A2190, 568a, 1999.

Cellular Morphology

In the past ALL lymphoblasts were classified using the French-American-British (FAB) criteria as having L1 morphology, L2 morphology, or L3 morphology.[65] Due to the lack of independent prognostic significance and the subjective nature of this classification system, it is no longer used in the United States. The FAB L3 morphology is morphologically and cytogenetically identical to that of Burkitt's lymphoma. B-cell ALL (surface immunoglobulin (Ig) expression, generally with FAB L3 morphology and c-myc gene translocation) is a systemic manifestation of Burkitt's and Burkitt's-like non-Hodgkin's lymphoma, and its treatment is completely different from that for other forms of childhood ALL. (NOTE: Rare cases of FAB L3 ALL with c-myc gene translocations lack surface immunoglobulin expression, and these cases are appropriately treated as B-cell ALL).[66] Conversely, rare cases of ALL that express surface Ig but that lack L3 morphology and lack c-myc gene translocations are appropriately treated as B-precursor ALL rather than B-cell ALL.[67] (Refer to the PDQ summary on Childhood Non-Hodgkin's Lymphoma for more information.)

Molecular and Biological Characteristics of Leukemia Cells at Diagnosis

Molecular and biological characteristics of leukemia cells at diagnosis which are associated with outcome include:

Immunophenotype

B-precursor ALL: B-cell precursor (or B-lineage) ALL, defined by the expression of CD19, HLA-DR, CD10 (cALLa), and other B-cell associated antigens, represents 80% to 85% of childhood ALL. Approximately 80% of B-precursor ALL express the cALLa, CD10 antigen. The lack of cALLa expression has also been shown in some series to be associated with a worse

---

[65] Bennett M, Catovsky D, Daniel MT, et al.: The morphological classification of acute lymphoblastic leukemia: concordance among observers and clinical correlations. British Journal of Haematology 47(4): 553-561, 1981.

[66] Navid F, Mosijczuk AD, Head D, et al.: Acute lymphoblastic leukemia with (8:14)(q24:q32) translocation and FAB L3 morphology associated with a B-precursor immunophenotype: the Pediatric Oncology Group experience. Leukemia 13(1): 135-141, 1999.

[67] Behm FG, Head DR, Pui CH, et al.: B-precursor ALL with unexpected expression of surface immunoglobulin (sig) mu and lambda. Laboratory Investigation 72: A-613, 106a, 1995.

prognosis. For example, CD10 negativity is observed in a higher proportion of infants with B-precursor ALL and is associated with poor outcome.[68]

Stage of B-Cell Maturation

There are 3 major subtypes of B-lineage ALL: early pre-B (no surface or cytoplasmic immunoglobulin), pre-B (presence of cytoplasmic immunoglobulin), and B-cell (presence of surface immunoglobulin). Approximately three quarters of patients with B-precursor ALL have the early pre-B phenotype and have the best prognosis. The leukemic cells of patients with pre-B ALL contain cytoplasmic immunoglobulin (cIg), an intermediate stage of B-cell differentiation. Twenty-five percent of patients with pre-B ALL have the t(1;19) translocation (see below).[69] Approximately 2% of patients present with B-cell ALL (surface Ig expression, generally with FAB L3 morphology and c-myc gene translocation).[70] B-cell ALL is a systemic manifestation of Burkitt's and Burkitt's-like non-Hodgkin's lymphoma, and its treatment is completely different from that for other forms of childhood ALL. (NOTE: Rare cases of FAB L3 ALL with c-myc gene translocations lack surface immunoglobulin expression, and these cases are appropriately treated as B-cell ALL).[71] Conversely, rare cases of ALL that express surface Ig but that lack L3 morphology and lack c-myc gene translocations are appropriately treated as B-precursor ALL rather than B-cell ALL.[72] (Refer to the PDQ summary on Childhood Non-Hodgkin's Lymphoma for more information on the treatment of children with B-cell ALL.)

---

[68] Reaman GH, Sposto R, Sensel MG, et al.: Treatment outcome and prognostic factors for infants with acute lymphoblastic leukemia treated on two consecutive trials of the Children's Cancer Group. Journal of Clinical Oncology 17(2): 445-455, 1999.

[69] Crist WM, Carroll AJ, Shuster JJ, et al.: Poor prognosis of children with pre-B acute lymphoblastic leukemia is associated with the t(1;19)(q23;p13): a Pediatric Oncology Group study. Blood 76(1): 117-122, 1990.

[70] Pui CH, Evans WE: Acute lymphoblastic leukemia. New England Journal of Medicine 339(9): 605-615, 1998.

[71] Navid F, Mosijczuk AD, Head D, et al.: Acute lymphoblastic leukemia with (8:14)(q24:q32) translocation and FAB L3 morphology associated with a B-precursor immunophenotype: the Pediatric Oncology Group experience. Leukemia 13(1): 135-141, 1999.

[72] Behm FG, Head DR, Pui CH, et al.: B-precursor ALL with unexpected expression of surface immunoglobulin (sig) mu and lambda. Laboratory Investigation 72: A-613, 106a, 1995.

T-Cell ALL

T-cell ALL is defined by the leukemic cell expression of the T-cell-associated antigens CD2, CD7, CD5, or CD3 and is frequently associated with a constellation of clinical features including male sex, older age, leukocytosis, and mediastinal mass.[73] Approximately 15% of children with newly diagnosed ALL have the T-cell phenotype. With appropriately intensive therapy, however, children with T-cell ALL have an outcome similar to that for children with B-precursor ALL, when matched for age and WBC count.[74] Cytogenetic abnormalities common in B-cell lineage ALL (e.g. hyperdiploidy) are uncommon in T-cell ALL and when present, are not associated with prognostic significance.[75]

Myeloid Antigen Expression

A minority of childhood ALL cases have leukemia cells that express myeloid surface antigens. Myeloid antigen expression appears to be associated with specific ALL subgroups, notably those with MLL gene rearrangements and those with the TEL-AML1 gene rearrangement.[76] Early reports suggested a poorer prognosis for these patients,[77] but reports from large patient populations indicate no adverse prognostic significance for myeloid surface antigen expression.[78]

---

[73] Uckun FM, Sensel MG, Sun L, et al.: Biology and treatment of childhood T-lineage acute lymphoblastic leukemia. Blood 91(3): 735-746, 1998.
[74] Uckun FM, Sensel MG, Sun L, et al.: Biology and treatment of childhood T-lineage acute lymphoblastic leukemia. Blood 91(3): 735-746, 1998.
[75] Schneider NR, Carroll AJ, Shuster JJ, et al.: New recurring cytogenetic abnormalities and association of blast cell karyotypes with prognosis in childhood T-cell acute lymphoblastic leukemia: a Pediatric Oncology Group report of 343 cases. Blood 96(7): 2543-2549, 2000.
[76] Pui CH, Rubnitz JE, Hancock ML, et al.: Reappraisal of the clinical and biologic significance of myeloid-associated antigen expression in childhood acute lymphoblastic leukemia. Journal of Clinical Oncology 16(12): 3768-3773, 1998.
[77] Fink FM, Koller U, et al, for the Austrian Pediatric Oncology Group: Prognostic significance of myeloid-associated antigen expression on blast cells in children with acute lymphoblastic leukemia. Medical and Pediatric Oncology 21(5): 340-346, 1993.
[78] Pui CH, Rubnitz JE, Hancock ML, et al.: Reappraisal of the clinical and biologic significance of myeloid-associated antigen expression in childhood acute lymphoblastic leukemia. Journal of Clinical Oncology 16(12): 3768-3773, 1998.
Putti MC, Rondelli R, Cocito MG, et al.: Expression of myeloid markers lacks prognostic impact in children treated for acute lymphoblastic leukemia: Italian experience in AIEOP-ALL 88-91 studies. Blood 92(3): 795-801, 1998.
Uckun FM, Sather H, Gaynon PS, et al.: Clinical features and treatment outcome of children with myeloid antigen positive acute lymphoblastic leukemia: a report from the Children's Cancer Group. Blood 90(1): 28-35, 1997.

Chromosome Number

Hyperdiploidy

Hyperdiploidy (> 50 chromosomes per cell or DNA index > 1.16) is the presence of additional copies of whole chromosomes and occurs in 20% to 25% of cases of B-precursor ALL but very rarely in cases of T-cell ALL.[79] Hyperdiploidy can be evaluated by measuring the DNA content of cells (DNA index) or by karyotyping. Hyperdiploidy generally occurs in cases with favorable prognostic factors (age 1-9 years and low WBC count), and is itself associated with favorable prognosis.[80] Hyperdiploid leukemia cells are particularly susceptible to undergoing apoptosis, which may explain the favorable outcome commonly observed for these cases.[81]

Trisomies

For the treatment approaches utilized by both the Pediatric Oncology Group (POG) and the Children's Cancer Group (CCG), extra copies of certain chromosomes appear to be specifically associated with favorable prognosis among hyperdiploid ALL cases. In POG studies, patients whose leukemia cells have extra copies of both chromosome 4 and chromosome 10 appear to have particularly favorable outcome.[82] In CCG studies, children with trisomies of chromosomes 10 and 17 have an excellent prognosis.[83]

---

[79] Pui CH, Evans WE: Acute lymphoblastic leukemia. New England Journal of Medicine 339(9): 605-615, 1998.

[80] Trueworthy R, Shuster J, Look T, et al.: Ploidy of lymphoblasts is the strongest predictor of treatment outcome in B-progenitor cell acute lymphoblastic leukemia of childhood: a Pediatric Oncology Group study. Journal of Clinical Oncology 10(4): 606-613, 1992.
Raimondi SC, Pui CH, Hancock ML, et al.: Heterogeneity of hyperdiploid (51-67) childhood acute lymphoblastic leukemia. Leukemia 10(2): 213-224, 1996.
Hann I, Vora A, Harrison G, et al.: Determinants of outcome after intensified therapy of childhood lymphoblastic leukaemia: results from Medical Research Council United Kingdom acute lymphoblastic leukaemia XI protocol. British Journal of Haematology 113(1): 103-114, 2001.

[81] Ito C, Kumagai M, Manabe A, et al.: Hyperdiploid acute lymphoblastic leukemia with 51 to 65 chromosomes: a distinct biological entity with a marked propensity to undergo apoptosis. Blood 93(1): 315-320, 1999.

[82] Harris MB, Shuster JJ, Carroll A, et al.: Trisomy of leukemic cell chromosomes 4 and 10 identifies children with B-progenitor cell acute lymphoblastic leukemia with a very low risk of treatment failure: a Pediatric Oncology Group study. Blood 79(12): 3316-3324, 1992.

[83] Heerema NA, Sather HN, Sensel MG, et al.: Prognostic impact of trisomies of chromosomes 10, 17, and 5 among children with acute lymphoblastic leukemia and high hyperdiploidy (>50 chromosomes). Journal of Clinical Oncology 18(9): 1876-1887, 2000.

Hypodiploidy

Approximately 1% of children with ALL have leukemia cells showing hypodiploidy with less than 45 chromosomes. These patients are at high risk for treatment failure.[84]

Recurring Chromosomal Translocations

Recurring chromosomal translocations can be detected in a substantial number of cases of childhood ALL, and some of these translocations, as described below, have prognostic significance.

TEL-AML1 (t(12;21) Cryptic Translocation)

Fusion of the TEL (ETV6) gene on chromosome 12 to the AML1 (CBFA2) gene on chromosome 21 can be detected in 20% to 25% of cases of B-precursor ALL, but is rarely observed in T-cell ALL.[85] Children with the t(12;21) cryptic translocation resulting in the TEL-AML1 fusion are generally 2 to 9 years of age.[86] Patients with the TEL-AML1 fusion have very good outcomes,[87] although there is controversy about whether the ultimate cure

---

[84] Pui CH, Carroll AJ, Raimondi SC, et al.: Clinical presentation, karyotypic characterization, and treatment outcome of childhood acute lymphoblastic leukemia with a near-haploid or hypodiploid less than 45 line. Blood 75(5): 1170-1177, 1990.
Heerema NA, Nachman JB, Sather HN, et al.: Hypodiploidy with less than 45 chromosomes confers adverse risk in childhood acute lymphoblastic leukemia: a report from the Children's Cancer Group. Blood 94(12): 4036-4045, 1999.
Hann I, Vora A, Harrison G, et al.: Determinants of outcome after intensified therapy of childhood lymphoblastic leukaemia: results from Medical Research Council United Kingdom acute lymphoblastic leukaemia XI protocol. British Journal of Haematology 113(1): 103-114, 2001.
[85] Pui CH, Evans WE: Acute lymphoblastic leukemia. New England Journal of Medicine 339(9): 605-615, 1998.
McLean TW, Ringold S, Neuberg D, et al.: TEL/AML-1 dimerizes and is associated with a favorable outcome in childhood acute lymphoblastic leukemia. Blood 88(11): 4252-4258, 1996.
[86] McLean TW, Ringold S, Neuberg D, et al.: TEL/AML-1 dimerizes and is associated with a favorable outcome in childhood acute lymphoblastic leukemia. Blood 88(11): 4252-4258, 1996.
[87] McLean TW, Ringold S, Neuberg D, et al.: TEL/AML-1 dimerizes and is associated with a favorable outcome in childhood acute lymphoblastic leukemia. Blood 88(11): 4252-4258, 1996.
Rubnitz JE, Shuster JJ, Land VJ, et al.: Case-control study suggests a favorable impact of TEL rearrangement in patients with B-lineage acute lymphoblastic leukemia treated with

rate is actually superior to that of other patients with B-precursor ALL or whether the ultimate cure rate is similar but the timing of relapse is significantly later for patients with the TEL-AML1 fusion compared to other patients with B-precursor ALL.[88]

The Philadelphia chromosome t(9;22) is present in approximately 4% of pediatric ALL patients and confers an unfavorable prognosis, especially when it is associated with either a high WBC count or slow early response to initial therapy.[89] Philadelphia-positive ALL is more common in older patients with B-precursor ALL and high WBC count.

---

antimetabolite-based therapy: a Pediatric Oncology Group study. Blood 89(4): 1143-1146, 1997.

Borkhardt A, Cazzaniga G, Viehmann S, et al.: Incidence and clinical relevance of TEL/AML1 fusion genes in children with acute lymphoblastic leukemia enrolled in the German and Italian Multicenter Therapy Trials. Blood 90(2): 571-577, 1997.

[88] Hann I, Vora A, Harrison G, et al.: Determinants of outcome after intensified therapy of childhood lymphoblastic leukaemia: results from Medical Research Council United Kingdom acute lymphoblastic leukaemia XI protocol. British Journal of Haematology 113(1): 103-114, 2001.

Rubnitz JE, Shuster JJ, Land VJ, et al.: Case-control study suggests a favorable impact of TEL rearrangement in patients with B-lineage acute lymphoblastic leukemia treated with antimetabolite-based therapy: a Pediatric Oncology Group study. Blood 89(4): 1143-1146, 1997.

Rubnitz JE, Behm FG, Wichlan D, et al.: Low frequency of TEL-AML1 in relapsed acute lymphoblastic leukemia supports a favorable prognosis for this genetic subgroup. Leukemia 13(1): 19-21, 1999.

Seeger K, Adams HP, Buchwald D, et al.: TEL-AML1 fusion transcript in relapsed childhood acute lymphoblastic leukemia. The Berlin-Frankfurt-Munster Study Group. Blood 91(5): 1716-1722, 1998.

Seeger K, Buchwald D, Taube T, et al.: TEL-AML1 positivity in relapsed B cell precursor acute lymphoblastic leukemia in childhood. Berlin-Frankfurt-Munster Study Group. Leukemia 13(9): 1469-1470, 1999.

Hubeek I, Ramakers-van Woerden NI, Pieters R, et al.: TEL/AML1 fusion is not a prognostic factor in Dutch childhood acute lymphoblastic leukaemia. British Journal of Haematology 113(1): 254-255, 2001.

[89] Hann I, Vora A, Harrison G, et al.: Determinants of outcome after intensified therapy of childhood lymphoblastic leukaemia: results from Medical Research Council United Kingdom acute lymphoblastic leukaemia XI protocol. British Journal of Haematology 113(1): 103-114, 2001.

Arico M, Valsecchi MG, Camitta B, et al.: Outcome of treatment in children with Philadelphia chromosome-positive acute lymphoblastic leukemia. New England Journal of Medicine 342(14): 998-1006, 2000.

Schrappe M, Arico M, Harbott J, et al.: Philadelphia chromosome-positive (Ph+) childhood acute lymphoblastic leukemia: good initial steroid response allows early prediction of a favorable treatment outcome. Blood 92(8): 2730-2741, 1998.

Ribeiro RC, Broniscer A, Rivera GK, et al.: Philadelphia chromosome-positive acute lymphoblastic leukemia in children: durable responses to chemotherapy associated with low initial white blood cell counts. Leukemia 11(9): 1493-1496, 1997.

Translocations involving the MLL (11q23) gene occur in approximately 6% of childhood ALL cases, and are generally associated with increased risk for treatment failure.[90] The t(4;11) is the most common translocation involving the MLL gene in children with ALL and occurs in approximately 4% of cases.[91] Patients with t(4;11) generally present in infancy with high WBC count, and they are more likely than other children with ALL to have CNS disease and to have a poor response to initial therapy.[92] While both infants and adults with the t(4;11) are at high risk for treatment failure, children with the t(4;11) appear to have a better outcome than either infants or adults, although this observation is not consistent among all reports.[93] Another translocation involving the MLL gene in children with ALL is the t(11;19), which occurs in approximately 1% of cases and which occurs in both B-precursor and T-cell ALL.[94] Outcome for infants with t(11;19) is poor, but outcome appears relatively favorable for children with T-cell ALL and the t(11;19) translocation.[95]

The t(1;19) translocation occurs in 5% to 6% of childhood ALL, and involves fusion of the E2A gene on chromosome 19 to the PBX1 gene on chromosome 1.[96] The t(1;19) may occur as either a balanced translocation or as an

---

[90] Pui CH, Evans WE: Acute lymphoblastic leukemia. New England Journal of Medicine 339(9): 605-615, 1998.

[91] Rubnitz JE, Look AT: Molecular genetics of childhood leukemias. Journal of Pediatric Hematology/Oncology 20(1): 1-11, 1998.

[92] Pui CH, Frankel LS, Carroll AJ, et al.: Clinical characteristics and treatment outcome of childhood acute lymphoblastic leukemia with the t(4;11)(q21;q23): a collaborative study of 40 cases. Blood 77(3): 440-447, 1991.

[93] Hann I, Vora A, Harrison G, et al.: Determinants of outcome after intensified therapy of childhood lymphoblastic leukaemia: results from Medical Research Council United Kingdom acute lymphoblastic leukaemia XI protocol. British Journal of Haematology 113(1): 103-114, 2001.

Pui CH, Frankel LS, Carroll AJ, et al.: Clinical characteristics and treatment outcome of childhood acute lymphoblastic leukemia with the t(4;11)(q21;q23): a collaborative study of 40 cases. Blood 77(3): 440-447, 1991.

Pui CH, Carroll LA, Raimondi SC, et al.: Childhood acute lymphoblastic leukemia with the t(4;11)(q21;q23): an update. Blood 83(8): 2384-2385, 1994.

Johansson B, Moorman AV, et al, on behalf of the European 11q23 Workshop participants: Hematologic malignancies with t(4;11)(q21;q23) - a cytogenetic, morphologic, immunophenotypic and clinical study of 183 cases. Leukemia 12(5): 779-787, 1998.

[94] Rubnitz JE, Camitta BM, Mahmoud M, et al.: Childhood acute lymphoblastic leukemia with the MLL-ENL fusion and t(11;19)(q23;p13) translocation. Journal of Clinical Oncology 17(1): 191-196, 1999.

[95] Rubnitz JE, Camitta BM, Mahmoud M, et al.: Childhood acute lymphoblastic leukemia with the MLL-ENL fusion and t(11;19)(q23;p13) translocation. Journal of Clinical Oncology 17(1): 191-196, 1999.

[96] Crist WM, Carroll AJ, Shuster JJ, et al.: Poor prognosis of children with pre-B acute lymphoblastic leukemia is associated with the t(1;19)(q23;p13): a Pediatric Oncology Group study. Blood 76(1): 117-122, 1990.

unbalanced translocation and is primarily associated with pre-B ALL (cytoplasmic immunoglobulin positive). Its presence was initially associated with inferior outcome in the context of antimetabolite based therapy.[97] Studies have shown that the poorer prognosis associated with t(1;19) can be largely overcome by more intensive therapy.[98] The improved outcome, however, appears to be primarily for patients with the unbalanced t(1;19)(approximately three fourths of all t(1;19) cases), with patients who have the balanced t(1;19) remaining at increased risk for treatment failure.[99]

The rapidity with which leukemia cells are eliminated following onset of treatment is also associated with outcome. Various ways of evaluating the leukemia cell response to treatment have been utilized, including:

- Day 7 and day 14 bone marrow responses: Patients who have a rapid reduction in the leukemia cells in their bone marrow within 7 or 14 days following initiation of multiagent chemotherapy have a more favorable prognosis than do patients who have slower clearance of leukemia cells from the bone marrow.[100] This "response to treatment" prognostic factor

---

Pui CH, Evans WE: Acute lymphoblastic leukemia. New England Journal of Medicine 339(9): 605-615, 1998.
Hunger SP: Chromosomal translocations involving the E2A gene in acute lymphoblastic leukemia: clinical features and molecular pathogenesis. Blood 87(4): 1211-1224, 1996.
[97] Crist WM, Carroll AJ, Shuster JJ, et al.: Poor prognosis of children with pre-B acute lymphoblastic leukemia is associated with the t(1;19)(q23;p13): a Pediatric Oncology Group study. Blood 76(1): 117-122, 1990.
[98] Uckun FM, Sensel MG, Sather HN, et al.: Clinical significance of translocation t(1;19) in childhood acute lymphoblastic leukemia in the context of contemporary therapies: a report from the Children's Cancer Group. Journal of Clinical Oncology 16(2): 527-535, 1998.
Raimondi SC, Behm FG, Roberson PK, et al.: Cytogenetics of pre-B-cell acute lymphoblastic leukemia with emphasis on prognostic implications of the t(1;19). Journal of Clinical Oncology 8(8): 1380-1388, 1990.
[99] Uckun FM, Sensel MG, Sather HN, et al.: Clinical significance of translocation t(1;19) in childhood acute lymphoblastic leukemia in the context of contemporary therapies: a report from the Children's Cancer Group. Journal of Clinical Oncology 16(2): 527-535, 1998.
Secker-Walker LM, Berger R, Fenaux P, et al.: Prognostic significance of the balanced t(1;19) and unbalanced der(19)t(1;19) translocations in acute lymphoblastic leukemia. Leukemia 6(5): 363-369, 1992.
[100] Hann I, Vora A, Harrison G, et al.: Determinants of outcome after intensified therapy of childhood lymphoblastic leukaemia: results from Medical Research Council United Kingdom acute lymphoblastic leukaemia XI protocol. British Journal of Haematology 113(1): 103-114, 2001.
Gaynon PS, Bleyer WA, Steinherz PG, et al.: Day 7 marrow response and outcome for children with acute lymphoblastic leukemia and unfavorable presenting features. Medical and Pediatric Oncology 18(4): 273-279, 1990.
Gaynon PS, Desai AA, Bostrom BC, et al.: Early response to therapy and outcome in childhood acute lymphoblastic leukemia: a review. Cancer 80(9): 1717-1726, 1997.

is used by the Children's Cancer Group to stratify patients into prognostic categories for treatment assignment.

- Peripheral blood response to steroid prephase: Patients with a reduction in peripheral blast count to less than 1000/mm3 after a 7-day induction prephase with prednisone and one dose of intrathecal methotrexate ("good prednisone response") have a more favorable prognosis than patients whose peripheral blast counts remain above 1000/mm3 ("poor prednisone response").[101] Treatment stratification for protocols of the German BFM clinical trials group is based on early response to the prednisone 7-day induction prephase.

- Peripheral blood response to multiagent induction therapy: Patients with persistent circulating leukemia cells at 7 to 10 days after the initiation of multiagent chemotherapy are at increased risk of relapse compared to patients who have clearance of peripheral blasts within 1 week of therapy initiation.[102] Rate of clearance of peripheral blasts has been found to be of prognostic significance in T-lineage as well as B-lineage ALL.[103]

- Minimal residual disease: Patients in clinical remission after induction therapy may have "minimal residual disease," i.e., leukemia cells that can only be detected by highly sensitive techniques such as polymerase chain reaction (PCR) or specialized flow cytometry. Numerous groups have reported an association between minimal residual disease and outcome with early absence of minimal residual disease being associated with

---

Steinherz PG, Gaynon PS, Breneman JC, et al.: Cytoreduction and prognosis in acute lymphoblastic leukemia - the importance of early marrow response: report from the Childrens Cancer Group. Journal of Clinical Oncology 14(2): 389-398, 1996.

[101] Dordelmann M, Reiter A, et al, for the ALL-BFM Group: Prednisone response is the strongest predictor of treatment outcome in infant acute lymphoblastic leukemia. Blood 94(4): 1209-1217, 1999.

Schrappe M, Arico M, Harbott J, et al.: Philadelphia chromosome-positive (Ph+) childhood acute lymphoblastic leukemia: good initial steroid response allows early prediction of a favorable treatment outcome. Blood 92(8): 2730-2741, 1998.

Arico M, Basso G, et al, for the Associazione Italiana Ematologia Oncologia Pediatrica (AIEOP): Good steroid response in vivo predicts a favorable outcome in children with T-cell acute lymphoblastic leukemia. Cancer 75(7): 1684-1693, 1995.

[102] Gajjar A, Ribeiro R, Hancock ML, et al.: Persistence of circulating blasts after 1 week of multiagent chemotherapy confers a poor prognosis in childhood acute lymphoblastic leukemia. Blood 86(4): 1292-1295, 1995.

Rautonen J, Hovi L, Siimes MA: Slow disappearance of peripheral blast cells: an independent risk factor indicating poor prognosis in children with acute lymphoblastic leukemia. Blood 71(4): 989-991, 1988.

[103] Griffin TC, Shuster JJ, Buchanan GR et al.: Slow disappearance of peripheral blood blasts is an adverse prognostic factor in childhood T cell acute lymphoblastic leukemia: a Pediatric Oncology Group study. Leukemia 14(5): 792-795, 2000.

better outcome and presence of minimal residual disease being associated with poor outcome.[104]

CCG makes initial assignment of patients as "standard risk" or "high risk" based on the NCI consensus age and WBC criteria.[105] The standard-risk category includes patients 1 to 9 years of age who have a WBC count at diagnosis less than 50,000/uL. The remaining patients are classified as having high-risk ALL. Final treatment assignment for CCG protocols is based on the early response to therapy (day 7 or day 14 bone marrow response), with slow early responders being assigned to receive more aggressive treatment.

POG defines its "low risk" group based on the NCI consensus age and WBC criteria for low risk, and additionally requires absence of adverse translocations, absence of CNS disease and testicular disease, and the presence of either the TEL/AML1 translocation or trisomy of chromosomes 4 and 10. The "high risk" group requires the absence of favorable translocations and the presence of CNS or testicular leukemia, or the presence of MLL gene rearrangement, or unfavorable age and WBC count.[106] The "standard risk" category includes patients not meeting the criteria for inclusion in any of the other risk group categories.

---

[104] Cave H, van der Werff ten Bosch J, Suciu S, et al.: Clinical significance of minimal residual disease in childhood acute lymphoblastic leukemia. European Organization for Research and Treatment of Cancer--Childhood Leukemia Cooperative Group. New England Journal of Medicine 339(9): 591-598, 1998.
Dibenedetto SP, Lo Nigro L, Mayer SP, et al.: Detectable molecular residual disease at the beginning of maintenance therapy indicates poor outcome in children with T-cell acute lymphoblastic leukemia. Blood 90(3): 1226-1232, 1997.
Roberts WM, Estrov Z, Ouspenskaia MV, et al.: Measurement of residual leukemia during remission in childhood acute lymphoblastic leukemia. New England Journal of Medicine 336(5): 317-323, 1997.
van Dongen JJ, Seriu T, Panzer-Grumayer ER, et al.: Prognostic value of minimal residual disease in acute lymphoblastic leukaemia in childhood. Lancet 352(9142): 1731-1738, 1998.
Panzer-Grumayer ER, Schneider M, Panzer S, et al.: Rapid molecular response during early induction chemotherapy predicts a good outcome in childhood acute lymphoblastic leukemia. Blood 95(3): 790-794, 2000.
Coustan-Smith E, Sancho J, Hancock ML, et al.: Clinical importance of minimal residual disease in childhood acute lymphoblastic leukemia. Blood 96(8): 2691-2696, 2000.
[105] Smith M, Arthur D, Camitta B, et al.: Uniform approach to risk classification and treatment assignment for children with acute lymphoblastic leukemia. Journal of Clinical Oncology 14(1): 18-24, 1996.
[106] Shuster JJ, Camitta BM, Pullen J, et al.: Identification of newly diagnosed children with acute lymphocytic leukemia at high risk for relapse. Cancer Research, Therapy and Control 9(1-2): 101-107, 1999.

The "very high-risk" category for both CCG and POG is defined by one of the following, taking precedence over all other considerations: presence of the t(9;22); M3 marrow on day 29 or M2 or M3 marrow on day 43; or hypodiploidy (DNA index < 0.95). Infants with ALL are considered "high risk" and are treated on special protocols designed specifically for infants.

Children with T-cell ALL are much more likely than children with B-precursor ALL to meet "high risk" age and WBC criteria (75% for T-cell ALL versus 32% for B-precursor ALL).[107] In POG, children with T-cell ALL are grouped together with children who have lymphoblastic lymphoma and are treated on T-cell specific protocols. In CCG, children with T-cell ALL are treated on the same protocols as children with B-precursor ALL, with protocol assignment based on the same risk factor criteria for both patient populations.

Treatment Option Overview

Risk-based treatment assignment is the key therapeutic strategy utilized for children with acute lymphoblastic leukemia (ALL). This approach allows children who historically have a very good outcome with modest therapy to be spared more intensive and toxic treatment, while allowing children with a historically lower probability of long-term survival to receive more intensive therapy that may increase their chance of cure. As discussed in the "Cellular Classification and Prognostic Variables" section of this summary, a number of clinical and laboratory features have demonstrated prognostic value. A subset of the known prognostic factors (e.g., age, white blood cell (WBC) count at diagnosis, presence of specific cytogenetic abnormalities) are used for the initial stratification of children with ALL into treatment groups with varying degrees of risk for treatment failure. Event-free survival (EFS) rates for children meeting "good risk" age and WBC criteria exceed 80%, while for children meeting "high risk" criteria, EFS rates are approximately 70% or greater.[108] Application of biological factors (e.g., specific chromosomal

---

[107] Smith M, Arthur D, Camitta B, et al.: Uniform approach to risk classification and treatment assignment for children with acute lymphoblastic leukemia. Journal of Clinical Oncology 14(1): 18-24, 1996.

[108] Gaynon PS, Trigg ME, Heerema NA, et al.: Children's Cancer Group trials in childhood acute lymphoblastic leukemia: 1983-1995. Leukemia 14(12): 2223-2233, 2000.
Schrappe M, Reiter A, Zimmermann M, et al.: Long-term results of four consecutive trials in childhood ALL performed by the ALL-BFM study group from 1981 to 1995. Leukemia 14(12): 2205-2222, 2000.
Silverman LB, Declerck L, Gelber RD, et al.: Results of Dana-Farber Cancer Institute consortium protocols for children with newly diagnosed acute lymphoblastic leukemia (1981-1995). Leukemia 14(12): 2247-2256, 2000.

translocations) can identify patient groups with expected outcome survival rates ranging from less than 40% to greater than 85%.[109]

Nationwide clinical trials are generally available for children with ALL, with specific protocols designed for children at standard (or low) risk of treatment failure and for children at higher risk for treatment failure. Clinical trials for children with ALL are generally designed to compare therapy that is currently accepted as standard for a particular risk group with a potentially better treatment approach that may improve survival outcome and/or diminish toxicities associated with the standard treatment regimen. Many of the improvements in therapy that have led to increased survival rates for children with ALL have been made through nationwide clinical trials,[110] and it is appropriate for children and adolescents with ALL to be offered participation in a clinical trial. In addition, treatment planning by a multidisciplinary team of pediatric cancer specialists with experience and expertise in treating leukemias of childhood is required to determine and implement optimum treatment. This treatment is best accomplished in a pediatric cancer center.[111]

Successful treatment of children with ALL requires the control of systemic disease (marrow, liver and spleen, lymph nodes, etc.) as well as the treatment (or prevention) of extramedullary disease particularly in the central nervous system (CNS). Only 3% of patients have detectable CNS involvement by accepted criteria at diagnosis (>/= 5 WBC/mm3 with lymphoblast cells present), however, unless specific therapy is directed toward the CNS (intrathecal medication, cranial irradiation, high-dose systemic chemotherapy with methotrexate or cytarabine) 50% to 70% or more of children will eventually develop overt CNS leukemia. Therefore all children with ALL should receive systemic combination chemotherapy together with some form of CNS prophylaxis. At present, patients with documented CNS leukemia at diagnosis receive intrathecal therapy followed by cranial irradiation with or without concurrent spinal radiation.

---

[109] Pui CH, Evans WE: Acute lymphoblastic leukemia. New England Journal of Medicine 339(9): 605-615, 1998.
Pui CH: Acute lymphoblastic leukemia in children. Current Opinion in Oncology 12(1): 3-12, 2000.
[110] Vietti TJ, Land V, et al, for the Pediatric Oncology Group: Progress against childhood cancer: the Pediatric Oncology Group experience. Pediatrics 89(4 pt 1): 597-600, 1992.
Bleyer WA: The U.S. pediatric cancer clinical trials programmes: international implications and the way forward. European Journal of Cancer 33(9): 1439-1447, 1997.
[111] Sanders J, Glader B, Cairo M, et al.: Guidelines for the pediatric cancer center and role of such centers in diagnosis and treatment. American Academy of Pediatrics Section Statement Section on Hematology/Oncology. Pediatrics 99(1): 139-141, 1997.

Treatment for children with ALL is divided into stages: remission induction, consolidation or intensification, and maintenance (continuation) therapy, with CNS sanctuary therapy generally provided in each stage. An intensification phase of therapy following remission induction is used for all patients. The intensity of both induction therapy and postinduction therapy is determined by the clinical and biologic prognostic factors utilized for risk-based treatment assignment. The average duration of maintenance therapy for children with ALL ranges between 2 and 3 years.

Subgroups of patients who have a poor prognosis with current standard therapy may require different treatment. For example, infants with ALL represent a distinct category of patients at higher risk for treatment failure, with the poorest prognosis for those with MLL gene rearrangements.[112] These children are generally treated with regimens designed specifically for infants.[113] Current regimens for infants employ intensified treatment approaches and may offer improved disease control compared to previously utilized, less intensive approaches, but long-term outcome and toxicity are unknown.[114] Certain children with ALL older than 1 year of age also have a

---

[112] Rubnitz JE, Link MP, Shuster JJ, et al.: Frequency and prognostic significance of HRX rearrangements in infant acute lymphoblastic leukemia: a Pediatric Oncology Group study. Blood 84(2): 570-573, 1994.
Hilden JM, Frestedt JL, Moore RO, et al.: Molecular analysis of infant acute lymphoblastic leukemia: MLL gene rearrangement and reverse transcriptase-polymerase chain reaction for t(4;11)(q21;q23). Blood 86(10): 3876-3882, 1995.
Pui C, Behm FG, Downing JR, et al.: 11q23/MLL rearrangement confers a poor prognosis in infants with acute lymphoblastic leukemia. Journal of Clinical Oncology 12(5): 909-915, 1994.
[113] Frankel LS, Ochs J, Shuster JJ, et al.: Therapeutic trial for infant acute lymphoblastic leukemia: the Pediatric Oncology Group experience (POG 8493). Journal of Pediatric Hematology/Oncology 19(1): 35-42, 1997.
Chessells JM, Eden OB, Bailey CC, et al.: Acute lymphoblastic leukaemia in infancy: experience in MRC UKALL trials. Report from the Medical Research Council Working Party on Childhood Leukaemia. Leukaemia 8(8): 1275-1279, 1994.
Ferster A, Bertrand Y, Benoit Y, et al.: Improved survival for acute lymphoblastic leukaemia in infancy: the experience of EORTC-Childhood Leukaemia Cooperative Group. British Journal of Haematology 86(2): 284-290, 1994.
Silverman LB, McLean TW, Gelber RD, et al.: Intensified therapy for infants with acute lymphoblastic leukemia: results from the Dana-Farber Cancer Institute Consortium. Cancer 80(12): 2285-2295, 1997.
[114] Silverman LB, McLean TW, Gelber RD, et al.: Intensified therapy for infants with acute lymphoblastic leukemia: results from the Dana-Farber Cancer Institute Consortium. Cancer 80(12): 2285-2295, 1997.
Dreyer ZE, Steuber CP, Bowman WP, et al.: High risk infant ALL--improved survival with intensive chemotherapy. Proceedings of the American Society of Clinical Oncology 17: A2032, 529a, 1998.

less than 50% likelihood of long-term remission with current therapy (e.g., t(9;22) Philadelphia chromosome positive ALL and patients with hypodiploid lymphoblasts). For these patients in first remission, allogeneic bone marrow transplantation from a HLA- matched sibling should be considered.[115] However, HLA-matched sibling donor transplant has not been proven to be of benefit in patients defined as high-risk solely by WBC count, gender, and age.[116]

Since myelosuppression and generalized immunosuppression are an anticipated consequence of both leukemia and its treatment with chemotherapy, it is imperative that patients be closely monitored during treatment. Adequate facilities must be immediately available both for hematologic support and for the treatment of infectious complications throughout all phases of leukemia treatment.

The designations in PDQ that treatments are "standard" or "under clinical evaluation" are not to be used as a basis for reimbursement determinations.

Treatment Options for Untreated Childhood ALL

Induction Chemotherapy

Three-drug induction therapy using vincristine, prednisone/dexamethasone, plus L-asparaginase in conjunction with intrathecal therapy (IT) results in complete remission rates of greater than 95%.[117] For patients at high risk for treatment failure, a more intense

---

Reaman GH, Sposto R, Sensel MG, et al.: Treatment outcome and prognostic factors for infants with acute lymphoblastic leukemia treated on two consecutive trials of the Children's Cancer Group. Journal of Clinical Oncology 17(2): 445-455, 1999.
[115] Snyder DS, Nademanee AP, O'Donnell MR, et al.: Long-term follow-up of 23 patients with Philadelphia chromosome-positive acute lymphoblastic leukemia treated with allogeneic bone marrow transplant in first complete remission. Leukemia 13(12): 2053-2058, 1999.
Arico M, Valsecchi MG, Camitta B, et al.: Outcome of treatment in children with Philadelphia chromosome-positive acute lymphoblastic leukemia. New England Journal of Medicine 342(14): 998-1006, 2000.
[116] Wheeler KA, Richards SM, Bailey CC, et al.: Bone marrow transplantation versus chemotherapy in the treatment of very high-risk childhood acute lymphoblastic leukemia in first remission: results from Medical Research Council UKALL X and XI. Blood 96(7): 2412-2418, 2000.
[117] Pui CH, Evans WE: Acute lymphoblastic leukemia. New England Journal of Medicine 339(9): 605-615, 1998.

induction regimen (4 or 5 agents) may result in improved event-free survival,[118] and "high risk" patients generally receive induction therapy that includes an anthracycline (e.g., daunomycin) in addition to vincristine, prednisone/dexamethasone, plus L-asparaginase. For patients who are at standard or low risk of treatment failure, the addition of an anthracycline to 3-drug induction therapy does not appear necessary for favorable outcome provided that adequate postremission intensification therapy is administered.[119] Because of the likelihood of increased toxicity by the addition of an anthracycline to standard 3-drug induction therapy, most centers treat standard or lower risk patients with prednisone/dexamethasone, vincristine, and L-asparaginase and reserve the use of induction regimens using 4 or more agents for higher risk patients.[120]

Gaynon PS, Bleyer WA, Steinherz PG, et al.: Day 7 marrow response and outcome for children with acute lymphoblastic leukemia and unfavorable presenting features. Medical and Pediatric Oncology 18(4): 273-279, 1990.

[118] Tubergen DG, Gilchrist GS, O'Brien RT, et al.: Improved outcome with delayed intensification for children with acute lymphoblastic leukemia and intermediate presenting features: a Childrens Cancer Group phase III trial. Journal of Clinical Oncology 11(3): 527-537, 1993.

Gaynon PS, Steinherz PG, Bleyer WA, et al.: Improved therapy for children with acute lymphoblastic leukemia and unfavorable presenting features: a follow-up report of the Childrens Cancer Group Study CCG-106. Journal of Clinical Oncology 11(11): 2234-2242, 1993.

Schorin MA, Blattner S, Gelber RD, et al.: Treatment of childhood acute lymphoblastic leukemia: results of Dana-Farber Cancer Institute/Children's Hospital Acute Lymphoblastic Leukemia Consortium protocol 85-01. Journal of Clinical Oncology 12(4): 740-747, 1994.

[119] Tubergen DG, Gilchrist GS, O'Brien RT, et al.: Improved outcome with delayed intensification for children with acute lymphoblastic leukemia and intermediate presenting features: a Childrens Cancer Group phase III trial. Journal of Clinical Oncology 11(3): 527-537, 1993.

Veerman AJ, Hahlen K, Kamps WA, et al.: High cure rate with a moderately intensive treatment regimen in non-high-risk childhood acute lymphoblastic leukemia: results of protocol ALL VI from the Dutch Childhood Leukemia Study Group. Journal of Clinical Oncology 14(3): 911-918, 1996.

[120] Tubergen DG, Gilchrist GS, O'Brien RT, et al.: Improved outcome with delayed intensification for children with acute lymphoblastic leukemia and intermediate presenting features: a Childrens Cancer Group phase III trial. Journal of Clinical Oncology 11(3): 527-537, 1993.

Veerman AJ, Hahlen K, Kamps WA, et al.: High cure rate with a moderately intensive treatment regimen in non-high-risk childhood acute lymphoblastic leukemia: results of protocol ALL VI from the Dutch Childhood Leukemia Study Group. Journal of Clinical Oncology 14(3): 911-918, 1996.

Mahoney DH Jr, Shuster J, Nitschke R, et al.: Intermediate-dose intravenous methotrexate with intravenous mercaptopurine is superior to repetitive low-dose oral methotrexate with intravenous mercaptopurine for children with lower-risk Blineage acute lymphoblastic leukemia: a Pediatric Oncology Group phase III trial. Journal of Clinical Oncology 16(1): 246-254, 1998.

Dexamethasone is preferred over prednisone for younger patients with acute lymphoblastic leukemia (ALL) receiving 3-drug induction therapy based on data from a Children's Cancer Group (CCG) study in which dexamethasone was compared to prednisone for children 1 to 9 years of age with lower risk ALL.[121] Patients randomized to receive dexamethasone had significantly fewer CNS relapses and bone marrow relapses, and a significantly better event-free survival rate.[122] The benefit of using dexamethasone in induction therapy for adolescents requires investigation, because of the increased risk of steroid-induced aseptic necrosis in this age group.[123] Dexamethasone should be used with caution in patients receiving intensive induction therapy (more than 3 drugs) as its use appears to increase the frequency and severity of infectious complications.[124]

Several forms of L-asparaginase are available for use in the treatment of children with ALL, with E. coli L-asparaginase being most commonly used.[125] Pegaspargase is an alternative form of L-asparaginase in which the E. coli enzyme is modified by the covalent attachment of polyethylene glycol. Pegasparagase has a much longer serum half-life than native E. coli L-asparaginase, allowing it to produce asparagine depletion with less frequent administration.[126] A single intramuscular dose of pegaspargase given in conjunction with vincristine and prednisone during induction therapy appears to have similar activity and toxicity as 9 doses of intramuscular E. coli L-asparaginase (3 times a week for 3 weeks).[127]

---

[121] Bostrom B, Gaynon PS, Sather S, et al.: Dexamethasone (DEX) decreases central nervous system (CNS) relapse and improves event-free survival (EFS) in lower risk acute lymphoblastic leukemia (ALL). Proceedings of the American Society of Clinical Oncology 17: A2024, 527a, 1998.

[122] Bostrom B, Gaynon PS, Sather S, et al.: Dexamethasone (DEX) decreases central nervous system (CNS) relapse and improves event-free survival (EFS) in lower risk acute lymphoblastic leukemia (ALL). Proceedings of the American Society of Clinical Oncology 17: A2024, 527a, 1998.

[123] Ojala AE, Lanning FP, Paakko E, et al.: Osteonecrosis in children treated for acute lymphoblastic leukemia: a magnetic resonance imaging study after treatment. Medical and Pediatric Oncology 29(4): 260-265, 1997.

[124] Hurwitz CA, Silverman LB, Schorin MA, et al.: Substituting dexamethasone for prednisone complicates remission induction in children with acute lymphoblastic leukemia. Cancer 88(8): 1964-1969, 2000.

[125] Muller HJ, Boos J: Use of L-asparaginase in childhood ALL. Critical Reviews in Oncology/Hematology 28(2): 97-113, 1998.

[126] Asselin BL, Whitin JC, Coppola DJ, et al.: Comparative pharmacokinetic studies of three asparaginase preparations. Journal of Clinical Oncology 11(9): 1780-1786, 1993.

[127] Cohen A, Ettinger L, Ettinger P, et al.: Randomized trial of PEG-vs native-asparaginase in children with newly diagnosed acute lymphoblastic leukemia (ALL): CCG study 1962. Blood 94(10 pt 1): A-2790, 628a, 1999.

In general, patients will achieve a complete remission within the first 4 weeks. Patients who require more than 4 weeks to achieve remission have a poor prognosis.[128] Outcome is also less favorable for patients who demonstrate more than 25% blasts in the bone marrow or persistent blasts in the peripheral blood after 1 week of intensive induction therapy,[129] and protocols of the Children's Cancer Group base treatment decisions on the day 7 bone marrow response (for high-risk protocols) or day 14 bone marrow response (for standard-risk protocols).[130] (Information about ongoing clinical trials is available from the NCI (**http://cancer.gov/clinical_trials/**).

Central Nervous System Sanctuary Therapy

The early institution of adequate central nervous system (CNS) sanctuary therapy is critical in preventing CNS relapse. A current goal of ALL therapy design is to achieve effective CNS sanctuary therapy while minimizing neurotoxicity. Every patient with ALL receives intrathecal chemotherapy with methotrexate plus cytarabine and hydrocortisone. Intrathecal therapy may also have a significant systemic effect which could result in a decrease in marrow relapse rate.[131] Significant control of bone marrow relapse did not occur until CNS sanctuary therapy was instituted. Conversely, the type and extent of systemic intensification also appears to influence the efficacy of the CNS sanctuary therapy. Systemically administered drugs such as dexamethasone, L-asparaginase, high dose methotrexate, and high dose Ara-C may provide some degree of CNS protection. For example, in a recent CCG study for patients with standard risk ALL, dexamethasone decreased

---

[128] Silverman LB, Gelber RD, Young ML, et al.: Induction failure in acute lymphoblastic leukemia of childhood. Cancer 85(6): 1395-1404, 1999.

[129] Gaynon PS, Bleyer WA, Steinherz PG, et al.: Day 7 marrow response and outcome for children with acute lymphoblastic leukemia and unfavorable presenting features. Medical and Pediatric Oncology 18(4): 273-279, 1990.

Gajjar A, Ribeiro R, Hancock ML, et al.: Persistence of circulating blasts after 1 week of multiagent chemotherapy confers a poor prognosis in childhood acute lymphoblastic leukemia. Blood 86(4): 1292-1295, 1995.

Steinherz PG, Gaynon PS, Breneman JC, et al.: Cytoreduction and prognosis in acute lymphoblastic leukemia - the importance of early marrow response: report from the Childrens Cancer Group. Journal of Clinical Oncology 14(2): 389-398, 1996.

[130] Nachman JB, Sather HN, Sensel MG, et al.: Augmented post-induction therapy for children with high-risk acute lymphoblastic leukemia and a slow response to initial therapy. New England Journal of Medicine 338(23): 1663-1671, 1998.

[131] Thyss A, Suciu S, et al, for the European Organization for Research and Treatment of Cancer Children's Leukemia Cooperative Group: Systemic effect of intrathecal methotrexate during the initial phase of treatment of childhood acute lymphoblastic leukemia. Journal of Clinical Oncology 15(5): 1824-1830, 1997.

the CNS relapse rate by 50% compared to patients receiving prednisone (patients received IT methotrexate alone for CNS prophylaxis).[132]

Intrathecal chemotherapy may be the sole form of presymptomatic CNS therapy or it may be combined with systemic moderate to high dose infusion methotrexate with leucovorin rescue and/or cranial radiation (1200-1800 cGy). Appropriate systemic therapy combined with IT chemotherapy results in CNS relapse rates of less than 5% for children with standard risk ALL.[133] Whether patients at high risk of CNS relapse (for example, age greater than or equal to 10 years, presence of hyperleukocytosis, or T cell ALL) continue to require cranial radiation in addition to extended intrathecal therapy is controversial,[134] although patients designated as high risk generally receive cranial radiation as part of their CNS sanctuary therapy.[135] High-risk patients with rapid early response to therapy, however, appear to have adequate CNS prophylaxis with intrathecal therapy alone.[136] Children with ALL who

---

[132] Bostrom B, Gaynon PS, Sather S, et al.: Dexamethasone (DEX) decreases central nervous system (CNS) relapse and improves event-free survival (EFS) in lower risk acute lymphoblastic leukemia (ALL). Proceedings of the American Society of Clinical Oncology 17: A2024, 527a, 1998.

[133] Veerman AJ, Hahlen K, Kamps WA, et al.: High cure rate with a moderately intensive treatment regimen in non-high-risk childhood acute lymphoblastic leukemia: results of protocol ALL VI from the Dutch Childhood Leukemia Study Group. Journal of Clinical Oncology 14(3): 911-918, 1996.

Tubergen DG, Gilchrist GS, O'Brien RT, et al.: Prevention of CNS disease in intermediate-risk acute lymphoblastic leukemia: comparison of cranial radiation and intrathecal methotrexate and the importance of systemic therapy: a Childrens Cancer Group report. Journal of Clinical Oncology 11(3): 520-526, 1993.

Conter V, Arico M, Valsecchi MG, et al.: Extended intrathecal methotrexate may replace cranial irradiation for prevention of CNS relapse in children with intermediate-risk acute lymphoblastic leukemia treated with Berlin-Frankfurt-Munster-based intensive chemotherapy. Journal of Clinical Oncology 13(10): 2497-2502, 1995.

[134] Schrappe M, Reiter A, Riehm H: Prophylaxis and treatment of neoplastic meningeosis in childhood acute lymphoblastic leukemia. Journal of Neuro-Oncology 38(2-3): 159-165, 1998.

Laver JH, Barredo JC, Amylon M, et al.: Effects of cranial radiation in children with high risk T cell acute lymphoblastic leukemia: a Pediatric Oncology Group report. Leukemia 14(3): 369-373, 2000.

[135] Nachman JB, Sather HN, Sensel MG, et al.: Augmented post-induction therapy for children with high-risk acute lymphoblastic leukemia and a slow response to initial therapy. New England Journal of Medicine 338(23): 1663-1671, 1998.

Pui CH, Mahmoud HH, Rivera GK, et al.: Early intensification of intrathecal chemotherapy virtually eliminates central nervous system relapse in children with acute lymphoblastic leukemia. Blood 92(2): 411-415, 1998.

Waber DP, Shapiro BL, Carpentieri SC, et al.: Excellent therapeutic efficacy and minimal late neurotoxicity in children treated with 18 grays of cranial radiation therapy for high-risk acute lymphoblastic leukemia. Cancer 92(1): 15-22, 2001.

[136] Nachman J, Sather HN, Cherlow JM, et al.: Response of children with high-risk acute lymphoblastic leukemia treated with and without cranial irradiation: a report from the Children's Cancer Group. Journal of Clinical Oncology 16(3): 920-930, 1998.

present with CNS disease at diagnosis (defined as greater than or equal to 5 white cells per cubic millimeter in cerebral spinal fluid (CSF) with lymphoblasts present) generally receive cranial radiation with or without concurrent spinal radiation in addition to appropriate systemic and intrathecal chemotherapy.

Toxic effects of CNS-directed therapy for childhood ALL can be divided into two broad groups. Acute/subacute toxicities include seizures, stroke, somnolence syndrome, and ascending paralysis. Chronic toxicities include leukoencephalopathy and a range of behavioral and neuropsychological, and neuroendocrine disturbances.[137]

The long-term deleterious effects of cranial radiation when used for CNS prophylaxis, particularly at doses greater than 1800 cGy, have been recognized for years. Children receiving these higher doses of cranial radiation were at significant risk for neurocognitive and neuroendocrine sequelae.[138] Children receiving 1800 cGy of cranial radiation may be at diminished risk for neurologic toxicity compared to those receiving 2400 cGy,[139] although neurocognitive and neuroendocrine effects have been noted at this lower dose.[140]. In the German BFM studies, many patients receive only

---

[137] Moore IM, Espy KA, Kaufman P, et al.: Cognitive consequences and central nervous system injury following treatment for childhood leukemia. Seminars in Oncology Nursing 16(4): 279-290, 2000.

[138] Stubberfield TG, Byrne GC, Jones TW: Growth and growth hormone secretion after treatment for acute lymphoblastic leukemia in childhood. 18-Gy versus 24-Gy cranial irradiation. Journal of Pediatric Hematology/Oncology 17(2): 167-171, 1995.
Rowland JH, Glidewell OJ, Sibley RF, et al.: Effects of different forms of central nervous system prophylaxis on neuropsychologic function in childhood leukemia. Journal of Clinical Oncology 2(12): 1327-1335, 1984.
Halberg FE, Kramer JH, Moore IM, et al.: Prophylactic cranial irradiation dose effects on late cognitive function in children treated for acute lymphoblastic leukemia. International Journal of Radiation Oncology, Biology, Physics 22: 13-16, 1992.
Hill JM, Kornblith AB, Jones D, et al.: A comparative study of the long term psychosocial functioning of childhood acute lymphoblastic leukemia survivors treated by intrathecal methotrexate with or without cranial radiation. Cancer 82(1): 208-218, 1998.

[139] Waber DP, Shapiro BL, Carpentieri SC, et al.: Excellent therapeutic efficacy and minimal late neurotoxicity in children treated with 18 grays of cranial radiation therapy for high-risk acute lymphoblastic leukemia. Cancer 92(1): 15-22, 2001.

[140] Jankovic, M, Brouwers P, Valsecchi MG, et al.: Association of 1800 cGy cranial irradiation with intellectual function in children with acute lymphoblastic leukaemia. Lancet 344(8917): 224-227, 1994.
Butler RW, Hill JM, Steinherz PG, et al.: Neuropsychologic effects of cranial irradiation, intrathecal methotrexate, and systemic methotrexate in childhood cancer. Journal of Clinical Oncology 12(12): 2621-2629, 1994.

1200 cGy of central nervous system radiation.[141] Longer follow-up is needed to determine whether 1200 cGy will be associated with a lower incidence of neurologic sequelae. Young children (e.g., younger than four years) are at increased risk for neurocognitive decline and other sequelae following cranial radiation.[142] It appears that girls may be at a higher risk for radiation-induced neuropsychologic and neuroendocrine sequelae than boys.[143] In general, high-dose methotrexate should not be given following cranial radiation.

The most common toxicity associated with intrathecal therapy alone in the absence of cranial radiation is seizures. Approximately 5% to 10% of patients with ALL will have at least one seizure during therapy.[144] Patients with ALL who develop seizures during the course of treatment and who require anticonvulsant therapy should not receive phenobarbital or dilantin as anticonvulsant treatment, as these drugs may increase the clearance of some chemotherapeutic drugs. Valproic acid or gabapentin are alternative anticonvulsants with less enzyme-inducing capabilities.[145] In general, patients who receive intrathecal therapy without cranial radiation as CNS prophylaxis appear to have a low incidence of neurocognitive sequelae, and the deficits that do develop represent relatively modest declines in a limited

---

[141] Schrappe M, Reiter A, Ludwig WD, et al.: Improved outcome in childhood acute lymphoblastic leukemia despite reduced use of anthracyclines and cranial radiotherapy: results of trial ALL-BFM 90. Blood 95(11): 3310-3322, 2000.

[142] Jankovic, M, Brouwers P, Valsecchi MG, et al.: Association of 1800 cGy cranial irradiation with intellectual function in children with acute lymphoblastic leukaemia. Lancet 344(8917): 224-227, 1994.
Sklar C, Mertens A, Walter A, et al.: Final height after treatment for childhood acute lymphoblastic leukemia: comparison of no cranial irradiation with 1800 and 2400 centigrays of cranial irradiation. Journal of Pediatrics 123(1): 59-64, 1993.
Christie D, Leiper AD, Chessells JM, et al.: Intellectual performance after presymptomatic cranial radiotherapy for leukaemia: effects of age and sex. Archives of Disease in Childhood 73(2): 136-140, 1995.

[143] Sklar C, Mertens A, Walter A, et al.: Final height after treatment for childhood acute lymphoblastic leukemia: comparison of no cranial irradiation with 1800 and 2400 centigrays of cranial irradiation. Journal of Pediatrics 123(1): 59-64, 1993.
Christie D, Leiper AD, Chessells JM, et al.: Intellectual performance after presymptomatic cranial radiotherapy for leukaemia: effects of age and sex. Archives of Disease in Childhood 73(2): 136-140, 1995.
Waber DP, Tarbell NJ, Kahn CM, et al.: The relationship of sex and treatment modality to neuropsychologic outcome in childhood acute lymphoblastic leukemia. Journal of Clinical Oncology 10(5): 810-817, 1992.

[144] Ochs JJ, Bowman WP, Pui CH, et al.: Seizures in childhood lymphoblastic leukaemia patients. Lancet 2(8417-8418): 1422-1424, 1984.

[145] Relling MV, Pui CH, Sandlund JT, et al.: Adverse effect of anticonvulsants on efficacy of chemotherapy for acute lymphoblastic leukaemia. Lancet 356(9226): 285-290, 2000.

number of domains of neuropsychological functioning.[146] However, regimens that utilize a bi-weekly schedule of 12 doses of intravenous high-dose methotrexate with leucovorin rescue and intrathecal chemotherapy in the off-week have been associated with excessive neurologic toxicity.[147] There is controversy regarding whether patients who receive dexamethasone are at risk for neurocognitive disturbances.[148]

Treatment Options for Childhood ALL in Remission

Consolidation/Intensification

Once remission has been achieved, systemic treatment in conjunction with central nervous system (CNS) sanctuary therapy follows. The intensity of the postinduction chemotherapy varies considerably, but all patients receive some form of "intensification" following achievement of remission and before beginning continuous maintenance therapy. "Intensification" may involve the use of intermediate- or high-dose methotrexate,[149] the use of

---

[146] Espy KA, Moore IM, Kaufmann PM, et al.: Chemotherapeutic CNS prophylaxis and neuropsychologic change in children with acute lymphoblastic leukemia: a prospective study. Journal of Pediatric Psychology 26(1): 1-9, 2001.
Butler RW, Hill JM, Steinherz PG, et al.: Neuropsychologic effects of cranial irradiation, intrathecal methotrexate, and systemic methotrexate in childhood cancer. Journal of Clinical Oncology 12(12): 2621-2629, 1994.
Copeland DR, Moore BD III, Francis DJ, et al.: Neuropsychologic effects of chemotherapy on children with cancer: a longitudinal study. Journal of Clinical Oncology 14(10): 2826-2835, 1996.
[147] Mahoney DH, Shuster JJ, Nitschke R, et al.: Acute neurotoxicity in children with B precursor acute lymphoid leukemia: an association with intermediate-dose intravenous methotrexate and intrathecal triple therapy. Journal of Clinical Oncology 16(5): 1712-1722, 1998.
[148] Waber DP, Carpentieri SC, Klar N, et al.: Cognitive sequelae in children treated for acute lymphoblastic leukemia with dexamethasone or prednisone. Journal of Pediatric Hematology/Oncology 22(3): 206-213, 2000.
[149] Harris MB, Shuster JJ, Pullen DJ, et al.: Consolidation therapy with antimetabolite-based therapy in standard-risk acute lymphocytic leukemia of childhood: a Pediatric Oncology Group study. Journal of Clinical Oncology 16(8): 2840-2847, 1998.
Reiter A, Schrappe M, Ludwig W, et al.: Chemotherapy in 998 unselected childhood acute lymphoblastic leukemia patients: results and conclusions of the multicenter trial ALL-BFM 86. Blood 84(9): 3122-3133, 1994.
Veerman AJ, Hahlen K, Kamps WA, et al.: High cure rate with a moderately intensive treatment regimen in non-high-risk childhood acute lymphoblastic leukemia: results of protocol ALL VI from the Dutch Childhood Leukemia Study Group. Journal of Clinical Oncology 14(3): 911-918, 1996.
Mahoney DH Jr, Shuster JJ, Nitschke R, et al.: Intensification with intermediate-dose intravenous methotrexate is effective therapy for children with lower-risk B-precursor acute

similar drugs as those used to achieve remission,[150] the use of different drug combinations with little known cross resistance to the induction therapy drug combination,[151] the extended use of high-dose L-asparaginase,[152] or combinations of the above.[153]

In children with standard-risk disease, there has been an attempt to limit exposure to drugs, such as the anthracyclines and alkylating agents, which are associated with an increased risk of late toxic effects.[154] For example,

---

lymphoblastic leukemia: a Pediatric Oncology Group study. Journal of Clinical Oncology 18(6): 1285-1294, 2000.

[150] Reiter A, Schrappe M, Ludwig W, et al.: Chemotherapy in 998 unselected childhood acute lymphoblastic leukemia patients: results and conclusions of the multicenter trial ALL-BFM 86. Blood 84(9): 3122-3133, 1994.

Tubergen DG, Gilchrist GS, O'Brien RT, et al.: Improved outcome with delayed intensification for children with acute lymphoblastic leukemia and intermediate presenting features: a Childrens Cancer Group phase III trial. Journal of Clinical Oncology 11(3): 527-537, 1993.

[151] Reiter A, Schrappe M, Ludwig W, et al.: Chemotherapy in 998 unselected childhood acute lymphoblastic leukemia patients: results and conclusions of the multicenter trial ALL-BFM 86. Blood 84(9): 3122-3133, 1994.

Richards S, Burrett J, et al, for the Medical Research Council Working Party on Childhood Leukaemia: Improved survival with early intensification: combined results from the Medical Research Council childhood ALL randomised trials, UKALL X and UKALL XI. Leukemia 12(7): 1031-1036, 1998.

[152] Silverman LB, Gelber RD, Dalton VK, et al.: Improved outcome for children with acute lymphoblastic leukemia: results of Dana-Farber Consortium Protocol 91-01. Blood 97(5): 1211-1218, 2001.

[153] Reiter A, Schrappe M, Ludwig W, et al.: Chemotherapy in 998 unselected childhood acute lymphoblastic leukemia patients: results and conclusions of the multicenter trial ALL-BFM 86. Blood 84(9): 3122-3133, 1994.

Hann I, Vora A, Richards S, et al.: Benefit of intensified treatment for all children with acute lymphoblastic leukaemia: results from MRC UKALL XI and MRC ALL97 randomised trials. Leukemia 14(3): 356-363, 2000.

Harris MB, Shuster JJ, Pullen J, et al.: Treatment of children with early pre-B and pre-B acute lymphocytic leukemia with antimetabolite-based intensification regimens: a Pediatric Oncology Group study. Leukemia 14(9): 1570-1576, 2000.

Rizzari C, Valsecchi MG, Arico M, et al.: Effect of protracted high-dose L-asparaginase given as a second exposure in a Berlin-Frankfurt-Munster-based treatment: results of the randomized 9102 intermediate risk childhood acute lymphoblastic leukemia study--a report from the Associazione Italiana Ematologia Oncologia Pediatrica. Journal of Clinical Oncology 19(5): 1297-1303, 2001.

[154] Veerman AJ, Hahlen K, Kamps WA, et al.: High cure rate with a moderately intensive treatment regimen in non-high-risk childhood acute lymphoblastic leukemia: results of protocol ALL VI from the Dutch Childhood Leukemia Study Group. Journal of Clinical Oncology 14(3): 911-918, 1996.

Camitta B, Leventhal B, Lauer S, et al.: Intermediate-dose intravenous methotrexate and mercaptopurine therapy for non-T, non-B acute lymphocytic leukemia of childhood: a Pediatric Oncology Group study. Journal of Clinical Oncology 7(10): 1539-1544, 1989.

Gustafsson G, Kreuger A, et al. for the Nordic Society of Paediatric Haematology and Oncology (NOPHO): Intensified treatment of acute childhood lymphoblastic leukaemia has

regimens utilizing a limited number of courses of intermediate- or high-dose methotrexate have been used with good results for treating children with standard-risk acute lymphoblastic leukemia (ALL).[155] Another treatment approach for decreasing late effects of therapy utilizes anthracyclines and alkylating agents, but limits their cumulative dose to an amount not associated with substantial long-term toxicity. An example of this approach is the use of "delayed intensification," in which patients receive an anthracycline-based "reinduction" regimen and a cyclophosphamide-containing "reconsolidation" regimen at approximately 3 months after remission is achieved. The use of "delayed intensification" improves outcome for children with standard-risk ALL, in comparison to that achieved without an intensification phase.[156] Two blocks of "delayed intensification" may improve outcome for some patients with standard-risk ALL, although further studies are needed to define those patients that benefit from the additional therapy.[157]

In high-risk patients, a number of different approaches have been used with comparable efficacy.[158] Treatment for high-risk patients generally includes

---

improved prognosis, especially in non-high-risk patients: the Nordic experience of 2648 patients diagnosed between 1981 and 1996. Acta Paediatrica 87(11): 1151-1161, 1998.

[155] Harris MB, Shuster JJ, Pullen DJ, et al.: Consolidation therapy with antimetabolite-based therapy in standard-risk acute lymphocytic leukemia of childhood: a Pediatric Oncology Group study. Journal of Clinical Oncology 16(8): 2840-2847, 1998.

Veerman AJ, Hahlen K, Kamps WA, et al.: High cure rate with a moderately intensive treatment regimen in non-high-risk childhood acute lymphoblastic leukemia: results of protocol ALL VI from the Dutch Childhood Leukemia Study Group. Journal of Clinical Oncology 14(3): 911-918, 1996.

Mahoney DH Jr, Shuster JJ, Nitschke R, et al.: Intensification with intermediate-dose intravenous methotrexate is effective therapy for children with lower-risk B-precursor acute lymphoblastic leukemia: a Pediatric Oncology Group study. Journal of Clinical Oncology 18(6): 1285-1294, 2000.

[156] Tubergen DG, Gilchrist GS, O'Brien RT, et al.: Improved outcome with delayed intensification for children with acute lymphoblastic leukemia and intermediate presenting features: a Childrens Cancer Group phase III trial. Journal of Clinical Oncology 11(3): 527-537, 1993.

Riehm H, Gadner H, Henze G, et al.: Results and significance of six randomized trials in four consecutive ALL-BFM studies. Haematologie und Bluttransfusion 33(Suppl): 439-450, 1990.

[157] Lange BJ, Bostrom BC, Cherlow JM, et al.: Double-delayed intensification improves event-free survival for children with intermediate-risk acute lymphoblastic leukemia: a report from the Children's Cancer Group. Blood 99(3): 825-833, 2002.

[158] Richards S, Burrett J, et al, for the Medical Research Council Working Party on Childhood Leukaemia: Improved survival with early intensification: combined results from the Medical Research Council childhood ALL randomised trials, UKALL X and UKALL XI. Leukemia 12(7): 1031-1036, 1998.

blocks of intensified therapy, such as the "delayed intensification" blocks (reinduction/reconsolidation) used by the Children's Cancer Group (CCG) and by the German Berlin-Frankfurt-Munster (BFM) group.[159] For high-risk patients with slow early response to therapy (M3 marrow on day 7 of induction therapy), augmented BFM therapy has been shown to improve outcome.[160] The augmented BFM regimen utilizes 2 courses of "delayed intensification", while also intensifying therapy with repeated courses of intravenous methotrexate (without leucovorin rescue) given with vincristine and asparaginase. The augmented BFM regimen is now being evaluated for other groups of high-risk patients. The incidence of osteonecrosis is increased with the use of steroids in this treatment approach.[161]

Silverman LB, Gelber RD, Dalton VK, et al.: Improved outcome for children with acute lymphoblastic leukemia: results of Dana-Farber Consortium Protocol 91-01. Blood 97(5): 1211-1218, 2001.

Gaynon PS, Steinherz PG, Bleyer WA, et al.: Improved therapy for children with acute lymphoblastic leukemia and unfavorable presenting features: a follow-up report of the Childrens Cancer Group Study CCG-106. Journal of Clinical Oncology 11(11): 2234-2242, 1993.

Rivera GK, Pui CH, Hancock ML, et al.: Update of St Jude Study XI for childhood acute lymphoblastic leukemia. Leukemia 6(suppl 2): 153-156, 1992.

Lauer SJ, Shuster JJ, Mahoney DH Jr, et al.: A comparison of early intensive methotrexate/mercaptopurine with early intensive alternating combination chemotherapy for high-risk B-precursor acute lymphoblastic leukemia: a Pediatric Oncology Group phase III randomized trial. Leukemia 15(7): 1038-1045, 2001.

[159] Reiter A, Schrappe M, Ludwig W, et al.: Chemotherapy in 998 unselected childhood acute lymphoblastic leukemia patients: results and conclusions of the multicenter trial ALL-BFM 86. Blood 84(9): 3122-3133, 1994.

Hann I, Vora A, Richards S, et al.: Benefit of intensified treatment for all children with acute lymphoblastic leukaemia: results from MRC UKALL XI and MRC ALL97 randomised trials. Leukemia 14(3): 356-363, 2000.

Gaynon PS, Steinherz PG, Bleyer WA, et al.: Improved therapy for children with acute lymphoblastic leukemia and unfavorable presenting features: a follow-up report of the Childrens Cancer Group Study CCG-106. Journal of Clinical Oncology 11(11): 2234-2242, 1993.

[160] Nachman J, Sather HN, Gaynon PS, et al.: Augmented Berlin-Frankfurt-Munster therapy abrogates the adverse prognostic significance of slow early response to induction chemotherapy for children and adolescents with acute lymphoblastic leukemia and unfavorable presenting features: a report from the Children's Cancer Group. Journal of Clinical Oncology 15(6): 2222-2230, 1997.

[161] Mattano LA Jr, Sather HN, Trigg ME, et al.: Osteonecrosis as a complication of treating acute lymphoblastic leukemia in children: a report from the Children's Cancer Group. Journal of Clinical Oncology 18(18): 3262-3272, 2000.

Maintenance

The backbone of maintenance therapy in most protocols includes daily oral mercaptopurine and weekly oral methotrexate. If the patient has not had cranial irradiation, intrathecal chemotherapy for CNS sanctuary therapy is generally given during maintenance therapy. Clinical trials generally call for giving oral mercaptopurine in the evening, which is supported by evidence that this practice may improve event-free survival.[162] It is imperative to carefully monitor children on maintenance therapy for both drug-related toxicity and for compliance with the oral chemotherapy agents used during maintenance therapy.[163] It is also important for treating physicians to recognize that some patients may develop severe hematopoietic toxicity when receiving conventional dosages of mercaptopurine because of an inherited deficiency of thiopurine S-methyltransferase, an enzyme that inactivates mercaptopurine.[164] These patients are able to tolerate mercaptopurine only if dosages much lower than those conventionally used are administered.[165] Patients who are heterozygous for this mutant enzyme gene generally tolerate mercaptopurine without excessive toxicity, but do require more frequent dose reductions for hematopoietic toxicity than patients who are homozygous for the normal allele.[166]

Pulses of vincristine and prednisone/dexamethasone are often added to the standard maintenance regimen. A CCG randomized trial demonstrated improved outcome for patients receiving vincristine/prednisone pulses,[167]

---

[162] Schmieglow K, Glomstein A, Kristinsson J, et al.: Impact of morning versus evening schedule for oral methotrexate and 6-mercaptopurine on relapse risk for children with acute lymphoblastic leukemia. Journal of Pediatric Hematology/Oncology 19(2): 102-109, 1997.

[163] Davies HA, Lilleyman JS: Compliance with oral chemotherapy in childhood lymphoblastic leukaemia. Cancer Treatment Reviews 21(2): 93-103, 1995.

[164] Relling MV, Hancock ML, Rivera GK, et al.: Mercaptopurine therapy intolerance and heterozygosity at the thiopurine Smethyltransferase gene locus. Journal of the National Cancer Institute 91(23): 2001-2008, 1999.

Andersen JB, Szumlanski C, Weinshilboum RM, et al.: Pharmacokinetics, dose adjustments, and 6-mercaptopurine/methotrexate drug interactions in two patients with thiopurine methyltransferase deficiency. Acta Paediatrica 87(1): 108-111, 1998.

[165] Relling MV, Hancock ML, Rivera GK, et al.: Mercaptopurine therapy intolerance and heterozygosity at the thiopurine Smethyltransferase gene locus. Journal of the National Cancer Institute 91(23): 2001-2008, 1999.

Andersen JB, Szumlanski C, Weinshilboum RM, et al.: Pharmacokinetics, dose adjustments, and 6-mercaptopurine/methotrexate drug interactions in two patients with thiopurine methyltransferase deficiency. Acta Paediatrica 87(1): 108-111, 1998.

[166] Relling MV, Hancock ML, Rivera GK, et al.: Mercaptopurine therapy intolerance and heterozygosity at the thiopurine Smethyltransferase gene locus. Journal of the National Cancer Institute 91(23): 2001-2008, 1999.

[167] Bleyer WA, Sather HN, Nickerson HJ, et al.: Monthly pulses of vincristine and prednisone prevent bone marrow and testicular relapse in low-risk childhood acute

and a meta-analysis combining data from 6 clinical trials showed an event-free survival advantage for vincristine/prednisone pulses.[168] Dexamethasone is preferred over prednisone for younger patients with ALL based on data from a CCG study, in which dexamethasone was compared to prednisone for children 1 to 9 years of age with lower risk ALL.[169] Patients randomized to receive dexamethasone had significantly fewer CNS relapses and a significantly better event-free survival rate.[170] The benefit of using dexamethasone in adolescents requires investigation, because of the increased risk of steroid-induced aseptic necrosis and a higher incidence of bone fractures in this age group.[171]

Maintenance chemotherapy generally continues until 2 to 3 years of continuous complete remission. Extending the duration of maintenance therapy to 5 years does not improve outcome.[172]

---

lymphoblastic leukemia: a report of the CCG-161 study by the Childrens Cancer Study Group. Journal of Clinical Oncology 9(6): 1012-1021, 1991.

[168] Bleyer WA, Sather HN, Nickerson HJ, et al.: Monthly pulses of vincristine and prednisone prevent bone marrow and testicular relapse in low-risk childhood acute lymphoblastic leukemia: a report of the CCG-161 study by the Childrens Cancer Study Group. Journal of Clinical Oncology 9(6): 1012-1021, 1991.
Richards S, Gray R, Peto R, et al.: Duration and intensity of maintenance chemotherapy in acute lymphoblastic leukaemia: overview of 42 trials involving 12 000 randomised children. Childhood ALL Collaborative Group. Lancet 347(9018): 1783-1788, 1996.

[169] Bostrom B, Gaynon PS, Sather H, et al.: Dexamethasone decreases central nervous system relapse and improves event-free survival in lower risk acute lymphoblastic leukemia. Proceedings of the American Society of Clinical Oncology 17: A2024, 1998.

[170] Bostrom B, Gaynon PS, Sather H, et al.: Dexamethasone decreases central nervous system relapse and improves event-free survival in lower risk acute lymphoblastic leukemia. Proceedings of the American Society of Clinical Oncology 17: A2024, 1998.

[171] Ojala AE, Lanning FP, Paakko E, et al.: Osteonecrosis in children treated for acute lymphoblastic leukemia: a magnetic resonance imaging study after treatment. Medical and Pediatric Oncology 29(4): 260-265, 1997.
Strauss AJ, Su JT, Dalton VM, et al.: Bony morbidity in children treated for acute lymphoblastic leukemia. Journal of Clinical Oncology 19(12): 3066-3072, 2001.

[172] Richards S, Gray R, Peto R, et al.: Duration and intensity of maintenance chemotherapy in acute lymphoblastic leukaemia: overview of 42 trials involving 12 000 randomised children. Childhood ALL Collaborative Group. Lancet 347(9018): 1783-1788, 1996.
Miller DL, Leikin SL, Albo VC, et al.: Three versus five years of maintenance therapy are equivalent in childhood acute lymphoblastic leukemia: a report of the Childrens Cancer Study Group. Journal of Clinical Oncology 7(3): 316-325, 1989.

Role of Bone Marrow Transplant for Philadelphia Chromosome-Positive ALL

Bone marrow transplant (BMT) using a HLA-matched sibling as a donor appears to improve disease-free survival in Philadelphia chromosome-positive ALL. The outcome of BMT using an unrelated or partially matched donor may be inferior to chemotherapy.[173]

Treatment Options Under Clinical Evaluation

Risk-based treatment assignment is a key therapeutic strategy utilized for children with ALL, and protocols are designed for specific patient populations that have varying degrees of risk for treatment failure. The "Cellular Classification and Prognostic Variables" section of this summary describes the clinical and laboratory features used for the initial stratification of children with ALL into risk-based treatment groups.

Children with Standard or Lower Risk of Relapse

- The Pediatric Oncology Group (POG) is evaluating whether high-dose methotrexate can be administered as a more convenient 4-hour infusion rather than as the standard 24-hour infusion and is also evaluating whether delayed intensification with a multiagent regimen improves outcome when added to a treatment backbone that includes sequential courses of high-dose methotrexate.

- The CCG protocol for standard-risk patients is comparing oral methotrexate versus escalating-dose intravenous methotrexate without leucovorin rescue following remission induction therapy. The protocol also addresses the question of whether 2 courses of delayed intensification improves outcome compared to a single course of delayed intensification.

Children with Higher Risk of Relapse

- POG is evaluating the augmented BFM regimen in comparison to its previously utilized therapy for children with ALL at high risk for relapse.

---

[173] Arico M, Valsecchi MG, Camitta B, et al.: Outcome of treatment in children with Philadelphia chromosome-positive acute lymphoblastic leukemia. New England Journal of Medicine 342(14): 998-1006, 2000.

- The CCG protocol for children with higher risk of relapse is stratified based on whether patients have a rapid response or a slow response to the first 7 days of induction therapy. For children with a rapid early response, the primary question of therapy is to determine whether components of the augmented BFM regimen, a regimen previously identified as effective for children with slow early response to induction therapy,[174] can improve outcome in comparison to standard therapy with delayed intensification. For children with a slow early response to induction therapy, the primary question of therapy is whether intensification of therapy with idarubicin and cyclophosphamide can improve outcome in comparison to treatment with the augmented BFM regimen.

Children with T-Cell ALL

- CCG treats children with T-cell ALL on the same protocols as children with B-precursor ALL. Protocol and treatment assignment are based on the clinical characteristics of the patient (e.g., age and WBC) and their response to initial therapy.

- POG treats children with T-cell ALL distinctly from children with B-precursor ALL. The POG protocol for patients with T-cell ALL was designed to evaluate the role of high-dose methotrexate and the role of the cardioprotectant dexrazoxane. The multi-agent chemotherapy backbone for this protocol is based on an effective leukemia regimen developed at the Dana Farber Cancer Institute (DFCI) that produced a 5-year event-free survival (EFS) rate of 79% in a relatively small number of children with T-cell ALL (n=29).[175] Results of an interim analysis of the POG protocol led investigators to conclude that the addition of high-dose methotrexate to the DFCI-based chemotherapy regimen results in significantly improved EFS, due in large measure to a decrease in the rate of CNS relapse.[176] The POG study is the first clinical trial to provide convincing evidence that high-dose methotrexate can improve outcome

---

[174] Nachman JB, Sather HN, Sensel MG, et al.: Augmented post-induction therapy for children with high-risk acute lymphoblastic leukemia and a slow response to initial therapy. New England Journal of Medicine 338(23): 1663-1671, 1998.

[175] Silverman LB, Gelber RD, Dalton VK, et al.: Improved outcome for children with acute lymphoblastic leukemia: results of Dana-Farber Consortium Protocol 91-01. Blood 97(5): 1211-1218, 2001.

[176] Asselin B, Shuster J, Amylon M, et al.: Improved event-free survival (EFS) with high dose methotrexate (HDM) in T-cell lymphoblastic leukemia (T-ALL) and advanced lymphoblastic lymphoma (T-NHL): a Pediatric Oncology Group (POG) study. Proceedings of the American Society of Clinical Oncology A-1464, 2001.

for children with T-cell ALL, and based on these results, all patients entered onto the POG protocol now receive high-dose methotrexate.

Infants with ALL

Because of their distinctive biological characteristics and their high risk for leukemia recurrence, infants with ALL are treated on protocols specifically designed for this patient population.

- Currently under evaluation is the role of intensive induction and consolidation chemotherapy including high-dose methotrexate.

- For infants with ALL whose leukemia cells have chromosome 11q23 abnormalities and who therefore have a very high risk of treatment failure, the role of bone marrow transplantation with HLA-matched related or unrelated donors is under evaluation.

Recurrent Childhood Acute Lymphoblastic Leukemia

The prognosis for a child with acute lymphoblastic leukemia (ALL) whose disease recurs depends on the time and site of relapse.[177] If the recurrence occurs in the bone marrow either during front-line therapy or within 6 months of discontinuation of initial therapy, the prognosis for long-term survival is poor with a less than 10% to 20% likelihood of long-term survival using chemotherapy alone.[178] However, if relapse occurs more than a year

---

[177] Gaynon PS, Qu RP, Chappell RJ, et al.: Survival after relapse in childhood acute lymphoblastic leukemia: impact of site and time to first relapse--the Children's Cancer Group Experience. Cancer 82(7): 1387-1395, 1998.
Uderzo C, Conter V, Dini G, et al.: Treatment of childhood acute lymphoblastic leukemia after the first relapse: curative strategies. Haematologica 86(1): 1-7, 2001.
[178] Gaynon PS, Qu RP, Chappell RJ, et al.: Survival after relapse in childhood acute lymphoblastic leukemia: impact of site and time to first relapse--the Children's Cancer Group Experience. Cancer 82(7): 1387-1395, 1998.
Henze G, Fengler R, Hartmann B, et al.: Six-year experience with a comprehensive approach to the treatment of recurrent childhood acute lymphoblastic leukemia (ALL-REZ BFM 85): a relapse study of the BFM group. Blood 78(5): 1166-1172, 1991.
Schroeder H, Garwicz S, Kristinsson J, et al.: Outcome after first relapse in children with acute lymphoblastic leukemia: a population-based study of 315 patients from the Nordic Society of Pediatric Hematology and Oncology (NOPHO). Medical and Pediatric Oncology 25(5): 372-378, 1995.
Wheeler K, Richards S, et al. for the Medical Research Council Working Party on Childhood Leukaemia: Comparison of bone marrow transplant and chemotherapy for relapsed childhood acute lymphoblastic leukemia: the MRC UKALL X experience. British Journal of Haematology 101(1): 94-103, 1998.

after discontinuation of initial therapy, the prognosis is better with 30% to 40% of these patients achieving long-term, disease-free survival in large studies using aggressive salvage chemotherapy.[179] Children with T-cell ALL who relapse also have survival rates less than 20%.[180]

The selection of therapy for the child whose disease recurs on or shortly after therapy depends on many factors including prior treatment, whether the recurrence is medullary or extramedullary, and individual patient considerations. Aggressive approaches including bone marrow transplantation should be strongly considered for patients with marrow relapse occurring while on treatment or within 6 months of termination of therapy, or late marrow relapse with high tumor load as indicated by a peripheral blast count of 10,000/uL or more.[181] For patients with an early marrow relapse, allogeneic transplant from an HLA identical sibling or matched unrelated donor that is performed in second remission has resulted in longer leukemia free survival when compared with a chemotherapy approach.[182] A retrospective case control study suggests that transplant

---

Buchanan GR, Rivera GK, Pollock BH, et al.: Alternating drug pairs with or without periodic reinduction in children with acute lymphoblastic leukemia in second bone marrow remission: a Pediatric Oncology Group study. Cancer 88(5): 1166-1174, 2000.
[179] Rivera GK, Hudson MM, Liu Q, et al.: Effectiveness of intensified rotational combination chemotherapy for late hematologic relapse of childhood acute lymphoblastic leukemia. Blood 88(3): 831-837, 1996.
Buhrer C, Hartmann R, Fengler R, et al.: Peripheral blast counts at diagnosis of late isolated bone marrow relapse of childhood acute lymphoblastic leukemia predict response to salvage chemotherapy and outcome. Journal of Clinical Oncology 14(10): 2812-2817, 1996.
Sadowitz PD, Smith SD, Shuster J, et al.: Treatment of late bone marrow relapse in children with acute lymphoblastic leukemia: a Pediatric Oncology Group study. Blood 81(3): 602-609, 1993.
[180] Schroeder H, Garwicz S, Kristinsson J, et al.: Outcome after first relapse in children with acute lymphoblastic leukemia: a population-based study of 315 patients from the Nordic Society of Pediatric Hematology and Oncology (NOPHO). Medical and Pediatric Oncology 25(5): 372-378, 1995.
Abshire TC, Buchanan GR, Jackson JF, et al.: Morphologic, immunologic and cytogenetic studies in children with acute lymphoblastic leukemia at diagnosis and relapse: a Pediatric Oncology Group study. Leukemia 6(5): 357-362, 1992.
[181] Buhrer C, Hartmann R, Fengler R, et al.: Peripheral blast counts at diagnosis of late isolated bone marrow relapse of childhood acute lymphoblastic leukemia predict response to salvage chemotherapy and outcome. Journal of Clinical Oncology 14(10): 2812-2817, 1996.
[182] Wheeler K, Richards S, et al. for the Medical Research Council Working Party on Childhood Leukaemia: Comparison of bone marrow transplant and chemotherapy for relapsed childhood acute lymphoblastic leukemia: the MRC UKALL X experience. British Journal of Haematology 101(1): 94-103, 1998.
Barrett AJ, Horowitz MM, Pollock BH, et al.: Bone marrow transplants from HLA-identical siblings as compared with chemotherapy for children with acute lymphoblastic leukemia in a second remission. New England Journal of Medicine 331(19): 1253-1258, 1994.

conditioning regimens which include total body irradiation (TBI) produce higher cure rates than chemotherapy only preparative regimens.[183] The potential neurotoxic effects of TBI should be considered, particularly for very young patients. For patients with a late marrow relapse, a primary chemotherapy approach should be considered with bone marrow transplantation reserved for a subsequent marrow relapse.[184] The value of matched unrelated stem cell transplantation in the therapy of children with recurrent ALL is under investigation.[185]

With the improved success of treatment of children with ALL, the incidence of isolated extramedullary relapse has decreased. The incidence of both isolated central nervous system (CNS) and testicular relapse is less than 10%. While the prognosis for children with isolated CNS relapse had been quite poor in the past, aggressive systemic and intrathecal therapy combined with craniospinal irradiation has improved the outlook particularly for patients

---

Uderzo C, Valsecchi MG, Bacigalupo A, et al.: Treatment of childhood acute lymphoblastic leukemia in second remission with allogeneic bone marrow transplantation and chemotherapy: ten-year experience of the Italian Bone Marrow Transplantation Group and the Italian Pediatric Hematology Oncology Association. Journal of Clinical Oncology 13(2): 352-358, 1995.

Harrison G, Richards S, Lawson S, et al.: Comparison of allogeneic transplant versus chemotherapy for relapsed childhood acute lymphoblastic leukaemia in the MRC UKALL R1 trial. Annals of Oncology 11(8): 999-1006, 2000.

[183] Davies SM, Ramsay NK, Klein JP, et al.: Comparison of preparative regimens in transplants for children with acute lymphoblastic leukemia. Journal of Clinical Oncology 18(2): 340-347, 2000.

[184] Rivera GK, Hudson MM, Liu Q, et al.: Effectiveness of intensified rotational combination chemotherapy for late hematologic relapse of childhood acute lymphoblastic leukemia. Blood 88(3): 831-837, 1996.

Borgmann A, Baumgarten E, Schmid H, et al.: Allogeneic bone marrow transplantation for a subset of children with acute lymphoblastic leukemia in third remission: a conceivable alternative? Bone Marrow Transplantation 20(11): 939-944, 1997.

Schroeder H, Gustafsson G, Saarinen-Pihkala UM, et al.: Allogeneic bone marrow transplantation in second remission of childhood acute lymphoblastic leukemia: a population-based case control study from the Nordic countries. Bone Marrow Transplantation 23(6): 555-560, 1999.

[185] Hongeng S, Krance RA, Bowman LC, et al.: Outcomes of transplantation with matched-sibling and unrelated-donor bone marrow in children with leukaemia. Lancet 350(9080): 767-771, 1997.

Casper J, Camitta B, Truitt R, et al.: Unrelated bone marrow donor transplants for children with leukemia or myelodysplasia. Blood 85(9): 2354-2363, 1995.

Weisdorf DJ, Billett AL, Hannan P, et al.: Autologous versus unrelated donor allogeneic marrow transplantation for acute lymphoblastic leukemia. Blood 90(8): 2962-2968, 1997.

Saarinen-Pihkala UM, Gustafsson G, Ringden O, et al.: No disadvantage in outcome of using matched unrelated donors as compared with matched sibling donors for bone marrow transplantation in children with acute lymphoblastic leukemia in second remission. Journal of Clinical Oncology 19(14): 3406-3414, 2001.

who did not receive cranial irradiation during their first remission.[186] For children whose initial remission was 18 months or greater, 4-year event-free survival (EFS) rates of approximately 80% have been observed using this strategy, compared to EFS rates of approximately 45% for children with CNS relapse within 18 months of diagnosis.[187] The results of treatment of isolated testicular relapse depend on the timing of the relapse. The 3-year event-free survival (EFS) of boys with overt testicular relapse during therapy is approximately 40%, and it is approximately 85% for boys with late testicular relapse.[188] A study that looked at testicular biopsy at the end of therapy failed to demonstrate a survival benefit for patients with early detection of occult disease.[189]

Treatment Options under Clinical Evaluation

Clinical trials investigating new agents and new combinations of agents are available for children with recurrent ALL and should be considered. Targeted therapies specific for ALL are being developed, including monoclonal antibody based therapies and using drugs that inhibit signal transduction pathways required for leukemia cell growth and survival. Information about ongoing clinical trials is available from the NCI (**http://cancer.gov/clinical_trials/**).

---

[186] Ribeiro RC, Rivera GK, Hudson M, et al.: An intensive re-treatment protocol for children with an isolated CNS relapse of acute lymphoblastic leukemia. Journal of Clinical Oncology 13(2): 333-338, 1995.

Kumar P, Kun LE, Hustu HO, et al.: Survival outcome following isolated central nervous system relapse treated with additional chemotherapy and craniospinal irradiation in childhood acute lymphoblastic leukemia. International Journal of Radiation Oncology, Biology, Physics 31(3): 477-483, 1995.

Ritchey AK, Pollock BH, Lauer SJ, et al.: Improved survival of children with isolated CNS relapse of acute lymphoblastic leukemia: a Pediatric Oncology Group study. Journal of Clinical Oncology 17(12): 3745-3752, 1999.

[187] Ritchey AK, Pollock BH, Lauer SJ, et al.: Improved survival of children with isolated CNS relapse of acute lymphoblastic leukemia: a Pediatric Oncology Group study. Journal of Clinical Oncology 17(12): 3745-3752, 1999.

[188] Wofford MM, Smith SD, Shuster JJ, et al.: Treatment of occult or late overt testicular relapse in children with acute lymphoblastic leukemia: a Pediatric Oncology Group study. Journal of Clinical Oncology 10(4): 624-630, 1992.

[189] Trigg ME, Steinherz PG, Chappell R, et al.: Early testicular biopsy in males with acute lymphoblastic leukemia: lack of impact on subsequent event-free survival. Journal of Pediatric Hematology/Oncology 22(1): 27-33, 2000.

NIH Databases

In addition to the various Institutes of Health that publish professional guidelines, the NIH has designed a number of databases for professionals.[190] Physician-oriented resources provide a wide variety of information related to the biomedical and health sciences, both past and present. The format of these resources varies. Searchable databases, bibliographic citations, full text articles (when available), archival collections, and images are all available. The following are referenced by the National Library of Medicine:[191]

- **Bioethics:** Access to published literature on the ethical, legal and public policy issues surrounding healthcare and biomedical research. This information is provided in conjunction with the Kennedy Institute of Ethics located at Georgetown University, Washington, D.C.: **http://www.nlm.nih.gov/databases/databases_bioethics.html**

- **HIV/AIDS Resources:** Describes various links and databases dedicated to HIV/AIDS research: **http://www.nlm.nih.gov/pubs/factsheets/aidsinfs.html**

- **NLM Online Exhibitions:** Describes "Exhibitions in the History of Medicine": **http://www.nlm.nih.gov/exhibition/exhibition.html**. Additional resources for historical scholarship in medicine: **http://www.nlm.nih.gov/hmd/hmd.html**

- **Biotechnology Information:** Access to public databases. The National Center for Biotechnology Information conducts research in computational biology, develops software tools for analyzing genome data, and disseminates biomedical information for the better understanding of molecular processes affecting human health and disease: **http://www.ncbi.nlm.nih.gov/**

- **Population Information:** The National Library of Medicine provides access to worldwide coverage of population, family planning, and related health issues, including family planning technology and programs, fertility, and population law and policy: **http://www.nlm.nih.gov/databases/databases_population.html**

- **Cancer Information:** Access to caner-oriented databases: **http://www.nlm.nih.gov/databases/databases_cancer.html**

---

[190] Remember, for the general public, the National Library of Medicine recommends the databases referenced in MEDLINE*plus* (**http://medlineplus.gov/** or **http://www.nlm.nih.gov/medlineplus/databases.html**).
[191] See **http://www.nlm.nih.gov/databases/databases.html**.

- **Profiles in Science:** Offering the archival collections of prominent twentieth-century biomedical scientists to the public through modern digital technology: **http://www.profiles.nlm.nih.gov/**

- **Chemical Information:** Provides links to various chemical databases and references: **http://sis.nlm.nih.gov/Chem/ChemMain.html**

- **Clinical Alerts:** Reports the release of findings from the NIH-funded clinical trials where such release could significantly affect morbidity and mortality: **http://www.nlm.nih.gov/databases/alerts/clinical_alerts.html**

- **Space Life Sciences:** Provides links and information to space-based research (including NASA):
http://www.nlm.nih.gov/databases/databases_space.html

- **MEDLINE:** Bibliographic database covering the fields of medicine, nursing, dentistry, veterinary medicine, the healthcare system, and the pre-clinical sciences:
http://www.nlm.nih.gov/databases/databases_medline.html

- **Toxicology and Environmental Health Information (TOXNET):** Databases covering toxicology and environmental health:
http://sis.nlm.nih.gov/Tox/ToxMain.html

- **Visible Human Interface:** Anatomically detailed, three-dimensional representations of normal male and female human bodies:
http://www.nlm.nih.gov/research/visible/visible_human.html

While all of the above references may be of interest to physicians who study and treat childhood acute lymphoblastic leukemia, the following are particularly noteworthy.

The Combined Health Information Database

A comprehensive source of information on clinical guidelines written for professionals is the Combined Health Information Database. You will need to limit your search to "Brochure/Pamphlet," "Fact Sheet," or "Information Package" and childhood acute lymphoblastic leukemia using the "Detailed Search" option. Go directly to the following hyperlink: **http://chid.nih.gov/detail/detail.html**. To find associations, use the drop boxes at the bottom of the search page where "You may refine your search by." For the publication date, select "All Years," select your preferred language, and the format option "Fact Sheet." By making these selections and typing "childhood acute lymphoblastic leukemia" (or synonyms) into the "For these words:" box above, you will only receive results on fact sheets dealing with childhood acute lymphoblastic leukemia.

The NLM Gateway[192]

The NLM (National Library of Medicine) Gateway is a Web-based system that lets users search simultaneously in multiple retrieval systems at the U.S. National Library of Medicine (NLM). It allows users of NLM services to initiate searches from one Web interface, providing "one-stop searching" for many of NLM's information resources or databases.[193] One target audience for the Gateway is the Internet user who is new to NLM's online resources and does not know what information is available or how best to search for it. This audience may include physicians and other healthcare providers, researchers, librarians, students, and, increasingly, parents and the public.[194] To use the NLM Gateway, simply go to the search site at **http://gateway.nlm.nih.gov/gw/Cmd**. Type "childhood acute lymphoblastic leukemia" (or synonyms) into the search box and click "Search." The results will be presented in a tabular form, indicating the number of references in each database category.

Results Summary

Category	Items Found
Journal Articles	350247
Books / Periodicals / Audio Visual	2584
Consumer Health	294
Meeting Abstracts	2575
Other Collections	87
Total	355787

---

[192] Adapted from NLM: **http://gateway.nlm.nih.gov/gw/Cmd?Overview.x**.
[193] The NLM Gateway is currently being developed by the Lister Hill National Center for Biomedical Communications (LHNCBC) at the National Library of Medicine (NLM) of the National Institutes of Health (NIH).
[194] Other users may find the Gateway useful for an overall search of NLM's information resources. Some searchers may locate what they need immediately, while others will utilize the Gateway as an adjunct tool to other NLM search services such as PubMed® and MEDLINEplus®. The Gateway connects users with multiple NLM retrieval systems while also providing a search interface for its own collections. These collections include various types of information that do not logically belong in PubMed, LOCATORplus, or other established NLM retrieval systems (e.g., meeting announcements and pre-1966 journal citations). The Gateway will provide access to the information found in an increasing number of NLM retrieval systems in several phases.

HSTAT[195]

HSTAT is a free, Web-based resource that provides access to full-text documents used in healthcare decision-making.[196] HSTAT's audience includes healthcare providers, health service researchers, policy makers, insurance companies, consumers, and the information professionals who serve these groups. HSTAT provides access to a wide variety of publications, including clinical practice guidelines, quick-reference guides for clinicians, consumer health brochures, evidence reports and technology assessments from the Agency for Healthcare Research and Quality (AHRQ), as well as AHRQ's Put Prevention Into Practice.[197] Simply search by "childhood acute lymphoblastic leukemia" (or synonyms) at the following Web site: **http://text.nlm.nih.gov**.

Coffee Break: Tutorials for Biologists[198]

Some parents may wish to have access to a general healthcare site that takes a scientific view of the news and covers recent breakthroughs in biology that may one day assist physicians in developing treatments. To this end, we recommend "Coffee Break," a collection of short reports on recent biological discoveries. Each report incorporates interactive tutorials that demonstrate how bioinformatics tools are used as a part of the research process. Currently, all Coffee Breaks are written by NCBI staff.[199] Each report is about 400 words and is usually based on a discovery reported in one or more articles from recently published, peer-reviewed literature.[200] This site has

---

[195] Adapted from HSTAT: **http://www.nlm.nih.gov/pubs/factsheets/hstat.html**.
[196] The HSTAT URL is **http://hstat.nlm.nih.gov/**.
[197] Other important documents in HSTAT include: the National Institutes of Health (NIH) Consensus Conference Reports and Technology Assessment Reports; the HIV/AIDS Treatment Information Service (ATIS) resource documents; the Substance Abuse and Mental Health Services Administration's Center for Substance Abuse Treatment (SAMHSA/CSAT) Treatment Improvement Protocols (TIP) and Center for Substance Abuse Prevention (SAMHSA/CSAP) Prevention Enhancement Protocols System (PEPS); the Public Health Service (PHS) Preventive Services Task Force's *Guide to Clinical Preventive Services*; the independent, nonfederal Task Force on Community Services *Guide to Community Preventive Services*; and the Health Technology Advisory Committee (HTAC) of the Minnesota Health Care Commission (MHCC) health technology evaluations.
[198] Adapted from **http://www.ncbi.nlm.nih.gov/Coffeebreak/Archive/FAQ.html**.
[199] The figure that accompanies each article is frequently supplied by an expert external to NCBI, in which case the source of the figure is cited. The result is an interactive tutorial that tells a biological story.
[200] After a brief introduction that sets the work described into a broader context, the report focuses on how a molecular understanding can provide explanations of observed biology and lead to therapies for diseases. Each vignette is accompanied by a figure and hypertext

new articles every few weeks, so it can be considered an online magazine of sorts, and intended for general background information. Access the Coffee Break Web site at **http://www.ncbi.nlm.nih.gov/Coffeebreak/**.

Other Commercial Databases

In addition to resources maintained by official agencies, other databases exist that are commercial ventures addressing medical professionals. Here are a few examples that may interest you:

- **CliniWeb International:** Index and table of contents to selected clinical information on the Internet; see **http://www.ohsu.edu/cliniweb/**.

- **Image Engine:** Multimedia electronic medical record system that integrates a wide range of digitized clinical images with textual data stored in the University of Pittsburgh Medical Center's MARS electronic medical record system; see the following Web site: **http://www.cml.upmc.edu/cml/imageengine/imageEngine.html**.

- **Medical World Search:** Searches full text from thousands of selected medical sites on the Internet; see **http://www.mwsearch.com/**.

- **MedWeaver:** Prototype system that allows users to search differential diagnoses for any list of signs and symptoms, to search medical literature, and to explore relevant Web sites; see **http://www.med.virginia.edu/ wmd4n/medweaver.html**.

- **Metaphrase:** Middleware component intended for use by both caregivers and medical records personnel. It converts the informal language generally used by caregivers into terms from formal, controlled vocabularies; see the following Web site: **http://www.lexical.com/Metaphrase.html**.

---

links that lead to a series of pages that interactively show how NCBI tools and resources are used in the research process.

The Genome Project and Childhood Acute Lymphoblastic Leukemia

With all the discussion in the press about the Human Genome Project, it is only natural that physicians, researchers, and parents want to know about how human genes relate to childhood acute lymphoblastic leukemia. In the following section, we will discuss databases and references used by physicians and scientists who work in this area.

Online Mendelian Inheritance in Man (OMIM)

The Online Mendelian Inheritance in Man (OMIM) database is a catalog of human genes and genetic disorders authored and edited by Dr. Victor A. McKusick and his colleagues at Johns Hopkins and elsewhere. OMIM was developed for the World Wide Web by the National Center for Biotechnology Information (NCBI).[201] The database contains textual information, pictures, and reference information. It also contains copious links to NCBI's Entrez database of MEDLINE articles and sequence information.

Go to **http://www.ncbi.nlm.nih.gov/Omim/searchomim.html** to search the database. Type "childhood acute lymphoblastic leukemia" (or synonyms) in the search box, and click "Submit Search." If too many results appear, you can narrow the search by adding the word "clinical." Each report will have additional links to related research and databases. By following these links, especially the link titled "Database Links," you will be exposed to numerous specialized databases that are largely used by the scientific community. These databases are overly technical and seldom used by the general public, but offer an abundance of information. The following is an example of the results you can obtain from the OMIM for childhood acute lymphoblastic leukemia:

- **Abelson Murine Leukemia Viral Oncogene Homolog 1**
  Web site: http://www.ncbi.nlm.nih.gov/htbin-post/Omim/dispmim?189980

---

[201] Adapted from **http://www.ncbi.nlm.nih.gov/**. Established in 1988 as a national resource for molecular biology information, NCBI creates public databases, conducts research in computational biology, develops software tools for analyzing genome data, and disseminates biomedical information--all for the better understanding of molecular processes affecting human health and disease.

- **Ataxia-telangiectasia**
  Web site: http://www.ncbi.nlm.nih.gov/htbin-post/Omim/dispmim?208900

- **Breakpoint Cluster Region**
  Web site: http://www.ncbi.nlm.nih.gov/htbin-post/Omim/dispmim?151410

- **Chondroitin Sulfate Proteoglycan 4**
  Web site: http://www.ncbi.nlm.nih.gov/htbin-post/Omim/dispmim?601172

- **Cyclic Hematopoiesis**
  Web site: http://www.ncbi.nlm.nih.gov/htbin-post/Omim/dispmim?162800

- **Cyclin-dependent Kinase Inhibitor 1b**
  Web site: http://www.ncbi.nlm.nih.gov/htbin-post/Omim/dispmim?600778

- **Ets Variant Gene 6**
  Web site: http://www.ncbi.nlm.nih.gov/htbin-post/Omim/dispmim?600618

- **Ewing Sarcoma Breakpoint Region 1**
  Web site: http://www.ncbi.nlm.nih.gov/htbin-post/Omim/dispmim?133450

- **Homco Box 11**
  Web site: http://www.ncbi.nlm.nih.gov/htbin-post/Omim/dispmim?186770

- **Homocystinuria due to Deficiency of N(5,10)-methylenetetrahydrofolate Reductase Activity**
  Web site: http://www.ncbi.nlm.nih.gov/htbin-post/Omim/dispmim?236250

Genes and Disease (NCBI - Map)

The Genes and Disease database is produced by the National Center for Biotechnology Information of the National Library of Medicine at the National Institutes of Health. This Web site categorizes each disorder by the system of the body associated with it. Go to **http://www.ncbi.nlm.nih.gov/disease/**, and browse the system pages to have a full view of important conditions linked to human genes. Since this site is regularly updated, you may wish to re-visit it from time to time. The following systems and associated disorders are addressed:

- **Cancer:** Uncontrolled cell division.
  Examples: Breast And Ovarian Cancer, Burkitt lymphoma, chronic myeloid leukemia, colon cancer, lung cancer, malignant melanoma, multiple endocrine neoplasia, neurofibromatosis, p53 tumor suppressor, pancreatic cancer, prostate cancer, Ras oncogene, RB: retinoblastoma, von Hippel-Lindau syndrome.
  Web site: **http://www.ncbi.nlm.nih.gov/disease/Cancer.html**

Entrez

Entrez is a search and retrieval system that integrates several linked databases at the National Center for Biotechnology Information (NCBI). These databases include nucleotide sequences, protein sequences, macromolecular structures, whole genomes, and MEDLINE through PubMed. Entrez provides access to the following databases:

- **PubMed:** Biomedical literature (PubMed),
  Web site: **http://www.ncbi.nlm.nih.gov/entrez/query.fcgi?db=PubMed**

- **Nucleotide Sequence Database (Genbank):**
  Web site:
  http://www.ncbi.nlm.nih.gov/entrez/query.fcgi?db=Nucleotide

- **Protein Sequence Database:**
  Web site: **http://www.ncbi.nlm.nih.gov/entrez/query.fcgi?db=Protein**

- **Structure:** Three-dimensional macromolecular structures,
  Web site: **http://www.ncbi.nlm.nih.gov/entrez/query.fcgi?db=Structure**

- **Genome:** Complete genome assemblies,
  Web site: **http://www.ncbi.nlm.nih.gov/entrez/query.fcgi?db=Genome**

- **PopSet:** Population study data sets,
  Web site: **http://www.ncbi.nlm.nih.gov/entrez/query.fcgi?db=Popset**

- **OMIM:** Online Mendelian Inheritance in Man,
  Web site: **http://www.ncbi.nlm.nih.gov/entrez/query.fcgi?db=OMIM**

- **Taxonomy:** Organisms in GenBank,
  Web site: **http://www.ncbi.nlm.nih.gov/entrez/query.fcgi?db=Taxonomy**

- **Books:** Online books,
  Web site: **http://www.ncbi.nlm.nih.gov/entrez/query.fcgi?db=books**

- **ProbeSet:** Gene Expression Omnibus (GEO),
  Web site: **http://www.ncbi.nlm.nih.gov/entrez/query.fcgi?db=geo**

- **3D Domains:** Domains from Entrez Structure,
  Web site: **http://www.ncbi.nlm.nih.gov/entrez/query.fcgi?db=geo**

- **NCBI's Protein Sequence Information Survey Results:**
  Web site: **http://www.ncbi.nlm.nih.gov/About/proteinsurvey/**

To access the Entrez system at the National Center for Biotechnology Information, go to **http://www.ncbi.nlm.nih.gov/entrez/**, and then select the database that you would like to search. The databases available are listed in the drop box next to "Search." In the box next to "for," enter "childhood acute lymphoblastic leukemia" (or synonyms) and click "Go."

Jablonski's Multiple Congenital Anomaly/Mental Retardation (MCA/MR) Syndromes Database[202]

This online resource can be quite useful. It has been developed to facilitate the identification and differentiation of syndromic entities. Special attention is given to the type of information that is usually limited or completely omitted in existing reference sources due to space limitations of the printed form.

At the following Web site you can also search across syndromes using an index: **http://www.nlm.nih.gov/mesh/jablonski/syndrome_toc/toc_a.html**. You can search by keywords at this Web site: **http://www.nlm.nih.gov/mesh/jablonski/syndrome_db.html**.

---

[202] Adapted from the National Library of Medicine: http://www.nlm.nih.gov/mesh/jablonski/about_syndrome.html.

The Genome Database[203]

Established at Johns Hopkins University in Baltimore, Maryland in 1990, the Genome Database (GDB) is the official central repository for genomic mapping data resulting from the Human Genome Initiative. In the spring of 1999, the Bioinformatics Supercomputing Centre (BiSC) at the Hospital for Sick Children in Toronto, Ontario assumed the management of GDB. The Human Genome Initiative is a worldwide research effort focusing on structural analysis of human DNA to determine the location and sequence of the estimated 100,000 human genes. In support of this project, GDB stores and curates data generated by researchers worldwide who are engaged in the mapping effort of the Human Genome Project (HGP). GDB's mission is to provide scientists with an encyclopedia of the human genome which is continually revised and updated to reflect the current state of scientific knowledge. Although GDB has historically focused on gene mapping, its focus will broaden as the Genome Project moves from mapping to sequence, and finally, to functional analysis.

To access the GDB, simply go to the following hyperlink: **http://www.gdb.org/**. Search "All Biological Data" by "Keyword." Type "childhood acute lymphoblastic leukemia" (or synonyms) into the search box, and review the results. If more than one word is used in the search box, then separate each one with the word "and" or "or" (using "or" might be useful when using synonyms). This database is extremely technical as it was created for specialists. The articles are the results which are the most accessible to non-professionals and often listed under the heading "Citations." The contact names are also accessible to non-professionals.

Specialized References

The following books are specialized references written for professionals interested in childhood acute lymphoblastic leukemia (sorted alphabetically by title; hyperlinks provide rankings, information, and reviews at Amazon.com):

- **Advanced and Critical Care Oncology Nursing: Managing Primary Complications** by Cynthia C. Chernecky (Editor), et al; Paperback - 736 pages (September 18, 1997), W B Saunders Co; ISBN: 0721668607; http://www.amazon.com/exec/obidos/ASIN/0721668607/icongroupinterna

---

[203] Adapted from the Genome Database:
http://gdbwww.gdb.org/gdb/aboutGDB.html#mission.

- **Atlas of Pediatric Physical Diagnosis** by Basil J. Zitelli, Holly W. Davis (Editor); Hardcover, 3rd edition (March 1997), Mosby-Year Book; ISBN: 0815199309;
  http://www.amazon.com/exec/obidos/ASIN/0815199309/icongroupinterna

- **Cancer: Etiology, Diagnosis, and Treatment** by Walter J. Burdette; Paperback - 287 pages, 1st edition (January 15, 1998), McGraw Hill Text; ISBN: 0070089922;
  http://www.amazon.com/exec/obidos/ASIN/0070089922/icongroupinterna

- **Cancer Management: A Multidisciplinary Approach: Medical, Surgical & Radiation** by Richard Pazdur (Editor), et al; Paperback - 982 pages, 5th edition (June 15, 2001), Publisher Research & Representation, Inc.; ISBN: 1891483080;
  http://www.amazon.com/exec/obidos/ASIN/1891483080/icongroupinterna

- **The Child with Cancer: Family-Centered Care in Practice** by Helen Langton (Editor); Paperback - 404 pages; 1st edition (January 15, 2000), W B Saunders Co; ISBN: 0702023000;
  http://www.amazon.com/exec/obidos/ASIN/0702023000/icongroupinterna

- **Familial Cancer and Prevention: Molecular Epidemiology: A New Strategy Toward Cancer Control** by Joji Utsunomiya (Editor), et al; Hardcover (April 1999), Wiley-Liss; ISBN: 0471249378;
  http://www.amazon.com/exec/obidos/ASIN/0471249378/icongroupinterna

- **The 5-Minute Pediatric Consult** by M. William Schwartz (Editor); Hardcover - 1050 pages, 2nd edition (January 15, 2000), Lippincott, Williams & Wilkins; ISBN: 0683307444;
  http://www.amazon.com/exec/obidos/ASIN/0683307444/icongroupinterna

- **Fundamentals of Cancer Epidemiology** by Philip C. Nasca, Ph.D. (Editor), Pastides Harris, Ph.D., MPH (Editor); Hardcover - 368 pages, 1st edition (February 15, 2001), Aspen Publishers, Inc.; ISBN: 0834217767;
  http://www.amazon.com/exec/obidos/ASIN/0834217767/icongroupinterna

- **Helping Cancer Patients Cope: A Problem-Solving Approach** by Arthur M. Nezu (Editor), et al; Hardcover - 314 pages (December 15, 1998), American Psychological Association (APA); ISBN: 1557985332;
  http://www.amazon.com/exec/obidos/ASIN/1557985332/icongroupinterna

- **Nelson Textbook of Pediatrics** by Richard E. Behrman (Editor), et al; Hardcover - 2414 pages, 16th edition (January 15, 2000), W B Saunders Co; ISBN: 0721677673;
  http://www.amazon.com/exec/obidos/ASIN/0721677673/icongroupinterna

- **Quantitative Estimation and Prediction of Human Cancer Risks (Iarc Scientific Publications, 131)** by Suresh H. Moolgavkar (Editor), et al;

Paperback (September 1999), Oxford University Press; ISBN: 9283221311;
http://www.amazon.com/exec/obidos/ASIN/9283221311/icongroupinterna

- **Textbook of Cancer Epidemiology** by ADAMI, et al; Hardcover - 385 pages, 1st edition (July 15, 2002), Oxford University Press; ISBN: 0195109694;
http://www.amazon.com/exec/obidos/ASIN/0195109694/icongroupinterna

Vocabulary Builder

Anthracycline: A member of a family of anticancer drugs that are also antibiotics. [NIH]

Antibody: A type of protein made by certain white blood cells in response to a foreign substance (antigen). Each antibody can bind to only a specific antigen. The purpose of this binding is to help destroy the antigen. Antibodies can work in several ways, depending on the nature of the antigen. Some antibodies destroy antigens directly. Others make it easier for white blood cells to destroy the antigen. [NIH]

Anticonvulsants: Drugs that prevent, reduce, or stop convulsions or seizures. [NIH]

Antimetabolite: A chemical that is very similar to one required in a normal biochemical reaction in cells. Antimetabolites can stop or slow down the reaction. [NIH]

Aseptic: Free from infection or septic material; sterile. [EU]

Ataxia: Loss of muscle coordination. [NIH]

Cerebral: Of or pertaining of the cerebrum or the brain. [EU]

CSF: Cerebrospinal fluid. The fluid flowing around the brain and spinal cord. CSF is produced in the ventricles of the brain. [NIH]

Cyclic: Pertaining to or occurring in a cycle or cycles; the term is applied to chemical compounds that contain a ring of atoms in the nucleus. [EU]

Cyclophosphamide: An anticancer drug that belongs to the family of drugs called alkylating agents. [NIH]

Cytarabine: An anticancer drug that belongs to the family of drugs called antimetabolites. [NIH]

Dexamethasone: A synthetic steroid (similar to steroid hormones produced naturally in the adrenal gland). Dexamethasone is used to treat leukemia and lymphoma and may be used to treat some of the problems caused by other cancers and their treatment. [NIH]

Hematologist: A doctor who specializes in treating diseases of the blood. [NIH]

Hematopoiesis: The forming of new blood cells. [NIH]

Hydrocortisone: A drug used to relieve the symptoms of certain hormone shortages and to suppress an immune response. [NIH]

Idarubicin: An anticancer drug that belongs to the family of drugs called antitumor antibiotics. Also called 4-demethoxydaunorubicin. [NIH]

Immunoglobulin: A protein that acts as an antibody. [NIH]

Intramuscular: IM. Within or into muscle. [NIH]

Intravenous: IV. Into a vein. [NIH]

Leukocytosis: A transient increase in the number of leukocytes in a body fluid. [NIH]

Millimeter: A measure of length. A millimeter is approximately 26-times smaller than an inch. [NIH]

Myelosuppression: A condition in which bone marrow activity is decreased, resulting in fewer red blood cells, white blood cells, and platelets. Myelosuppression is a side effect of some cancer treatments. [NIH]

Neuroendocrine: Having to do with the interactions between the nervous system and the endocrine system. Describes certain cells that release hormones into the blood in response to stimulation of the nervous system. [NIH]

Neurotoxicity: The tendency of some treatments to cause damage to the nervous system. [NIH]

Occult: Obscure; concealed from observation, difficult to understand. [EU]

Osteonecrosis: Death of a bone or part of a bone, either atraumatic or posttraumatic. [NIH]

Paralysis: Loss of ability to move all or part of the body. [NIH]

Pegaspargase: A modified form of asparaginase, an anticancer drug that belongs to the family of drugs derived from enzymes. [NIH]

Phenobarbital: A sedative/anticonvulsant barbiturate that has been used to treat diarrhea and to increase the antitumor effect of other therapies. [NIH]

Polyethylene: A vinyl polymer made from ethylene. It can be branched or linear. Branched or low-density polyethylene is tough and pliable but not to the same degree as linear polyethylene. Linear or high-density polyethylene has a greater hardness and tensile strength. Polyethylene is used in a variety of products, including implants and prostheses. [NIH]

Proteoglycan: A molecule that contains both protein and glycosaminoglycans, which are a type of polysaccharide. Proteoglycans are found in cartilage and other connective tissues. [NIH]

Retrospective: Looking back at events that have already taken place. [NIH]

Seizures: Convulsions; sudden, involuntary movements of the muscles. [NIH]

Serum: The clear liquid part of the blood that remains after blood cells and clotting proteins have been removed. [NIH]

Somnolence: Sleepiness; also unnatural drowsiness. [EU]

Subacute: Somewhat acute; between acute and chronic. [EU]

Telangiectasia: The permanent enlargement of blood vessels, causing redness in the skin or mucous membranes. [NIH]

Testicular: Pertaining to a testis. [EU]

Trisomy: The possession of a third chromosome of any one type in an otherwise diploid cell. [NIH]

Vincristine: An anticancer drug that belongs to the family of plant drugs called vinca alkaloids. [NIH]

CHAPTER 8. DISSERTATIONS ON CHILDHOOD ACUTE LYMPHOBLASTIC LEUKEMIA

Overview

University researchers are active in studying almost all known medical conditions. The result of research is often published in the form of Doctoral or Master's dissertations. You should understand, therefore, that applied diagnostic procedures and/or therapies can take many years to develop after the thesis that proposed the new technique or approach was written.

In this chapter, we will give you a bibliography on recent dissertations relating to childhood acute lymphoblastic leukemia. You can read about these in more detail using the Internet or your local medical library. We will also provide you with information on how to use the Internet to stay current on dissertations.

Dissertations on Childhood Acute Lymphoblastic Leukemia

ProQuest Digital Dissertations is the largest archive of academic dissertations available. From this archive, we have compiled the following list covering dissertations devoted to childhood acute lymphoblastic leukemia. You will see that the information provided includes the dissertation's title, its author, and the author's institution. To read more about the following, simply use the Internet address indicated. The following covers recent dissertations dealing with childhood acute lymphoblastic leukemia:

- **Race: a Risk Factor for Childhood Acute Lymphoblastic Leukemia** by Mallios, Ronna Reuben; MPh from California State University, Fresno, 2001, 75 pages
  http://wwwlib.umi.com/dissertations/fullcit/1405743

Keeping Current

As previously mentioned, an effective way to stay current on dissertations dedicated to childhood acute lymphoblastic leukemia is to use the database called *ProQuest Digital Dissertations* via the Internet, located at the following Web address: **http://wwwlib.umi.com/dissertations.** The site allows you to freely access the last two years of citations and abstracts. Ask your medical librarian if the library has full and unlimited access to this database. From the library, you should be able to do more complete searches than with the limited 2-year access available to the general public.

PART III. APPENDICES

ABOUT PART III

Part III is a collection of appendices on general medical topics relating to childhood acute lymphoblastic leukemia and related conditions.

Appendix A. Researching Your Child's Medications

Overview

There are a number of sources available on new or existing medications which could be prescribed to treat childhood acute lymphoblastic leukemia. While a number of hard copy or CD-Rom resources are available to parents and physicians for research purposes, a more flexible method is to use Internet-based databases. In this chapter, we will begin with a general overview of medications. We will then proceed to outline official recommendations on how you should view your child's medications. You may also want to research medications that your child is currently taking for other conditions as they may interact with medications for childhood acute lymphoblastic leukemia. Research can give you information on the side effects, interactions, and limitations of prescription drugs used in the treatment of childhood acute lymphoblastic leukemia. Broadly speaking, there are two sources of information on approved medications: public sources and private sources. We will emphasize free-to-use public sources.

Your Child's Medications: The Basics[204]

The Agency for Health Care Research and Quality has published extremely useful guidelines on the medication aspects of childhood acute lymphoblastic leukemia. Giving your child medication can involve many steps and decisions each day. The AHCRQ recommends that parents take part in treatment decisions. Do not be afraid to ask questions and talk about your concerns. By taking a moment to ask questions, your child may be spared from possible problems. Here are some points to cover each time a new medicine is prescribed:

- Ask about all parts of your child's treatment, including diet changes, exercise, and medicines.
- Ask about the risks and benefits of each medicine or other treatment your child might receive.
- Ask how often you or your child's doctor will check for side effects from a given medication.

Do not hesitate to tell the doctor about preferences you have for your child's medicines. You may want your child to have a medicine with the fewest side effects, or the fewest doses to take each day. You may care most about cost. Or, you may want the medicine the doctor believes will work the best. Sharing your concerns will help the doctor select the best treatment for your child.

Do not be afraid to "bother" the doctor with your questions about medications for childhood acute lymphoblastic leukemia. You can also talk to a nurse or a pharmacist. They can help you better understand your child's treatment plan. Talking over your child's options with someone you trust can help you make better choices. Specifically, ask the doctor the following:

- The name of the medicine and what it is supposed to do.
- How and when to give your child the medicine, how much, and for how long.
- What food, drinks, other medicines, or activities your child should avoid while taking the medicine.
- What side effects your child may experience, and what to do if they occur.
- If there are any refills, and how often.
- About any terms or directions you do not understand.

---
[204] This section is adapted from AHCRQ: **http://www.ahcpr.gov/consumer/ncpiebro.htm**.

- What to do if your child misses a dose.
- If there is written information you can take home (most pharmacies have information sheets on prescription medicines; some even offer large-print or Spanish versions).

Do not forget to tell the doctor about all the medicines your child is currently taking (not just those for childhood acute lymphoblastic leukemia). This includes prescription medicines and the medicines that you buy over the counter. When talking to the doctor, you may wish to prepare a list of medicines your child is currently taking including why and in what forms. Be sure to include the following information for each:

- Name of medicine
- Reason taken
- Dosage
- Time(s) of day

Also include any over-the-counter medicines, such as:

- Laxatives
- Diet pills
- Vitamins
- Cold medicine
- Aspirin or other pain, headache, or fever medicine
- Cough medicine
- Allergy relief medicine
- Antacids
- Sleeping pills
- Others (include names)

Learning More about Your Child's Medications

Because of historical investments by various organizations and the emergence of the Internet, it has become rather simple to learn about the medications the doctor has recommended for childhood acute lymphoblastic leukemia. One such source is the United States Pharmacopeia. In 1820, eleven physicians met in Washington, D.C. to establish the first compendium of standard drugs for the United States. They called this compendium the

"U.S. Pharmacopeia (USP)." Today, the USP is a non-profit organization consisting of 800 volunteer scientists, eleven elected officials, and 400 representatives of state associations and colleges of medicine and pharmacy. The USP is located in Rockville, Maryland, and its home page is located at **www.usp.org**. The USP currently provides standards for over 3,700 medications. The resulting USP DI® Advice for the Patient® can be accessed through the National Library of Medicine of the National Institutes of Health. The database is partially derived from lists of federally approved medications in the Food and Drug Administration's (FDA) Drug Approvals database.[205]

While the FDA database is rather large and difficult to navigate, the Phamacopeia is both user-friendly and free to use. It covers more than 9,000 prescription and over-the-counter medications. To access this database, simply type the following hyperlink into your Web browser: **http://www.nlm.nih.gov/medlineplus/druginformation.html**. To view examples of a given medication (brand names, category, description, preparation, proper use, precautions, side effects, etc.), simply follow the hyperlinks indicated within the United States Pharmacopoeia (USP). It is important to read the disclaimer by the USP (**http://www.nlm.nih.gov/medlineplus/drugdisclaimer.html**) before using the information provided.

Of course, we as editors cannot be certain as to what medications your child is taking. Therefore, we have compiled a list of medications associated with the treatment of childhood acute lymphoblastic leukemia. Once again, due to space limitations, we only list a sample of medications and provide hyperlinks to ample documentation (e.g. typical dosage, side effects, drug-interaction risks, etc.). The following drugs have been mentioned in the Pharmacopeia and other sources as being potentially applicable to childhood acute lymphoblastic leukemia:

Ifosfamide
- **Systemic - U.S. Brands:** IFEX
  http://www.nlm.nih.gov/medlineplus/druginfo/ifosfamidesystemic202293.html

---

[205] Though cumbersome, the FDA database can be freely browsed at the following site: **www.fda.gov/cder/da/da.htm**.

Commercial Databases

In addition to the medications listed in the USP above, a number of commercial sites are available by subscription to physicians and their institutions. You may be able to access these sources from your local medical library or your child's doctor's office.

Reuters Health Drug Database

The Reuters Health Drug Database can be searched by keyword at the hyperlink: **http://www.reutershealth.com/frame2/drug.html**.

Mosby's GenRx

Mosby's GenRx database (also available on CD-Rom and book format) covers 45,000 drug products including generics and international brands. It provides information on prescribing and drug interactions. Information can be obtained at the following hyperlink: **http://www.genrx.com/Mosby/PhyGenRx/group.html**.

Physicians Desk Reference

The Physicians Desk Reference database (also available in CD-Rom and book format) is a full-text drug database. The database is searchable by brand name, generic name or by indication. It features multiple drug interactions reports. Information can be obtained at the following hyperlink: **http://physician.pdr.net/physician/templates/en/acl/psuser_t.htm**.

Other Web Sites

A number of additional Web sites discuss drug information. As an example, you may like to look at **www.drugs.com** which reproduces the information in the Pharmacopeia as well as commercial information. You may also want to consider the Web site of the Medical Letter, Inc. which allows users to download articles on various drugs and therapeutics for a nominal fee: **http://www.medletter.com/**.

Drug Development and Approval

The following Web sites can be valuable resources when conducting research on the development and approval of new cancer drugs:

- FDA Home Page: Search for drugs currently in development or those which have been recently approved by the FDA.
  http://redir.nci.nih.gov/cgi-bin/redir.pl?section=Cancerinfo&destURI=http://www.fda.gov/

- Cancer Liaison Program: Answers questions from the public about drug approval processes, cancer clinical trials, and access to investigational therapies.
  http://redir.nci.nih.gov/cgi-bin/redir.pl?section=Cancerinfo&destURI=http://www.fda.gov/oashi/cancer/cancer.html

- Center for Drug Evaluation and Research
  http://redir.nci.nih.gov/cgi-bin/redir.pl?section=Cancerinfo&destURI=http://www.fda.gov/cder/

- Drug Approvals by Cancer Indications (Alphabetical List)
  http://redir.nci.nih.gov/cgi-bin/redir.pl?section=Cancerinfo&destURI=http://www.fda.gov/oashi/cancer/cdrugalpha.html

- Drug Approvals by Cancer Indications (Cancer Type)
  http://redir.nci.nih.gov/cgi-bin/redir.pl?section=Cancerinfo&destURI=http://www.fda.gov/oashi/cancer/cdrugind.html

- Electronic Orange Book of Approved Drug Products
  http://redir.nci.nih.gov/cgi-bin/redir.pl?section=Cancerinfo&destURI=http://www.fda.gov/cder/ob/default.htm

- Guidance Documents for Industry: Contains an archive of documents describing FDA policies on specific topics.
  http://redir.nci.nih.gov/cgi-bin/redir.pl?section=Cancerinfo&destURI=http://www.fda.gov/cder/guidance/index.htm

- Industry Collaboration: Provides information to industry on the process for getting new drugs into clinical trials.
  http://ctep.cancer.gov/industry/index.html

- Investigator's Handbook: Provides information to investigators on specific procedures related to clinical trial development.
  http://ctep.cancer.gov/handbook/index.html

- Questions and Answers About NCI's Natural Products Branch: A fact sheet that describes the functions of this branch, which collects and analyzes specimens of plant, marine, and microbial origin for possible anticancer properties.
  http://cis.nci.nih.gov/fact/7_33.htm

Understanding the Approval Process for New Cancer Drugs[206]

Since June 1996, about 80 new cancer-related drugs, or new uses for drugs already on the market, have been approved by the U.S. Food and Drug Administration (FDA), the division of the U.S. Department of Health and Human Services charged with ensuring the safety and effectiveness of new drugs before they can go on the market. (The FDA maintains an annotated online list of drugs approved for use with cancer since 1996.) Some of these drugs treat cancer, some alleviate pain and other symptoms, and, in one case, reduce the risk of invasive cancer in people who are considered high-risk. The FDA relied on the results of clinical trials in making every one of these approvals. Without reliable information about a drug's effects on humans, it would be impossible to approve any drug for widespread use.

When considering a new drug, the FDA faces two challenges:

- First, making sure that the drug is safe and effective before it is made widely available;

- Second, ensuring that drugs which show promise are made available as quickly as possible to the people they can help.

To deal with these challenges, the FDA maintains a rigorous review process but also has measures in place to make some drugs available in special cases. This aim of this section is to acquaint you with the drug approval process and point you to other resources for learning more about it.

---

[206] Adapted from the NCI:
http://www.cancer.gov/clinical_trials/doc_header.aspx?viewid=d94cbfac-e478-4704-9052-d8e8a3372b56.

The Role of the Federal Drug Administration (FDA)

Approval is only one step in the drug development process. In fact, the FDA estimates that, on average, it takes eight and a half years to study and test a new drug before it can be approved for the general public. That includes early laboratory and animal testing, as well as the clinical trials that evaluate the drugs in humans. The FDA plays a key role at three main points in this process:

- Determining whether or not a new drug shows enough promise to be given to people in clinical trials

- Once clinical trials begin, deciding whether or not they should continue, based on reports of efficacy and adverse reactions

- When clinical trials are completed, deciding whether or not the drug can be sold to the public and what its label should say about directions for use, side effects, warnings, and the like.

To make these decisions, the FDA must review studies submitted by the drug's sponsor (usually the manufacturer), evaluate any adverse reports from preclinical studies and clinical trials (that is, reports of side effects or complications), and review the adequacy of the chemistry and manufacturing. This process is lengthy, but it is meant to ensure that only beneficial drugs with acceptable side effects will make their way into the hands of the public. At the same time, recent legislative mandates and streamlined procedures within the FDA have accelerated the approval of effective drugs, especially for serious illnesses such as cancer. In addition, specific provisions make some drugs available to patients with special needs even before the approval process is complete.

From Lab to Patient Care

By law, the Food and Drug Administration (FDA) must review all test results for new drugs to ensure that products are safe and effective for specific uses. "Safe" does not mean that the drug is free of possible adverse side effects; rather, it means that the potential benefits have been determined to outweigh any risks. The testing process begins long before the first person takes the drug, with preliminary research and animal testing.

If a drug proves promising in the lab, the drug company or sponsor must apply for FDA approval to test it in clinical trials involving people. For drugs, the application, called an Investigational New Drug (IND)

Application, is sent through the Center for Drug Evaluation and Research's (CDER) IND Review Process; for biological agents, the IND is sent to the Center for Biologics Evaluation and Research (CBER). Once the IND is approved by CDER or CBER, clinical trials can begin.

If the drug makes it through the clinical trials process—that is, the studies show that it is superior to current drugs—the manufacturer must submit a New Drug Application (NDA) or (for biological agents) a Biologics License Application (BLA) to the FDA. (Biological agents, such as serums, vaccines, and cloned proteins, are manufactured from substances taken from living humans or animals.) This application must include:

- The exact chemical makeup of the drug or biologic and the mechanisms by which it is effective
- Results of animal studies
- Results of clinical trials
- How the drug or biologic is manufactured, processed, and packaged
- Quality control standards
- Samples of the product in the form(s) in which it is to be administered.

Once the FDA receives the NDA or BLA from the manufacturer or developer, the formal New Drug Application Review Process or Biologics/Product License Application Review Process begins.

For an overview of the entire process from start to finish, see the CDER's visual representation of The New Drug Development Process: Steps from Test Tube to New Drug Application Review, which is available for public viewing at the following Web address: **http://www.fda.gov/cder/handbook/develop.htm**.

Speed versus Safety in the Approval Process

The FDA's current goal is that no more than ten months will pass between the time that a complete application is submitted and the FDA takes action on it. But the process is not always smooth. Sometimes FDA's external advisory panels call for additional research or data. In other cases, the FDA staff asks for more information or revised studies. Some new drug approvals have taken as little as 42 days; other more difficult NDAs have spent years in the approval process.

Setting Priorities

The order in which NDAs are assessed by the FDA is determined by a classification system designed to give priority to drugs with the greatest potential benefits. All drugs that offer significant medical advances over existing therapies for any disease are considered "priority" drugs in the approval process. NDAs for cancer treatment drugs are reviewed for this status primarily by the Division of Oncology Drug Products in the FDA's Center for Drug Evaluation and Research (CDER). For Biologic License Applications (vaccines, blood products, and medicines made from animal products), the Center for Biologics Evaluation and Research (CBER) provides additional regulation and oversight.

Expert Advice

The FDA relies on a system of independent advisory committees, made up of professionals from outside the agency, for expert advice and guidance in making sound decisions about drug approval. Each committee meets as needed to weigh available evidence and assess the safety, effectiveness, and appropriate use of products considered for approval. In addition, these committees provide advice about general criteria for evaluation and scientific issues not related to specific products. The Oncologic Drugs Advisory Committee (ODAC) meets regularly to provide expert advice on cancer-related treatments and preventive drugs.

Each committee is composed of representatives from the research science and medical fields. At least one member on every advisory committee must represent the consumer perspective.

Final Approval

As the FDA looks at all the data submitted and the results of its own review, it applies two benchmark questions to each application for drug approval:

- Do the results of well-controlled studies provide substantial evidence of effectiveness?

- Do the results show the product is safe under the conditions of use in the proposed labeling? In this context, "safe" means that potential benefits have been determined to outweigh any risks.

Continued Vigilance

The FDA's responsibility for new drug treatments does not stop with final approval. The Office of Compliance in the Center for Drug Evaluation and Research (CDER) implements and tracks programs to make sure manufacturers comply with current standards and practice regulations. CDER's Office of Drug Marketing, Advertising, and Communication monitors new drug advertising to make sure it is truthful and complete. At the Center for Biologic Evaluation and Research, biologics are followed with the same vigilance after approval. And through a system called MedWatch, the FDA gets feedback from health professionals and consumers on how the new drugs are working, any adverse reactions, and potential problems in labeling and dosage.

Online FDA Resources

The following information from the FDA should help you better understand the drug approval process:

- Center for Drug Evaluation and Research:
  http://www.fda.gov/cder/handbook
- From Test Tube to Patient: New Drug Development in the U.S. – a special January 1995 issue of the magazine FDA Consumer:
  http://www.fda.gov/fdac/special/newdrug/ndd_toc.html
- Milestones in U.S. Food and Drug Law History:
  http://www.fda.gov/opacom/backgrounders/miles.html
- Drug Approvals for Cancer Indications:
  http://www.fda.gov/oashi/cancer/cdrug.html

Getting Drugs to Patients Who Need Them

Clinical trials provide the most important information used by the FDA in determining whether a new drug shows "substantial evidence of effectiveness," or whether an already-approved drug can be used effectively in new ways (for example, to treat or prevent other types of cancer, or at a different dosage). The FDA must certify that a drug has shown promise in laboratory and animal trials before human testing can begin. The trials process includes three main stages and involves continuous review, which ensures that the sponsor can stop the study early if major problems develop or unexpected levels of treatment benefit are found. As with all clinical trials, benefits and risks must be carefully weighed by the researchers conducting the study and the patients who decide to participate.

Not everyone is eligible to participate in a clinical trial. Some patients do not fit the exact requirements for studies, some have rare forms of cancer for which only a limited number of studies are underway, and others are too ill to participate. Working with the NCI and other sponsors, the FDA has established special conditions under which a patient and his or her physician can apply to receive cancer drugs that have not yet been through the approval process. In the past, these special case applications for new drugs were grouped under the name "compassionate uses." More recently, such uses have expanded to include more patients and more categories of investigational drugs.

Access to Investigational Drugs

The process of new drug development has many parts. In the United States, until a drug has been approved by the FDA, it can generally be obtained only through several mechanisms: enrollment in a clinical trial studying the drug, an expanded access program or special exemption/compassionate use programs. For more information about investigational drugs, see "Questions and Answers: Access to Investigational Drugs" at **http://www.cancer.gov/cancer_information/doc_img.aspx?viewid=74b62d8 4-e135-451f-9bc9-d54358ede947**.

"Group C" Drugs

In the 1970s, researchers from the NCI became concerned about the lag between the date when an investigational drug was found to have anti-tumor activity and the time that drug became available on the market. Working with the FDA, the NCI established the "Group C" classification to allow access to drugs with reproducible activity. Group C drugs are provided to properly trained physicians who have registered using a special form to assure that their patient qualifies under guideline protocols for the drug. Each Group C drug protocol specifies patient eligibility, reporting methodology, and drug use. Not only does Group C designation (now called Group C/Treatment INDs) speed new drugs to patients who need them most, but the process also allows the NCI to gather important information on the safety as well as activity of the drugs in the settings in which they will be most used after final FDA approval. Drugs are placed in the Group C category by agreement between the FDA and the NCI. Group C drugs are always provided free of charge, and the Health Care Financing Administration provides coverage for care associated with Group C therapy.

Treatment INDs

In 1987, the FDA began authorizing the use of new drugs still in the development process to treat certain seriously ill patients. In these cases, the process is referred to as a treatment investigational new drug application (Treatment IND). Clinical trials of the new drug must already be underway and have demonstrated positive results that are reproducible. The FDA sets guidelines about what constitutes serious and life-threatening illnesses, how much must already be known about a drug's side effects and benefits, and where physicians can obtain the drug for treatment. For many seriously ill patients, the risks associated with taking a not-yet-completely proven drug are outweighed by the possible benefits.

Accelerated Approval

"Accelerated approval" is the short-hand term for the FDA's new review system which, in the 1990s, has been used to ensure rapid approval while at the same time putting new safeguards into place. Accelerated approval is based on "surrogate endpoint" judgments: FDA can grant marketing approval to drugs and treatments that, according to certain indicators, prove they are likely to have beneficial effects on a disease or condition, even before such direct benefits have been shown clinically. Accelerated approval does NOT mean that additional clinical trials are not needed or that FDA stops gathering information about the effects of the drug; a follow-up study is required to demonstrate activity by more conventional endpoints.

Contraindications and Interactions (Hidden Dangers)

Some of the medications mentioned in the previous discussions can be problematic for children with childhood acute lymphoblastic leukemia--not because they are used in the treatment process, but because of contraindications, or side effects. Medications with contraindications are those that could react with drugs used to treat childhood acute lymphoblastic leukemia or potentially create deleterious side effects in patients with childhood acute lymphoblastic leukemia. You should ask the physician about any contraindications, especially as these might apply to other medications that your child may be taking for common ailments.

Drug-drug interactions occur when two or more drugs react with each other. This drug-drug interaction may cause your child to experience an unexpected side effect. Drug interactions may make medications less effective, cause unexpected side effects, or increase the action of a particular drug. Some drug interactions can even be harmful to your child.

Be sure to read the label every time you give your child a nonprescription or prescription drug, and take the time to learn about drug interactions. These precautions may be critical to your child's health. You can reduce the risk of potentially harmful drug interactions and side effects with a little bit of knowledge and common sense.

Drug labels contain important information about ingredients, uses, warnings, and directions which you should take the time to read and understand. Labels also include warnings about possible drug interactions. Further, drug labels may change as new information becomes avaiable. This is why it's especially important to read the label every time you give your child a medication. When the doctor prescribes a new drug, discuss all over-the-counter and prescription medications, dietary supplements, vitamins, botanicals, minerals and herbals your child takes. Ask your pharmacist for the package insert for each drug prescribed. The package insert provides more information about potential drug interactions.

A Final Warning

At some point, you may hear of alternative medications from friends, relatives, or in the news media. Advertisements may suggest that certain alternative drugs can produce positive results for childhood acute lymphoblastic leukemia. Exercise caution--some of these drugs may have fraudulent claims, and others may actually hurt your child. The Food and Drug Administration (FDA) is the official U.S. agency charged with discovering which medications are likely to improve the health of patients with childhood acute lymphoblastic leukemia. The FDA warns to watch out for[207]:

- Secret formulas (real scientists share what they know)
- Amazing breakthroughs or miracle cures (real breakthroughs don't happen very often; when they do, real scientists do not call them amazing or miracles)
- Quick, painless, or guaranteed cures

---

[207] This section has been adapted from **http://www.fda.gov/opacom/lowlit/medfraud.html**

- If it sounds too good to be true, it probably isn't true.

If you have any questions about any kind of medical treatment, the FDA may have an office near you. Look for their number in the blue pages of the phone book. You can also contact the FDA through its toll-free number, 1-888-INFO-FDA (1-888-463-6332), or on the World Wide Web at **www.fda.gov**.

General References

In addition to the resources provided earlier in this chapter, the following general references describe medications (sorted alphabetically by title; hyperlinks provide rankings, information and reviews at Amazon.com):

- **Antifolate Drugs in Cancer Therapy (Cancer Drug Discovery and Development)** by Ann L. Jackman (Editor); Hardcover: 480 pages; (March 1999), Humana Press; ISBN: 0896035964;
  http://www.amazon.com/exec/obidos/ASIN/0896035964/icongroupinterna

- **Consumers Guide to Cancer Drugs** by Gail M. Wilkes, et al; Paperback - 448 pages, 1st edition (January 15, 2000), Jones & Bartlett Publishing; ISBN: 0763711705;
  http://www.amazon.com/exec/obidos/ASIN/0763711705/icongroupinterna

- **Patient Education Guide to Oncology Drugs (Book with CD-ROM)** by Gail M. Wilkes, et al; CD-ROM - 447 pages, 1st edition (January 15, 2000), Jones & Bartlett Publishing; ISBN: 076371173X;
  http://www.amazon.com/exec/obidos/ASIN/076371173X/icongroupinterna

- **The Role of Multiple Intensification in Medical Oncology** by M. S. Aapro (Editor), D. Maraninchi (Editor); Hardcover (June 1998), Springer Verlag; ISBN: 3540635432;
  http://www.amazon.com/exec/obidos/ASIN/3540635432/icongroupinterna

Vocabulary Builder

The following vocabulary builder gives definitions of words used in this chapter that have not been defined in previous chapters:

Aspirin: A drug that reduces pain, fever, inflammation, and blood clotting. Aspirin belongs to the family of drugs called nonsteroidal anti-inflammatory agents. It is also being studied in cancer prevention. [NIH]

Ifosfamide: An anticancer drug that belongs to the family of drugs called alkylating agents. [NIH]

Preclinical: Before a disease becomes clinically recognizable. [EU]

APPENDIX B. RESEARCHING ALTERNATIVE MEDICINE

Overview[208]

Research indicates that the use of complementary and alternative therapies is increasing. A large-scale study published in the November 11, 1998, issue of the Journal of the American Medical Association found that CAM use among the general public increased from 34 percent in 1990 to 42 percent in 1997.

Several surveys of CAM use by cancer patients have been conducted with small numbers of patients. One study published in the February 2000 issue of the journal *Cancer* reported that 37 percent of 46 patients with prostate cancer used one or more CAM therapies as part of their cancer treatment. These therapies included herbal remedies, old-time remedies, vitamins, and special diets. A larger study of CAM use in patients with different types of cancer was published in the July 2000 issue of the Journal of Clinical Oncology . That study found that 83 percent of 453 cancer patients had used at least one CAM therapy as part of their cancer treatment. The study included CAM therapies such as special diets, psychotherapy, spiritual practices, and vitamin supplements. When psychotherapy and spiritual practices were excluded, 69 percent of patients had used at least one CAM therapy in their cancer treatment.

In this chapter, we will begin by giving you a broad perspective on complementary and alternative therapies. Next, we will introduce you to official information sources on CAM relating to childhood acute lymphoblastic leukemia. Finally, at the conclusion of this chapter, we will provide a list of readings on childhood acute lymphoblastic leukemia from various authors. We will begin, however, with the National Center for

---

[208] Adapted from the NCI: **http://cis.nci.nih.gov/fact/9_14.htm**

Complementary and Alternative Medicine's (NCCAM) overview of complementary and alternative medicine.

What Is CAM?[209]

Complementary and alternative medicine (CAM) covers a broad range of healing philosophies, approaches, and therapies. Generally, it is defined as those treatments and healthcare practices which are not taught in medical schools, used in hospitals, or reimbursed by medical insurance companies. Many CAM therapies are termed "holistic," which generally means that the healthcare practitioner considers the whole person, including physical, mental, emotional, and spiritual health. Some of these therapies are also known as "preventive," which means that the practitioner educates and treats the person to prevent health problems from arising, rather than treating symptoms after problems have occurred.

People use CAM treatments and therapies in a variety of ways. Therapies are used alone (often referred to as alternative), in combination with other alternative therapies, or in addition to conventional treatment (sometimes referred to as complementary). Complementary and alternative medicine, or "integrative medicine," includes a broad range of healing philosophies, approaches, and therapies. Some approaches are consistent with physiological principles of Western medicine, while others constitute healing systems with non-Western origins. While some therapies are far outside the realm of accepted Western medical theory and practice, others are becoming established in mainstream medicine.

Complementary and alternative therapies are used in an effort to prevent illness, reduce stress, prevent or reduce side effects and symptoms, or control or cure disease. Some commonly used methods of complementary or alternative therapy include mind/body control interventions such as visualization and relaxation, manual healing including acupressure and massage, homeopathy, vitamins or herbal products, and acupuncture.

Should you wish to explore non-traditional types of treatment, be sure to discuss all issues concerning treatments and therapies with your child's healthcare provider, whether a physician or practitioner of complementary and alternative medicine. Competent healthcare management requires that the practitioner know of all conventional and alternative therapies that your child is taking.

---

[209] Adapted from the NCCAM: **http://nccam.nih.gov/nccam/fcp/faq/index.html#what-is**.

The decision to use complementary and alternative treatments is an important one. Consider before selecting an alternative therapy, the safety and effectiveness of the therapy or treatment, the expertise and qualifications of the healthcare practitioner, and the quality of delivery. These topics should be considered when selecting any practitioner or therapy.

What Are the Domains of Alternative Medicine?[210]

The list of CAM practices changes continually. The reason being is that these new practices and therapies are often proved to be safe and effective, and therefore become generally accepted as "mainstream" healthcare practices. Today, CAM practices may be grouped within five major domains: (1) alternative medical systems, (2) mind-body interventions, (3) biologically-based treatments, (4) manipulative and body-based methods, and (5) energy therapies. The individual systems and treatments comprising these categories are too numerous to list in this sourcebook. Thus, only limited examples are provided within each.

Alternative Medical Systems

Alternative medical systems involve complete systems of theory and practice that have evolved independent of, and often prior to, conventional biomedical approaches. Many are traditional systems of medicine that are practiced by individual cultures throughout the world, including a number of venerable Asian approaches.

Traditional oriental medicine emphasizes the balance or disturbances of qi (pronounced chi) or vital energy in health and illness, respectively. Traditional oriental medicine consists of a group of techniques and methods including acupuncture, herbal medicine, oriental massage, and qi gong (a form of energy therapy). Acupuncture involves stimulating specific anatomic points in the body for therapeutic purposes, usually by puncturing the skin with a thin needle.

Ayurveda is India's traditional system of medicine. Ayurvedic medicine (meaning "science of life") is a comprehensive system of medicine that places equal emphasis on body, mind, and spirit. Ayurveda strives to restore the innate harmony of the individual. Some of the primary Ayurvedic

---

[210] Adapted from the NCCAM: **http://nccam.nih.gov/nccam/fcp/classify/index.html**

treatments include diet, exercise, meditation, herbs, massage, exposure to sunlight, and controlled breathing.

Other traditional healing systems have been developed by the world's indigenous populations. These populations include Native American, Aboriginal, African, Middle Eastern, Tibetan, and Central and South American cultures. Homeopathy and naturopathy are also examples of complete alternative medicine systems.

Homeopathic medicine is an unconventional Western system that is based on the principle that "like cures like," i.e., that the same substance that in large doses produces the symptoms of an illness, in very minute doses cures it. Homeopathic health practitioners believe that the more dilute the remedy, the greater its potency. Therefore, they use small doses of specially prepared plant extracts and minerals to stimulate the body's defense mechanisms and healing processes in order to treat illness.

Naturopathic medicine is based on the theory that a medical condition is the manifestation of alterations in the processes by which the body naturally heals itself and emphasizes health restoration rather than treatment for the condition itself. Naturopathic physicians employ an array of healing practices, including the following: diet and clinical nutrition, homeopathy, acupuncture, herbal medicine, hydrotherapy (the use of water in a range of temperatures and methods of applications), spinal and soft-tissue manipulation, physical therapies (such as those involving electrical currents, ultrasound, and light), therapeutic counseling, and pharmacology.

Mind-Body Interventions

Mind-body interventions employ a variety of techniques designed to facilitate the mind's capacity to affect bodily function and symptoms. Only a select group of mind-body interventions having well-documented theoretical foundations are considered CAM. For example, patient education and cognitive-behavioral approaches are now considered "mainstream." On the other hand, complementary and alternative medicine includes meditation, certain uses of hypnosis, dance, music, and art therapy, as well as prayer and mental healing.

Biological-Based Therapies

This category of CAM includes natural and biological-based practices, interventions, and products, many of which overlap with conventional medicine's use of dietary supplements. This category includes herbal, special dietary, orthomolecular, and individual biological therapies.

Herbal therapy employs an individual herb or a mixture of herbs for healing purposes. An herb is a plant or plant part that produces and contains chemical substances that act upon the body. Special diet therapies, such as those proposed by Drs. Atkins, Ornish, Pritikin, and Weil, are believed to prevent and/or control illness as well as promote health. Orthomolecular therapies aim to treat medical conditions with varying concentrations of chemicals such as magnesium, melatonin, and mega-doses of vitamins. Biological therapies include, for example, the use of laetrile and shark cartilage to treat cancer and the use of bee pollen to treat autoimmune and inflammatory conditions.

Manipulative and Body-Based Methods

This category includes methods that are based on manipulation and/or movement of the body. For example, chiropractors focus on the relationship between structure and function, primarily pertaining to the spine, and how that relationship affects the preservation and restoration of health. Chiropractors use manipulative therapy as an integral treatment tool.

In contrast, osteopaths place particular emphasis on the musculoskeletal system and practice osteopathic manipulation. Osteopaths believe that all of the body's systems work together and that disturbances in one system may have an impact upon function elsewhere in the body. Massage therapists manipulate the soft tissues of the body to normalize those tissues.

Energy Therapies

Energy therapies focus on energy fields originating within the body (biofields) or those from other sources (electromagnetic fields). Biofield therapies are intended to affect energy fields (the existence of which is not yet experimentally proven) that surround and penetrate the human body. Some forms of energy therapy manipulate biofields by applying pressure and/or manipulating the body by placing the hands in or through these fields. Examples include Qi gong, Reiki and Therapeutic Touch.

Qi gong is a component of traditional oriental medicine that combines movement, meditation, and regulation of breathing to enhance the flow of vital energy (qi) in the body, improve blood circulation, and enhance immune function. Reiki, the Japanese word representing Universal Life Energy, is based on the belief that, by channeling spiritual energy through the practitioner, the spirit is healed and, in turn, heals the physical body. Therapeutic Touch is derived from the ancient technique of "laying-on of hands." It is based on the premises that the therapist's healing force affects recovery and that healing is promoted when the body's energies are in balance. By passing their hands over the patient, these healers identify energy imbalances.

Bioelectromagnetic-based therapies involve the unconventional use of electromagnetic fields to treat illnesses or manage pain. These therapies are often used to treat asthma, cancer, and migraine headaches. Types of electromagnetic fields which are manipulated in these therapies include pulsed fields, magnetic fields, and alternating current or direct current fields.

How Are Complementary and Alternative Approaches Evaluated?[211]

It is important that the same scientific evaluation which is used to assess conventional approaches be used to evaluate complementary and alternative therapies. A number of medical centers are evaluating complementary and alternative therapies by developing clinical trials (research studies with people) to test them.

Conventional approaches to cancer treatment have generally been studied for safety and effectiveness through a rigorous scientific process, including clinical trials with large numbers of patients. Often, less is known about the safety and effectiveness of complementary and alternative methods. Some of these complementary and alternative therapies have not undergone rigorous evaluation. Others, once considered unorthodox, are finding a place in cancer treatment—not as cures, but as complementary therapies that may help patients feel better and recover faster. One example is acupuncture. According to a panel of experts at a National Institutes of Health (NIH) Consensus Conference in November 1997, acupuncture has been found to be effective in the management of chemotherapy-associated nausea and vomiting and in controlling pain associated with surgery. Some approaches, such as laetrile, have been studied and found ineffective or potentially harmful.

---

[211] Adapted from the NCI: **http://cis.nci.nih.gov/fact/9_14.htm**

NCI-Sponsored Clinical Trials in Complementary and Alternative Medicine

The NCI is currently sponsoring several clinical trials (research studies with patients) that study complementary and alternative treatments for cancer. Current trials include enzyme therapy with nutritional support for the treatment of inoperable pancreatic cancer, shark cartilage therapy for the treatment of non-small cell lung cancer, and studies of the effects of diet on prostate and breast cancers. Some of these trials compare alternative therapies with conventional treatments, while others study the effects of complementary approaches used in addition to conventional treatments. Patients who are interested in taking part in these or any clinical trials should talk with their doctor.

More information about clinical trials sponsored by the NCI can be obtained from NCCAM (http://nccam.nih.gov, 1-888-644-6226), OCCAM (http://occam.nci.nih.gov), and the NCI's Cancer Information Service (CIS) (http://cis.nci.nih.gov, 1-800-4-CANCER).

Questions to Ask Your Child's Healthcare Provider about CAM

When considering complementary and alternative therapies, ask your child's healthcare provider the following questions:

- What benefits can be expected from this therapy?
- What are the risks associated with this therapy?
- Do the known benefits outweigh the risks?
- What side effects can be expected?
- Will the therapy interfere with conventional treatment?
- Is this therapy part of a clinical trial? If so, who is sponsoring the trial?
- Will the therapy be covered by health insurance?
- How can patients and their health care providers learn more about complementary and alternative therapies?

Levels of Evidence for Human Studies of CAM for Cancer[212]

A classification system has been developed by the National Cancer Institute's PDQ Adult Treatment Editorial Board to allow the ranking of human cancer treatment studies according to statistical strength of the study design and scientific strength of the treatment outcomes (i.e., endpoints) measured. This classification system has been adapted to allow the ranking of human studies of complementary and alternative medicine treatments for cancer. The purpose of classifying studies in this way is to assist readers in evaluating the strength of the evidence associated with particular treatments. However, not all human studies are classified. Only those reporting a therapeutic endpoint(s), such as tumor response, improvement in survival, or measured improvement in quality of life, are considered. In addition, anecdotal reports and individual case reports are not classified because important clinical details are often missing, the evidence from them is generally considered weak, and there is an increased probability that similar results (either positive or negative) will not be obtained with other patients. Furthermore, reports of case series are excluded when the description of clinical findings is so incomplete as to hinder proper assessment and interpretation.

Finding CAM References on Childhood Acute Lymphoblastic Leukemia

Having read the previous discussion, you may be wondering which complementary or alternative treatments might be appropriate for childhood acute lymphoblastic leukemia. For the remainder of this chapter, we will direct you to a number of official sources which can assist you in researching studies and publications. Some of these articles are rather technical, so some patience may be required.

National Center for Complementary and Alternative Medicine

The National Center for Complementary and Alternative Medicine (NCCAM) of the National Institutes of Health (http://nccam.nih.gov) has created a link to the National Library of Medicine's databases to allow parents to search for articles that specifically relate to childhood acute

---

[212] For more information, visit the NCI's Web page dedicated to this topic: http://www.cancer.gov/cancer_information/doc.aspx?viewid=47595A5D-AD15-4F7D-BAE6-DEA914E6C153

lymphoblastic leukemia and complementary medicine. To search the database, go to the following Web site: **www.nlm.nih.gov/nccam/camonpubmed.html**. Select "CAM on PubMed." Enter "childhood acute lymphoblastic leukemia" (or synonyms) into the search box. Click "Go." The following references provide information on particular aspects of complementary and alternative medicine (CAM) that are related to childhood acute lymphoblastic leukemia:

- **6-Mercaptopurine cumulative dose: a critical factor of maintenance therapy in average risk childhood acute lymphoblastic leukemia.**
  Author(s): Dibenedetto P, Guardabasso V, Ragusa R, Di Cataldo A, Miraglia V, D'Amico S, Ippolito AM.
  Source: Pediatric Hematology and Oncology. 1994 May-June; 11(3): 251-8.
  http://www.ncbi.nlm.nih.gov:80/entrez/query.fcgi?cmd=Retrieve&db=PubMed&list_uids=8060809&dopt=Abstract

- **Aggressive combination chemotherapy of bone marrow relapse in childhood acute lymphoblastic leukemia containing aclacinomycin-A: a multicentric trial.**
  Author(s): Fengler R, Buchmann S, Riehm H, Berthold F, Dopfer R, Graf N, Holldack J, Jobke A, Jurgens H, Klingebiel T, et al.
  Source: Hamatol Bluttransfus. 1987; 30: 493-6.
  http://www.ncbi.nlm.nih.gov:80/entrez/query.fcgi?cmd=Retrieve&db=PubMed&list_uids=3305216&dopt=Abstract

- **Allogeneic BMT versus autologous BMT in childhood acute lymphoblastic leukemia (ALL): an Italian cooperative study of vincristine (VCR), F-TBI and cyclophosphamide. AIEOP (Associazione Italiana Ematologia ed Oncologia Pediatrica) Italy.**
  Author(s): Uderzo C, Coleselli P, Messina C, Dini G, Bonetti F, Andolina M, Bagnulo S, Miniero R, Rondelli R, Paolucci P, et al.
  Source: Bone Marrow Transplantation. 1991; 7 Suppl 2: 132. No Abstract Available.
  http://www.ncbi.nlm.nih.gov:80/entrez/query.fcgi?cmd=Retrieve&db=PubMed&list_uids=1878677&dopt=Abstract

- **Allogeneic bone marrow transplantation for childhood acute lymphoblastic leukemia in second remission after intensive primary and relapse therapy according to the BFM- and CoALL-protocols: results of the German Cooperative Study.**
  Author(s): Dopfer R, Henze G, Bender-Gotze C, Ebell W, Ehninger G, Friedrich W, Gadner H, Klingebiel T, Peters C, Riehm H, et al.

Source: Blood. 1991 November 15; 78(10): 2780-4.
http://www.ncbi.nlm.nih.gov:80/entrez/query.fcgi?cmd=Retrieve&db=PubMed&list_uids=1824271&dopt=Abstract

- **An Italian study comparing allogeneic and autologous BMT in childhood acute lymphoblastic leukemia using HD-vincristine, F-TBI and cyclophosphamide.**
  Author(s): Uderzo C, Colleselli P, Dini G, Bonetti F, Andolina F, Bagnulo S, Miniero R, Rondelli R, Balduzzi A, Locasciulli A.
  Source: Bone Marrow Transplantation. 1991; 7 Suppl 3: 19-21. No Abstract Available.
  http://www.ncbi.nlm.nih.gov:80/entrez/query.fcgi?cmd=Retrieve&db=PubMed&list_uids=1855081&dopt=Abstract

- **Bioavailability and pharmacokinetic features of etoposide in childhood acute lymphoblastic leukemia patients.**
  Author(s): Chen CL, Rawwas J, Sorrell A, Eddy L, Uckun FM.
  Source: Leukemia & Lymphoma. 2001 July; 42(3): 317-27.
  http://www.ncbi.nlm.nih.gov:80/entrez/query.fcgi?cmd=Retrieve&db=PubMed&list_uids=11699396&dopt=Abstract

- **Biological characteristics and prognostic value of in vitro three-drug resistance to prednisolone, L-asparaginase, and vincristine in childhood acute lymphoblastic leukemia.**
  Author(s): Hongo T, Yamada S, Yajima S, Watanabe C, Fujii Y, Kawasaki H, Yazaki M, Hanada R, Horikoshi Y.
  Source: International Journal of Hematology. 1999 December; 70(4): 268-77.
  http://www.ncbi.nlm.nih.gov:80/entrez/query.fcgi?cmd=Retrieve&db=PubMed&list_uids=10643153&dopt=Abstract

- **Bone marrow necrosis and thrombotic complications in childhood acute lymphoblastic leukemia.**
  Author(s): Eguiguren JM, Pui CH.
  Source: Medical and Pediatric Oncology. 1992; 20(1): 58-60.
  http://www.ncbi.nlm.nih.gov:80/entrez/query.fcgi?cmd=Retrieve&db=PubMed&list_uids=1727213&dopt=Abstract

- **Cellular drug resistance profiles that might explain the prognostic value of immunophenotype and age in childhood acute lymphoblastic leukemia.**

Author(s): Pieters R, Kaspers GJ, van Wering ER, Huismans DR, Loonen AH, Hahlen K, Veerman AJ.
Source: Leukemia : Official Journal of the Leukemia Society of America, Leukemia Research Fund, U.K. 1993 March; 7(3): 392-7.
http://www.ncbi.nlm.nih.gov:80/entrez/query.fcgi?cmd=Retrieve&db=PubMed&list_uids=8445945&dopt=Abstract

- **Chemotherapy of childhood acute lymphoblastic leukemia.**
  Author(s): Bell BA, Whitehead VM.
  Source: Dev Pharmacol Ther. 1986; 9(3): 145-70. Review.
  http://www.ncbi.nlm.nih.gov:80/entrez/query.fcgi?cmd=Retrieve&db=PubMed&list_uids=3519131&dopt=Abstract

- **Chemotherapy with cyclophosphamide, vincristine, cytosine arabinoside, and prednisone (COAP) in childhood acute lymphoblastic leukemia (ALL).**
  Author(s): Sallan SE, Camitta BM, Chan DM, Traggis D, Jaffe N.
  Source: Medical and Pediatric Oncology. 1977; 3(4): 359-64.
  http://www.ncbi.nlm.nih.gov:80/entrez/query.fcgi?cmd=Retrieve&db=PubMed&list_uids=270608&dopt=Abstract

- **Childhood acute lymphoblastic leukemia (ALL): sister chromatid exchange (SCE) frequency and lymphocyte subpopulations during therapy.**
  Author(s): Mertens R, Rubbert F, Bussing A.
  Source: Leukemia : Official Journal of the Leukemia Society of America, Leukemia Research Fund, U.K. 1995 March; 9(3): 501-5.
  http://www.ncbi.nlm.nih.gov:80/entrez/query.fcgi?cmd=Retrieve&db=PubMed&list_uids=7885047&dopt=Abstract

- **Childhood acute lymphoblastic leukemia immunophenotypes and their prognostic significance: experience of the IGCI-study in 389 children. International Society for Chemo-immunotherapy (IGCI-Vienna) Cooperative Group.**
  Author(s): Holowiecki J, Koehler M, Zintl Z, Kardos G, Lutz D, Krzemien S, Rewesz T, Brugiatelli M, Callea V, Kachel L, et al.
  Source: Leukemia & Lymphoma. 1992 June; 7(3): 225-34.
  http://www.ncbi.nlm.nih.gov:80/entrez/query.fcgi?cmd=Retrieve&db=PubMed&list_uids=1477650&dopt=Abstract

- **Childhood acute lymphoblastic leukemia relapse in the uterine cervix.**
  Author(s): Tsuruchi N, Okamura J.

Source: Journal of Pediatric Hematology/Oncology : Official Journal of the American Society of Pediatric Hematology/Oncology. 1996 August; 18(3): 311-3.
http://www.ncbi.nlm.nih.gov:80/entrez/query.fcgi?cmd=Retrieve&db=PubMed&list_uids=8689350&dopt=Abstract

- **Childhood acute lymphoblastic leukemia. a survey of children treated between 1963 and 1972 at Children's Memorial Hospital, Chicago.**
  Author(s): Pierce M, Borges WH, Hackl E, Dyer A, Lipp V.
  Source: J Am Med Womens Assoc. 1974 December; 29(12): 527-8, 530-1, 534-43, 546. No Abstract Available.
  http://www.ncbi.nlm.nih.gov:80/entrez/query.fcgi?cmd=Retrieve&db=PubMed&list_uids=4374470&dopt=Abstract

- **Clinical and cytokinetic aspects of remission induction of childhood acute lymphoblastic leukemia (ALL): addition of an anthracycline to vincristine and prednisone.**
  Author(s): Sallan SE, Camitta BM, Frei E 3rd, Furman L, Leavitt P, Bishop Y, Jaffe N.
  Source: Medical and Pediatric Oncology. 1977; 3(3): 281-7.
  http://www.ncbi.nlm.nih.gov:80/entrez/query.fcgi?cmd=Retrieve&db=PubMed&list_uids=284168&dopt=Abstract

- **Clinical importance of minimal residual disease in childhood acute lymphoblastic leukemia.**
  Author(s): Coustan-Smith E, Sancho J, Hancock ML, Boyett JM, Behm FG, Raimondi SC, Sandlund JT, Rivera GK, Rubnitz JE, Ribeiro RC, Pui CH, Campana D.
  Source: Blood. 2000 October 15; 96(8): 2691-6.
  http://www.ncbi.nlm.nih.gov:80/entrez/query.fcgi?cmd=Retrieve&db=PubMed&list_uids=11023499&dopt=Abstract

- **Combination chemotherapy in relapsed childhood acute lymphoblastic leukemia.**
  Author(s): Amato KR, Sallan SE, Lipton JM.
  Source: Cancer Treat Rep. 1984 February; 68(2): 411-2.
  http://www.ncbi.nlm.nih.gov:80/entrez/query.fcgi?cmd=Retrieve&db=PubMed&list_uids=6583001&dopt=Abstract

- **Comparison of the therapeutic response of patients with childhood acute lymphoblastic leukemia in relapse to vindesine versus vincristine in combination with prednisone and L-asparaginase: a**

phase III trial.
Author(s): Anderson J, Krivit W, Chilcote R, Pyesmany A, Chard R, Hammond D.
Source: Cancer Treat Rep. 1981 November-December; 65(11-12): 1015-9.
http://www.ncbi.nlm.nih.gov:80/entrez/query.fcgi?cmd=Retrieve&db=PubMed&list_uids=6945911&dopt=Abstract

- **Cyclophosphamide (NSC-26271) maintenance therapy after a second remission of childhood acute lymphoblastic leukemia: comparative clinical trial (standard dose versus intermittent high dose versus cyclophosphamide plus cytosine arabinoside (NSC-63878)).**
  Author(s): Albo V, Movassaghi N, Sitarz AL, Hammond D, Weiner J, Reed A.
  Source: Cancer Chemother Rep. 1975 November-December; 59(6): 1097-102.
  http://www.ncbi.nlm.nih.gov:80/entrez/query.fcgi?cmd=Retrieve&db=PubMed&list_uids=769949&dopt=Abstract

- **Cytosine arabinoside/cyclophosphamide pulses during continuation therapy for childhood acute lymphoblastic leukemia. Potential selective effect in T-cell leukemia.**
  Author(s): Lauer SJ, Pinkel D, Buchanan GR, Sartain P, Cornet JM, Krance R, Borella LD, Casper JT, Kun LE, Hoffman RG, et al.
  Source: Cancer. 1987 November 15; 60(10): 2366-71.
  http://www.ncbi.nlm.nih.gov:80/entrez/query.fcgi?cmd=Retrieve&db=PubMed&list_uids=3499211&dopt=Abstract

- **Decrease in number of CD16(Leu 11)+CD45RA(2H4)+ cells and defective production of natural killer cytotoxic factor in childhood acute lymphoblastic leukemia.**
  Author(s): Yamada S, Komiyama A.
  Source: Leukemia Research. 1991; 15(9): 785-90.
  http://www.ncbi.nlm.nih.gov:80/entrez/query.fcgi?cmd=Retrieve&db=PubMed&list_uids=1833597&dopt=Abstract

- **Decreased cytotoxic potential of fresh and recombinant interleukin 2-cultured large granular lymphocytes in childhood acute lymphoblastic leukemia.**
  Author(s): Yamada S, Miyagawa Y, Komiyama A.

- **Demodicidosis in childhood acute lymphoblastic leukemia; an opportunistic infection occurring with immunosuppression.**
  Author(s): Ivy SP, Mackall CL, Gore L, Gress RE, Hartley AH.
  Source: The Journal of Pediatrics. 1995 November; 127(5): 751-4.
  http://www.ncbi.nlm.nih.gov:80/entrez/query.fcgi?cmd=Retrieve&db=PubMed&list_uids=7472831&dopt=Abstract

- **Deoxycytidine kinase mRNA expression in childhood acute lymphoblastic leukemia.**
  Author(s): Stammler G, Zintl F, Sauerbrey A, Volm M.
  Source: Anti-Cancer Drugs. 1997 June; 8(5): 517-21.
  http://www.ncbi.nlm.nih.gov:80/entrez/query.fcgi?cmd=Retrieve&db=PubMed&list_uids=9215616&dopt=Abstract

- **Early response to induction therapy as a predictor of disease-free survival and late recurrence of childhood acute lymphoblastic leukemia: a report from the Childrens Cancer Study Group.**
  Author(s): Miller DR, Coccia PF, Bleyer WA, Lukens JN, Siegel SE, Sather HN, Hammond GD.
  Source: Journal of Clinical Oncology : Official Journal of the American Society of Clinical Oncology. 1989 December; 7(12): 1807-15.
  http://www.ncbi.nlm.nih.gov:80/entrez/query.fcgi?cmd=Retrieve&db=PubMed&list_uids=2685179&dopt=Abstract

- **Effectiveness of intensified rotational combination chemotherapy for late hematologic relapse of childhood acute lymphoblastic leukemia.**
  Author(s): Rivera GK, Hudson MM, Liu Q, Benaim E, Ribeiro RC, Crist WM, Pui CH.
  Source: Blood. 1996 August 1; 88(3): 831-7.
  http://www.ncbi.nlm.nih.gov:80/entrez/query.fcgi?cmd=Retrieve&db=PubMed&list_uids=8704238&dopt=Abstract

- **Epidural spinal cord compression as an initial symptom in childhood acute lymphoblastic leukemia: rapid decompression by local irradiation and systemic chemotherapy.**
  Author(s): Kataoka A, Shimizu K, Matsumoto T, Shintaku N, Okuno T, Takahashi Y, Akaishi K.

- **Four-agent induction and intensive asparaginase therapy for treatment of childhood acute lymphoblastic leukemia.**
  Author(s): Clavell LA, Gelber RD, Cohen HJ, Hitchcock-Bryan S, Cassady JR, Tarbell NJ, Blattner SR, Tantravahi R, Leavitt P, Sallan SE.
  Source: The New England Journal of Medicine. 1986 September 11; 315(11): 657-63.
  http://www.ncbi.nlm.nih.gov:80/entrez/query.fcgi?cmd=Retrieve&db=PubMed&list_uids=2943992&dopt=Abstract

- **Four-agent induction/consolidation therapy for childhood acute lymphoblastic leukemia: an Indian experience.**
  Author(s): Advani SH, Iyer RS, Pai SK, Gopal R, Saikia TK, Nair CN, Kurkure PA, Nadkarni KS, Pai VR.
  Source: American Journal of Hematology. 1992 April; 39(4): 242-8.
  http://www.ncbi.nlm.nih.gov:80/entrez/query.fcgi?cmd=Retrieve&db=PubMed&list_uids=1553952&dopt=Abstract

- **High incidence of potential p53 inactivation in poor outcome childhood acute lymphoblastic leukemia at diagnosis.**
  Author(s): Marks DI, Kurz BW, Link MP, Ng E, Shuster JJ, Lauer SJ, Brodsky I, Haines DS.
  Source: Blood. 1996 February 1; 87(3): 1155-61.
  http://www.ncbi.nlm.nih.gov:80/entrez/query.fcgi?cmd=Retrieve&db=PubMed&list_uids=8562942&dopt=Abstract

- **Ifosfamide and etoposide in recurrent childhood acute lymphoblastic leukemia.**
  Author(s): Crooks GM, Sato JK.
  Source: Journal of Pediatric Hematology/Oncology: Official Journal of the American Society of Pediatric Hematology/Oncology. 1995 February; 17(1): 34-8.
  http://www.ncbi.nlm.nih.gov:80/entrez/query.fcgi?cmd=Retrieve&db=PubMed&list_uids=7743235&dopt=Abstract

- **Improved outcome in high-risk childhood acute lymphoblastic leukemia defined by prednisone-poor response treated with double Berlin-Frankfurt-Muenster protocol II.**

Author(s): Arico M, Valsecchi MG, Conter V, Rizzari C, Pession A, Messina C, Barisone E, Poggi V, De Rossi G, Locatelli F, Micalizzi MC, Basso G, Masera G.
Source: Blood. 2002 July 15; 100(2): 420-6.
http://www.ncbi.nlm.nih.gov:80/entrez/query.fcgi?cmd=Retrieve&db=PubMed&list_uids=12091331&dopt=Abstract

- **In vitro cellular drug resistance and prognosis in newly diagnosed childhood acute lymphoblastic leukemia.**
  Author(s): Kaspers GJ, Veerman AJ, Pieters R, Van Zantwijk CH, Smets LA, Van Wering ER, Van Der Does-Van Den Berg A.
  Source: Blood. 1997 October 1; 90(7): 2723-9.
  http://www.ncbi.nlm.nih.gov:80/entrez/query.fcgi?cmd=Retrieve&db=PubMed&list_uids=9326239&dopt=Abstract

- **In vitro drug sensitivity testing can predict induction failure and early relapse of childhood acute lymphoblastic leukemia.**
  Author(s): Hongo T, Yajima S, Sakurai M, Horikoshi Y, Hanada R.
  Source: Blood. 1997 April 15; 89(8): 2959-65.
  http://www.ncbi.nlm.nih.gov:80/entrez/query.fcgi?cmd=Retrieve&db=PubMed&list_uids=9108416&dopt=Abstract

- **Intact T-cell regenerative capacity in childhood acute lymphoblastic leukemia after remission induction therapy.**
  Author(s): Moritz B, Eder J, Meister B, Heitger A.
  Source: Medical and Pediatric Oncology. 2001 February; 36(2): 283-9.
  http://www.ncbi.nlm.nih.gov:80/entrez/query.fcgi?cmd=Retrieve&db=PubMed&list_uids=11452936&dopt=Abstract

- **Intellectual function in long-term survivors of childhood acute lymphoblastic leukemia: protective effect of pre-irradiation methotrexate? A Childrens Cancer Study Group study.**
  Author(s): Balsom WR, Bleyer WA, Robison LL, Heyn RM, Meadows AT, Sitarz A, Blatt J, Sather HN, Hammond GD.
  Source: Medical and Pediatric Oncology. 1991; 19(6): 486-92.
  http://www.ncbi.nlm.nih.gov:80/entrez/query.fcgi?cmd=Retrieve&db=PubMed&list_uids=1961135&dopt=Abstract

- **Intensive retreatment of childhood acute lymphoblastic leukemia in first bone marrow relapse. A Pediatric Oncology Group Study.**
  Author(s): Rivera GK, Buchanan G, Boyett JM, Camitta B, Ochs J, Kalwinsky D, Amylon M, Vietti TJ, Crist WM.

Source: The New England Journal of Medicine. 1986 July 31; 315(5): 273-8.
http://www.ncbi.nlm.nih.gov:80/entrez/query.fcgi?cmd=Retrieve&db=PubMed&list_uids=3523250&dopt=Abstract

- **Intermediate-dose methotrexate versus cranial irradiation in childhood acute lymphoblastic leukemia: a ten-year follow-up.**
  Author(s): Freeman AI, Boyett JM, Glicksman AS, Brecher ML, Leventhal BG, Sinks LF, Holland JF.
  Source: Medical and Pediatric Oncology. 1997 February; 28(2): 98-107.
  http://www.ncbi.nlm.nih.gov:80/entrez/query.fcgi?cmd=Retrieve&db=PubMed&list_uids=8986145&dopt=Abstract

- **Intermittent combination chemotherapy with adriamycin for childhood acute lymphoblastic leukemia: clinical results.**
  Author(s): Sallan SE, Cammita BM, Cassady JR, Nathan DG, Frei E 3rd.
  Source: Blood. 1978 March; 51(3): 425-33.
  http://www.ncbi.nlm.nih.gov:80/entrez/query.fcgi?cmd=Retrieve&db=PubMed&list_uids=272207&dopt=Abstract

- **Intermittent combined chemotherapy with doxorubicin in recurrent childhood acute lymphoblastic leukemia.**
  Author(s): Ward Platt MP, Mott MG, Eden OB.
  Source: Medical and Pediatric Oncology. 1982; 10(6): 563-8.
  http://www.ncbi.nlm.nih.gov:80/entrez/query.fcgi?cmd=Retrieve&db=PubMed&list_uids=6960230&dopt=Abstract

- **Isolated breast relapse after allogeneic bone marrow transplantation for childhood acute lymphoblastic leukemia.**
  Author(s): Conter V, D'Angelo P, Rovelli A, Uderzo C, Jankovic M, Bratina G, Masera G.
  Source: Medical and Pediatric Oncology. 1992; 20(2): 165-8.
  http://www.ncbi.nlm.nih.gov:80/entrez/query.fcgi?cmd=Retrieve&db=PubMed&list_uids=1734223&dopt=Abstract

- **Low-dose versus high-dose methotrexate during remission induction in childhood acute lymphoblastic leukemia (Protocol 81-01 update).**
  Author(s): Niemeyer CM, Gelber RD, Tarbell NJ, Donnelly M, Clavell LA, Blattner SR, Donahue K, Cohen HJ, Sallan SE.
  Source: Blood. 1991 November 15; 78(10): 2514-9.
  http://www.ncbi.nlm.nih.gov:80/entrez/query.fcgi?cmd=Retrieve&db=PubMed&list_uids=1824248&dopt=Abstract

- **Maintenance chemotherapy for childhood acute lymphoblastic leukemia: relation of bone-marrow and hepatotoxicity to the concentration of methotrexate in erythrocytes.**
  Author(s): Schmiegelow K, Schroder H, Pulczynska MK, Hejl M.
  Source: Cancer Chemotherapy and Pharmacology. 1989; 25(1): 65-9.
  http://www.ncbi.nlm.nih.gov:80/entrez/query.fcgi?cmd=Retrieve&db=PubMed&list_uids=2591003&dopt=Abstract

- **Medical Research Council leukaemia trial--UKALL V: an attempt to reduce the immunosuppressive effects of therapy in childhood acute lymphoblastic leukemia. Report to the Council by the Working Party on Leukaemia in Childhood.**
  Author(s): Chessells JM, Durrant J, Hardy RM, Richards S.
  Source: Journal of Clinical Oncology : Official Journal of the American Society of Clinical Oncology. 1986 December; 4(12): 1758-64.
  http://www.ncbi.nlm.nih.gov:80/entrez/query.fcgi?cmd=Retrieve&db=PubMed&list_uids=3537216&dopt=Abstract

- **Modified BFM protocol for childhood acute lymphoblastic leukemia: a retrospective analysis.**
  Author(s): Aziz Z, Zahid M, Mahmood R, Maqbool S.
  Source: Medical and Pediatric Oncology. 1997 January; 28(1): 48-53.
  http://www.ncbi.nlm.nih.gov:80/entrez/query.fcgi?cmd=Retrieve&db=PubMed&list_uids=8950336&dopt=Abstract

- **Molecular and clinical prognostic factors in BFM-treated childhood acute lymphoblastic leukemia patients: a single institution series.**
  Author(s): Ruano D, Diaz MA, Tutor O, Garcia-Sanchez F, Martinez P, Madero L.
  Source: Haematologica. 2000 August; 85(8): 877-8. No Abstract Available.
  http://www.ncbi.nlm.nih.gov:80/entrez/query.fcgi?cmd=Retrieve&db=PubMed&list_uids=10942942&dopt=Abstract

- **Monthly pulses of vincristine and prednisone prevent bone marrow and testicular relapse in low-risk childhood acute lymphoblastic leukemia: a report of the CCG-161 study by the Childrens Cancer Study Group.**
  Author(s): Bleyer WA, Sather HN, Nickerson HJ, Coccia PF, Finklestein JZ, Miller DR, Littman PS, Lukens JN, Siegel SE, Hammond GD.

Source: Journal of Clinical Oncology : Official Journal of the American Society of Clinical Oncology. 1991 June; 9(6): 1012-21.
http://www.ncbi.nlm.nih.gov:80/entrez/query.fcgi?cmd=Retrieve&db=PubMed&list_uids=2033414&dopt=Abstract

- **Motor nervous pathway function is impaired after treatment of childhood acute lymphoblastic leukemia: a study with motor evoked potentials.**
  Author(s): Harila-Saari AH, Huuskonen UE, Tolonen U, Vainionpaa LK, Lanning BM.
  Source: Medical and Pediatric Oncology. 2001 March; 36(3): 345-51.
  http://www.ncbi.nlm.nih.gov:80/entrez/query.fcgi?cmd=Retrieve&db=PubMed&list_uids=11241435&dopt=Abstract

- **Nerve lesions after therapy for childhood acute lymphoblastic leukemia.**
  Author(s): Harila-Saari AH, Vainionpaa LK, Kovala TT, Tolonen EU, Lanning BM.
  Source: Cancer. 1998 January 1; 82(1): 200-7.
  http://www.ncbi.nlm.nih.gov:80/entrez/query.fcgi?cmd=Retrieve&db=PubMed&list_uids=9428498&dopt=Abstract

Additional Web Resources

A number of additional Web sites offer encyclopedic information covering CAM and related topics. The following is a representative sample:

- Alternative Medicine Foundation, Inc.: **http://www.herbmed.org/**
- AOL: **http://search.aol.com/cat.adp?id=169&layer=&from=subcats**
- Chinese Medicine: **http://www.newcenturynutrition.com/**
- drkoop.com®:
  http://www.drkoop.com/InteractiveMedicine/IndexC.html
- Family Village: **http://www.familyvillage.wisc.edu/med_altn.htm**
- Google: **http://directory.google.com/Top/Health/Alternative/**
- Healthnotes: **http://www.thedacare.org/healthnotes/**
- Open Directory Project: **http://dmoz.org/Health/Alternative/**
- TPN.com: **http://www.tnp.com/**
- Yahoo.com: **http://dir.yahoo.com/Health/Alternative_Medicine/**
- WebMD®Health: **http://my.webmd.com/drugs_and_herbs**

- WellNet: **http://www.wellnet.ca/herbsa-c.htm**
- WholeHealthMD.com: **http://www.wholehealthmd.com/reflib/0,1529,,00.html**

The following is a specific Web list relating to childhood acute lymphoblastic leukemia; please note that any particular subject below may indicate either a therapeutic use, or a contraindication (potential danger), and does not reflect an official recommendation:

- **Herbs and Supplements**

    Aesculus
    Alternative names: Horse Chestnut; Aesculus hippocastanum L.
    Source: Alternative Medicine Foundation, Inc.;
    www.amfoundation.org
    Hyperlink: http://www.herbmed.org/

    Inhalant, Systemic, and Topical Corticosteroids
    Source: Integrative Medicine Communications;
    www.onemedicine.com
    Hyperlink:
    http://www.drkoop.com/interactivemedicine/ConsDepletions/AntiinflammatoryMedicationsInhalantSystemicandTopicalCorticosteroidscl.html

General References

A good place to find general background information on CAM is the National Library of Medicine. It has prepared within the MEDLINEplus system an information topic page dedicated to complementary and alternative medicine. To access this page, go to the MEDLINEplus site at: **www.nlm.nih.gov/medlineplus/alternativemedicine.html.** This Web site provides a general overview of various topics and can lead to a number of general sources. The following additional references describe, in broad terms, alternative and complementary medicine (sorted alphabetically by title; hyperlinks provide rankings, information, and reviews at Amazon.com):

- **Alternative Medicine Definitive Guide to Cancer** by W. John Diamond, et al; Hardcover - 1120 pages Package edition (March 18, 1997),

Alternativemedicine.Com Books; ISBN: 1887299017;
http://www.amazon.com/exec/obidos/ASIN/1887299017/icongroupinterna

- **Beating Cancer With Nutrition - Revised** by Patrick Quillin, Noreen Quillin (Contributor); Paperback - 352 pages; Book & CD edition (January 1, 2001), Bookworld Services; ISBN: 0963837281;
http://www.amazon.com/exec/obidos/ASIN/0963837281/icongroupinterna

- **Cancer: Increasing Your Odds for Survival - A Resource Guide for Integrating Mainstream, Alternative and Complementary Therapies** by David Bognar, Walter Cronkite; Paperback (August 1998), Hunter House; ISBN: 0897932471;
http://www.amazon.com/exec/obidos/ASIN/0897932471/icongroupinterna

- **Choices in Healing** by Michael Lerner; Paperback - 696 pages; (February 28, 1996), MIT Press; ISBN: 0262621045;
http://www.amazon.com/exec/obidos/ASIN/0262621045/icongroupinterna

- **The Gerson Therapy: The Amazing Nutritional Program for Cancer and Other Illnesses** by Charlotte Gerson, Morton Walker, D.P.M.; Paperback - 448 pages (October 2001), Kensington Publishing Corp.; ISBN: 1575666286;
http://www.amazon.com/exec/obidos/ASIN/1575666286/icongroupinterna

- **Natural Compounds in Cancer Therapy** by John C. Boik; Paperback - 520 pages (March 2001), Oregon Medical Press; ISBN: 0964828014;
http://www.amazon.com/exec/obidos/ASIN/0964828014/icongroupinterna

- **There's No Place Like Hope: A Guide to Beating Cancer in Mind-Sized Bites** by Vickie Girard, Dan Zadra (Editor); Hardcover - 161 pages (April 2001), Compendium Inc.; ISBN: 1888387416;
http://www.amazon.com/exec/obidos/ASIN/1888387416/icongroupinterna

- **Your Life in Your Hands** by Jane A. Plant, Ph.D; Hardcover - 272 pages (December 13, 2000), St. Martins Press (Trade); ISBN: 0312275617;
http://www.amazon.com/exec/obidos/ASIN/0312275617/icongroupinterna

For additional information on complementary and alternative medicine, ask your child's doctor or write to:

National Institutes of Health
National Center for Complementary and Alternative Medicine Clearinghouse
P. O. Box 8218
Silver Spring, MD 20907-8218

APPENDIX C. FINDING MEDICAL LIBRARIES

Overview

At a medical library you can find medical texts and reference books, consumer health publications, specialty newspapers and magazines, as well as medical journals. In this appendix, we show you how to quickly find a medical library in your area.

Preparation

Before going to the library, highlight the references mentioned in this sourcebook that you find interesting. Focus on those items that are not available via the Internet, and ask the reference librarian for help with your search. He or she may know of additional resources that could be helpful to you. Most importantly, your local public library and medical libraries have Interlibrary Loan programs with the National Library of Medicine (NLM), one of the largest medical collections in the world. According to the NLM, most of the literature in the general and historical collections of the National Library of Medicine is available on interlibrary loan to any library. NLM's interlibrary loan services are only available to libraries. If you would like to access NLM medical literature, then visit a library in your area that can request the publications for you.[213]

---

[213] Adapted from the NLM: http://www.nlm.nih.gov/psd/cas/interlibrary.html

Finding a Local Medical Library

The quickest method to locate medical libraries is to use the Internet-based directory published by the National Network of Libraries of Medicine (NN/LM). This network includes 4626 members and affiliates that provide many services to librarians, health professionals, and the public. To find a library in your area, simply visit **http://nnlm.gov/members/adv.html** or call 1-800-338-7657.

Medical Libraries Open to the Public

In addition to the NN/LM, the National Library of Medicine (NLM) lists a number of libraries that are generally open to the public and have reference facilities. The following is the NLM's list plus hyperlinks to each library Web site. These Web pages can provide information on hours of operation and other restrictions. The list below is a small sample of libraries recommended by the National Library of Medicine (sorted alphabetically by name of the U.S. state or Canadian province where the library is located):[214]

- **Alabama:** Health InfoNet of Jefferson County (Jefferson County Library Cooperative, Lister Hill Library of the Health Sciences), **http://www.uab.edu/infonet/**

- **Alabama:** Richard M. Scrushy Library (American Sports Medicine Institute), **http://www.asmi.org/LIBRARY.HTM**

- **Arizona:** Samaritan Regional Medical Center: The Learning Center (Samaritan Health System, Phoenix, Arizona), **http://www.samaritan.edu/library/bannerlibs.htm**

- **California:** Kris Kelly Health Information Center (St. Joseph Health System), **http://www.humboldt1.com/~kkhic/index.html**

- **California:** Community Health Library of Los Gatos (Community Health Library of Los Gatos), **http://www.healthlib.org/orgresources.html**

- **California:** Consumer Health Program and Services (CHIPS) (County of Los Angeles Public Library, Los Angeles County Harbor-UCLA Medical Center Library) - Carson, CA, **http://www.colapublib.org/services/chips.html**

- **California:** Gateway Health Library (Sutter Gould Medical Foundation)

- **California:** Health Library (Stanford University Medical Center), **http://www-med.stanford.edu/healthlibrary/**

---

[214] Adapted from http://www.nlm.nih.gov/medlineplus/libraries.html.

- **California:** Patient Education Resource Center - Health Information and Resources (University of California, San Francisco), **http://sfghdean.ucsf.edu/barnett/PERC/default.asp**
- **California:** Redwood Health Library (Petaluma Health Care District), **http://www.phcd.org/rdwdlib.html**
- **California:** San José PlaneTree Health Library, **http://planetreesanjose.org/**
- **California:** Sutter Resource Library (Sutter Hospitals Foundation), **http://go.sutterhealth.org/comm/resc-library/sac-resources.html**
- **California:** University of California, Davis. Health Sciences Libraries
- **California:** ValleyCare Health Library & Ryan Comer Cancer Resource Center (ValleyCare Health System), **http://www.valleycare.com/library.html**
- **California:** Washington Community Health Resource Library (Washington Community Health Resource Library), **http://www.healthlibrary.org/**
- **Colorado:** William V. Gervasini Memorial Library (Exempla Healthcare), **http://www.exempla.org/conslib.htm**
- **Connecticut:** Hartford Hospital Health Science Libraries (Hartford Hospital), **http://www.harthosp.org/library/**
- **Connecticut:** Healthnet: Connecticut Consumer Health Information Center (University of Connecticut Health Center, Lyman Maynard Stowe Library), **http://library.uchc.edu/departm/hnet/**
- **Connecticut:** Waterbury Hospital Health Center Library (Waterbury Hospital), **http://www.waterburyhospital.com/library/consumer.shtml**
- **Delaware:** Consumer Health Library (Christiana Care Health System, Eugene du Pont Preventive Medicine & Rehabilitation Institute), **http://www.christianacare.org/health_guide/health_guide_pmri_health_info.cfm**
- **Delaware:** Lewis B. Flinn Library (Delaware Academy of Medicine), **http://www.delamed.org/chls.html**
- **Georgia:** Family Resource Library (Medical College of Georgia), **http://cmc.mcg.edu/kids_families/fam_resources/fam_res_lib/frl.htm**
- **Georgia:** Health Resource Center (Medical Center of Central Georgia), **http://www.mccg.org/hrc/hrchome.asp**
- **Hawaii:** Hawaii Medical Library: Consumer Health Information Service (Hawaii Medical Library), **http://hml.org/CHIS/**

- **Idaho:** DeArmond Consumer Health Library (Kootenai Medical Center), http://www.nicon.org/DeArmond/index.htm
- **Illinois:** Health Learning Center of Northwestern Memorial Hospital (Northwestern Memorial Hospital, Health Learning Center), http://www.nmh.org/health_info/hlc.html
- **Illinois:** Medical Library (OSF Saint Francis Medical Center), http://www.osfsaintfrancis.org/general/library/
- **Kentucky:** Medical Library - Services for Patients, Families, Students & the Public (Central Baptist Hospital), http://www.centralbap.com/education/community/library.htm
- **Kentucky:** University of Kentucky - Health Information Library (University of Kentucky, Chandler Medical Center, Health Information Library), http://www.mc.uky.edu/PatientEd/
- **Louisiana:** Alton Ochsner Medical Foundation Library (Alton Ochsner Medical Foundation), http://www.ochsner.org/library/
- **Louisiana:** Louisiana State University Health Sciences Center Medical Library-Shreveport, http://lib-sh.lsuhsc.edu/
- **Maine:** Franklin Memorial Hospital Medical Library (Franklin Memorial Hospital), http://www.fchn.org/fmh/lib.htm
- **Maine:** Gerrish-True Health Sciences Library (Central Maine Medical Center), http://www.cmmc.org/library/library.html
- **Maine:** Hadley Parrot Health Science Library (Eastern Maine Healthcare), http://www.emh.org/hll/hpl/guide.htm
- **Maine:** Maine Medical Center Library (Maine Medical Center), http://www.mmc.org/library/
- **Maine:** Parkview Hospital, http://www.parkviewhospital.org/communit.htm#Library
- **Maine:** Southern Maine Medical Center Health Sciences Library (Southern Maine Medical Center), http://www.smmc.org/services/service.php3?choice=10
- **Maine:** Stephens Memorial Hospital Health Information Library (Western Maine Health), http://www.wmhcc.com/hil_frame.html
- **Manitoba, Canada:** Consumer & Patient Health Information Service (University of Manitoba Libraries), http://www.umanitoba.ca/libraries/units/health/reference/chis.html
- **Manitoba, Canada:** J.W. Crane Memorial Library (Deer Lodge Centre), http://www.deerlodge.mb.ca/library/libraryservices.shtml

- **Maryland:** Health Information Center at the Wheaton Regional Library (Montgomery County, Md., Dept. of Public Libraries, Wheaton Regional Library), http://www.mont.lib.md.us/healthinfo/hic.asp
- **Massachusetts:** Baystate Medical Center Library (Baystate Health System), http://www.baystatehealth.com/1024/
- **Massachusetts:** Boston University Medical Center Alumni Medical Library (Boston University Medical Center), http://medlibwww.bu.edu/library/lib.html
- **Massachusetts:** Lowell General Hospital Health Sciences Library (Lowell General Hospital), http://www.lowellgeneral.org/library/HomePageLinks/WWW.htm
- **Massachusetts:** Paul E. Woodard Health Sciences Library (New England Baptist Hospital), http://www.nebh.org/health_lib.asp
- **Massachusetts:** St. Luke's Hospital Health Sciences Library (St. Luke's Hospital), http://www.southcoast.org/library/
- **Massachusetts:** Treadwell Library Consumer Health Reference Center (Massachusetts General Hospital), http://www.mgh.harvard.edu/library/chrcindex.html
- **Massachusetts:** UMass HealthNet (University of Massachusetts Medical School), http://healthnet.umassmed.edu/
- **Michigan:** Botsford General Hospital Library - Consumer Health (Botsford General Hospital, Library & Internet Services), http://www.botsfordlibrary.org/consumer.htm
- **Michigan:** Helen DeRoy Medical Library (Providence Hospital and Medical Centers), http://www.providence-hospital.org/library/
- **Michigan:** Marquette General Hospital - Consumer Health Library (Marquette General Hospital, Health Information Center), http://www.mgh.org/center.html
- **Michigan:** Patient Education Resouce Center - University of Michigan Cancer Center (University of Michigan Comprehensive Cancer Center), http://www.cancer.med.umich.edu/learn/leares.htm
- **Michigan:** Sladen Library & Center for Health Information Resources - Consumer Health Information, http://www.sladen.hfhs.org/library/consumer/index.html
- **Montana:** Center for Health Information (St. Patrick Hospital and Health Sciences Center), http://www.saintpatrick.org/chi/librarydetail.php3?ID=41

- **National:** Consumer Health Library Directory (Medical Library Association, Consumer and Patient Health Information Section), http://caphis.mlanet.org/directory/index.html
- **National:** National Network of Libraries of Medicine (National Library of Medicine) - provides library services for health professionals in the United States who do not have access to a medical library, http://nnlm.gov/
- **National:** NN/LM List of Libraries Serving the Public (National Network of Libraries of Medicine), http://nnlm.gov/members/
- **Nevada:** Health Science Library, West Charleston Library (Las Vegas Clark County Library District), http://www.lvccld.org/special_collections/medical/index.htm
- **New Hampshire:** Dartmouth Biomedical Libraries (Dartmouth College Library), http://www.dartmouth.edu/~biomed/resources.htmld/conshealth.htmld/
- **New Jersey:** Consumer Health Library (Rahway Hospital), http://www.rahwayhospital.com/library.htm
- **New Jersey:** Dr. Walter Phillips Health Sciences Library (Englewood Hospital and Medical Center), http://www.englewoodhospital.com/links/index.htm
- **New Jersey:** Meland Foundation (Englewood Hospital and Medical Center), http://www.geocities.com/ResearchTriangle/9360/
- **New York:** Choices in Health Information (New York Public Library) - NLM Consumer Pilot Project participant, http://www.nypl.org/branch/health/links.html
- **New York:** Health Information Center (Upstate Medical University, State University of New York), http://www.upstate.edu/library/hic/
- **New York:** Health Sciences Library (Long Island Jewish Medical Center), http://www.lij.edu/library/library.html
- **New York:** ViaHealth Medical Library (Rochester General Hospital), http://www.nyam.org/library/
- **Ohio:** Consumer Health Library (Akron General Medical Center, Medical & Consumer Health Library), http://www.akrongeneral.org/hwlibrary.htm
- **Oklahoma:** Saint Francis Health System Patient/Family Resource Center (Saint Francis Health System), http://www.sfh-tulsa.com/patientfamilycenter/default.asp

- **Oregon:** Planetree Health Resource Center (Mid-Columbia Medical Center), **http://www.mcmc.net/phrc/**
- **Pennsylvania:** Community Health Information Library (Milton S. Hershey Medical Center), **http://www.hmc.psu.edu/commhealth/**
- **Pennsylvania:** Community Health Resource Library (Geisinger Medical Center), **http://www.geisinger.edu/education/commlib.shtml**
- **Pennsylvania:** HealthInfo Library (Moses Taylor Hospital), **http://www.mth.org/healthwellness.html**
- **Pennsylvania:** Hopwood Library (University of Pittsburgh, Health Sciences Library System), **http://www.hsls.pitt.edu/chi/hhrcinfo.html**
- **Pennsylvania:** Koop Community Health Information Center (College of Physicians of Philadelphia), **http://www.collphyphil.org/kooppg1.shtml**
- **Pennsylvania:** Learning Resources Center - Medical Library (Susquehanna Health System), **http://www.shscares.org/services/lrc/index.asp**
- **Pennsylvania:** Medical Library (UPMC Health System), **http://www.upmc.edu/passavant/library.htm**
- **Quebec, Canada:** Medical Library (Montreal General Hospital), **http://ww2.mcgill.ca/mghlib/**
- **South Dakota:** Rapid City Regional Hospital - Health Information Center (Rapid City Regional Hospital, Health Information Center), **http://www.rcrh.org/education/LibraryResourcesConsumers.htm**
- **Texas:** Houston HealthWays (Houston Academy of Medicine-Texas Medical Center Library), **http://hhw.library.tmc.edu/**
- **Texas:** Matustik Family Resource Center (Cook Children's Health Care System), **http://www.cookchildrens.com/Matustik_Library.html**
- **Washington:** Community Health Library (Kittitas Valley Community Hospital), **http://www.kvch.com/**
- **Washington:** Southwest Washington Medical Center Library (Southwest Washington Medical Center), **http://www.swmedctr.com/Home/**

Appendix D. Your Child's Rights and Insurance

Overview

Parents face a series of issues related more to the healthcare industry than to their children's medical conditions. This appendix covers two important topics in this regard: your responsibilities and your child's rights as a patient, and how to get the most out of your child's medical insurance plan.

Your Child's Rights as a Patient

The President's Advisory Commission on Consumer Protection and Quality in the Healthcare Industry has created the following summary of your child's rights as a patient.[215]

---

[215] Adapted from Consumer Bill of Rights and Responsibilities: http://www.hcqualitycommission.gov/press/cbor.html#head1.

Information Disclosure

Consumers have the right to receive accurate, easily understood information. Some consumers require assistance in making informed decisions about health plans, health professionals, and healthcare facilities. Such information includes:

- *Health plans.* Covered benefits, cost-sharing, and procedures for resolving complaints, licensure, certification, and accreditation status, comparable measures of quality and consumer satisfaction, provider network composition, the procedures that govern access to specialists and emergency services, and care management information.

- *Health professionals.* Education, board certification, and recertification, years of practice, experience performing certain procedures, and comparable measures of quality and consumer satisfaction.

- *Healthcare facilities.* Experience in performing certain procedures and services, accreditation status, comparable measures of quality, worker, and consumer satisfaction, and procedures for resolving complaints.

- *Consumer assistance programs.* Programs must be carefully structured to promote consumer confidence and to work cooperatively with health plans, providers, payers, and regulators. Desirable characteristics of such programs are sponsorship that ensures accountability to the interests of consumers and stable, adequate funding.

Choice of Providers and Plans

Consumers have the right to a choice of healthcare providers that is sufficient to ensure access to appropriate high-quality healthcare. To ensure such choice, the Commission recommends the following:

- *Provider network adequacy.* All health plan networks should provide access to sufficient numbers and types of providers to assure that all covered services will be accessible without unreasonable delay -- including access to emergency services 24 hours a day and 7 days a week. If a health plan has an insufficient number or type of providers to provide a covered benefit with the appropriate degree of specialization, the plan should ensure that the consumer obtains the benefit outside the network at no greater cost than if the benefit were obtained from participating providers.

- *Access to specialists.* Consumers with complex or serious medical conditions who require frequent specialty care should have direct access to a qualified specialist of their choice within a plan's network of providers. Authorizations, when required, should be for an adequate number of direct access visits under an approved treatment plan.

- *Transitional care.* Consumers who are undergoing a course of treatment for a chronic or disabling condition at the time they involuntarily change health plans or at a time when a provider is terminated by a plan for other than cause should be able to continue seeing their current specialty providers for up to 90 days to allow for transition of care.
- *Choice of health plans.* Public and private group purchasers should, wherever feasible, offer consumers a choice of high-quality health insurance plans.

Access to Emergency Services

Consumers have the right to access emergency healthcare services when and where the need arises. Health plans should provide payment when a consumer presents to an emergency department with acute symptoms of sufficient severity--including severe pain--such that a "prudent layperson" could reasonably expect the absence of medical attention to result in placing that consumer's health in serious jeopardy, serious impairment to bodily functions, or serious dysfunction of any bodily organ or part.

Participation in Treatment Decisions

Consumers have the right and responsibility to fully participate in all decisions related to their healthcare. Consumers who are unable to fully participate in treatment decisions have the right to be represented by parents, guardians, family members, or other conservators. Physicians and other health professionals should:

- Provide parents with sufficient information and opportunity to decide among treatment options consistent with the informed consent process.
- Discuss all treatment options with a parent in a culturally competent manner, including the option of no treatment at all.
- Ensure that persons with disabilities have effective communications with members of the health system in making such decisions.
- Discuss all current treatments a consumer may be undergoing.
- Discuss all risks, benefits, and consequences to treatment or nontreatment.

- Give parents the opportunity to refuse treatment for their children and to express preferences about future treatment decisions.

- Discuss the use of advance directives -- both living wills and durable powers of attorney for healthcare -- with parents.

- Abide by the decisions made by parents consistent with the informed consent process.

Health plans, health providers, and healthcare facilities should:

- Disclose to consumers factors -- such as methods of compensation, ownership of or interest in healthcare facilities, or matters of conscience -- that could influence advice or treatment decisions.

- Assure that provider contracts do not contain any so-called "gag clauses" or other contractual mechanisms that restrict healthcare providers' ability to communicate with and advise parents about medically necessary treatment options for their children.

- Be prohibited from penalizing or seeking retribution against healthcare professionals or other health workers for advocating on behalf of their patients.

Respect and Nondiscrimination

Consumers have the right to considerate, respectful care from all members of the healthcare industry at all times and under all circumstances. An environment of mutual respect is essential to maintain a quality healthcare system. To assure that right, the Commission recommends the following:

- Consumers must not be discriminated against in the delivery of healthcare services consistent with the benefits covered in their policy, or as required by law, based on race, ethnicity, national origin, religion, sex, age, mental or physical disability, sexual orientation, genetic information, or source of payment.

- Consumers eligible for coverage under the terms and conditions of a health plan or program, or as required by law, must not be discriminated against in marketing and enrollment practices based on race, ethnicity, national origin, religion, sex, age, mental or physical disability, sexual orientation, genetic information, or source of payment.

Confidentiality of Health Information

Consumers have the right to communicate with healthcare providers in confidence and to have the confidentiality of their individually identifiable healthcare information protected. Consumers also have the right to review and copy their own medical records and request amendments to their records.

Complaints and Appeals

Consumers have the right to a fair and efficient process for resolving differences with their health plans, healthcare providers, and the institutions that serve them, including a rigorous system of internal review and an independent system of external review. A free copy of the Patient's Bill of Rights is available from the American Hospital Association.[216]

Parent Responsibilities

To underscore the importance of finance in modern healthcare as well as your responsibility for the financial aspects of your child's care, the President's Advisory Commission on Consumer Protection and Quality in the Healthcare Industry has proposed that parents understand the following "Consumer Responsibilities."[217] In a healthcare system that protects consumers' rights, it is reasonable to expect and encourage consumers to assume certain responsibilities. Greater involvement by parents in their children's care increases the likelihood of achieving the best outcome and helps support a quality-oriented, cost-conscious environment. Such responsibilities include:

- Take responsibility for maximizing your child's healthy habits.
- Work collaboratively with healthcare providers in developing and carrying out your child's agreed-upon treatment plans.
- Disclose relevant information and clearly communicate wants and needs.

---

[216] To order your free copy of the Patient's Bill of Rights, telephone 312-422-3000 or visit the American Hospital Association's Web site: **http://www.aha.org**. Click on "Resource Center," go to "Search" at bottom of page, and then type in "Patient's Bill of Rights." The Patient's Bill of Rights is also available from Fax on Demand, at 312-422-2020, document number 471124.

[217] Adapted from **http://www.hcqualitycommission.gov/press/cbor.html#head1**.

- Use the insurance company's internal complaint and appeal processes to address your concerns.

- Recognize the reality of risks, the limits of the medical science, and the human fallibility of the healthcare professional.

- Be aware of a healthcare provider's obligation to be reasonably efficient and equitable in providing care to the community.

- Become knowledgeable about health plan coverage and options (when available) including all covered benefits, limitations, and exclusions, rules regarding use of network providers, coverage and referral rules, appropriate processes to secure additional information, and the process to appeal coverage decisions.

- Make a good-faith effort to meet financial obligations.

- Abide by administrative and operational procedures of health plans, healthcare providers, and Government health benefit programs.

Choosing an Insurance Plan

There are a number of official government agencies that help consumers understand their healthcare insurance choices.[218] The U.S. Department of Labor, in particular, recommends ten ways to make your health benefits choices work best for your family.[219]

1. Your options are important. There are many different types of health benefit plans. Find out which one your employer offers, then check out the plan, or plans, offered. Your employer's human resource office, the health plan administrator, or your union can provide information to help you match your family's needs and preferences with the available plans. The more information you have, the better your healthcare decisions will be.

2. Reviewing the benefits available. Do the plans offered cover preventive care, well-baby care, vision or dental care? Are there deductibles? Answers to these questions can help determine the out-of-pocket expenses you may face. Cheapest may not always be best. Your goal is high quality health benefits.

---

[218] More information about quality across programs is provided at the following AHRQ Web site:
http://www.ahrq.gov/consumer/qntascii/qnthplan.htm.
[219] Adapted from the Department of Labor:
http://www.dol.gov/dol/pwba/public/pubs/health/top10-text.html.

3. Look for quality. The quality of healthcare services varies, but quality can be measured. You should consider the quality of healthcare in deciding among the healthcare plans or options available to your family. Not all health plans, doctors, hospitals and other providers give the highest quality care. Fortunately, there is quality information you can use right now to help you compare your healthcare choices. Find out how you can measure quality. Consult the U.S. Department of Health and Human Services publication "Your Guide to Choosing Quality Health Care" on the Internet at **www.ahcpr.gov/consumer**.

4. Your plan's summary plan description (SPD) provides a wealth of information. Your health plan administrator can provide you with a copy of your plan's SPD. It outlines your family's benefits and your legal rights under the Employee Retirement Income Security Act (ERISA), the federal law that protects your family's health benefits. It should contain information about the coverage of dependents, what services will require a co-pay, and the circumstances under which your employer can change or terminate a health benefits plan. Save the SPD and all other health plan brochures and documents, along with memos or correspondence from your employer relating to health benefits.

5. Assess your benefit coverage as your family status changes. Marriage, divorce, childbirth or adoption, and the death of a spouse are all life events that may signal a need to change your health benefits. You, your spouse and dependent children may be eligible for a special enrollment period under provisions of the Health Insurance Portability and Accountability Act (HIPAA). Even without life-changing events, the information provided by your employer should tell you how you can change benefits or switch plans, if more than one plan is offered. If your spouse's employer also offers a health benefits package, consider coordinating both plans for maximum coverage.

6. Changing jobs and other life events can affect your family's health benefits. Under the Consolidated Omnibus Budget Reconciliation Act (COBRA), you, your covered spouse, and your dependent children may be eligible to purchase extended health coverage under your employer's plan if you lose your job, change employers, get divorced, or upon occurrence of certain other events. Coverage can range from 18 to 36 months depending on your situation. COBRA applies to most employers with 20 or more workers and requires your plan to notify you of your rights. Most plans require eligible individuals to make their COBRA election within 60 days of the plan's notice. Be sure to follow up with your plan sponsor if you don't receive notice, and make sure you respond within the allotted time.

7. HIPAA can also help if you are changing jobs, particularly if you have a medical condition. HIPAA generally limits pre-existing condition exclusions to a maximum of 12 months (18 months for late enrollees). HIPAA also requires this maximum period to be reduced by the length of time you had prior "creditable coverage." You should receive a certificate documenting your prior creditable coverage from your old plan when coverage ends.

8. Plan for retirement. Before you retire, find out what health benefits, if any, extend to you and your spouse during your retirement years. Consult with your employer's human resources office, your union, the plan administrator, and check your SPD. Make sure there is no conflicting information among these sources about the benefits your family will receive or the circumstances under which they can change or be eliminated. With this information in hand, you can make other important choices, like finding out if you are eligible for Medicare and Medigap insurance coverage.

9. Know how to file an appeal if a health benefits claim is denied. Understand how your plan handles grievances and where to make appeals of the plan's decisions. Keep records and copies of correspondence. Check your health benefits package and your SPD to determine who is responsible for handling problems with benefit claims. Contact PWBA for customer service assistance if you are unable to obtain a response to your complaint.

10. You can take steps to improve the quality of the healthcare and the health benefits your family receives. Look for and use things like Quality Reports and Accreditation Reports whenever you can. Quality reports may contain consumer ratings -- how satisfied consumers are with the doctors in their plan, for instance-- and clinical performance measures -- how well a healthcare organization prevents and treats illness. Accreditation reports provide information on how accredited organizations meet national standards, and often include clinical performance measures. Look for these quality measures whenever possible. Consult "Your Guide to Choosing Quality Health Care" on the Internet at **www.ahcpr.gov/consumer**.

Medicaid

Illness strikes both rich and poor families. For low-income families, Medicaid is available to defer the costs of treatment. In the following pages, you will learn the basics about Medicaid as well as useful contact information on how to find more in-depth information.

Medicaid is a joint federal and state program that helps pay medical costs for some people with low incomes and limited resources. Medicaid programs vary from state to state. You can find more information about Medicaid on the HCFA.gov Web site at **http://www.hcfa.gov/medicaid/medicaid.htm**.

Financial Assistance for Cancer Care[220]

Cancer can impose heavy economic burdens. For many parents, a portion of their children's medical expenses is paid by their health insurance plan. For individuals who do not have health insurance or who need financial assistance to cover health care costs, resources are available, including government-sponsored programs and services supported by voluntary organizations.

Parents should discuss any concerns they may have about healthcare costs with the physician, medical social worker, or the business office of their hospital or clinic.

The organizations and resources listed below may offer financial assistance. Organizations that provide publications in Spanish or have Spanish-speaking staff have been identified.

- The American Cancer Society (ACS) office can provide the telephone number of the local ACS office serving your area. The local ACS office may offer reimbursement for expenses related to cancer treatment including transportation, medicine, and medical supplies. The ACS also offers programs that help cancer patients, family members, and friends cope with the emotional challenges they face. Some publications are available in Spanish. Spanish-speaking staff are available. Telephone: 1-800-ACS-2345 (1-800-227-2345). Web site: **http://www.cancer.org**

- The Candlelighters Childhood Cancer Foundation (CCCF) is a nonprofit organization that provides information, peer support, and advocacy through publications, an information clearinghouse, and a network of local support groups. CCCF maintains a list of organizations to which eligible families may apply for financial assistance. Telephone: 1-800-366-CCCF (1-800-366-2223). Web site: **http://www.candlelighters.org**.

Community voluntary agencies and service organizations such as the Salvation Army, Lutheran Social Services, Jewish Social Services, Catholic Charities, and the Lions Club may offer help. These organizations are listed

---

[220] Adapted from the NCI: **http://cis.nci.nih.gov/fact/8_3.htm**.

in your local phone directory. Some churches and synagogues may provide financial help or services to their members.

Fundraising is another mechanism to consider. Some parents find that friends, family, and community members are willing to contribute financially if they are aware of a difficult situation. Contact your local library for information about how to organize fundraising efforts.

General assistance programs provide food, housing, prescription drugs, and other medical expenses for those who are not eligible for other programs. Funds are often limited. Information can be obtained by contacting your state or local Department of Social Services; this number is found in the local telephone directory.

Hill-Burton is a program through which hospitals receive construction funds from the Federal Government. Hospitals that receive Hill-Burton funds are required by law to provide some services to people who cannot afford to pay for their hospitalization. Information about which facilities are part of this program is available by calling the toll-free number or visiting the Web site shown below. A brochure about the program is available in Spanish. Telephone: 1-800-638-0742. Web site: **http://www.hrsa.gov/osp/dfcr/obtain/consfaq.htm**.

Income Tax Deductions

Medical costs that are not covered by insurance policies sometimes can be deducted from annual income before taxes. Examples of tax deductible expenses might include mileage for trips to and from medical appointments, out-of-pocket costs for treatment, prescription drugs or equipment, and the cost of meals during lengthy medical visits. The local Internal Revenue Service office, tax consultants, or certified public accountants can determine medical costs that are tax deductible. These telephone numbers are available in the local telephone directory. Web site: **http://www.irs.ustreas.gov**.

The Patient Advocate Foundation

The Patient Advocate Foundation (PAF) is a national nonprofit organization that provides education, legal counseling, and referrals to cancer patients and survivors concerning managed care, insurance, financial issues, job discrimination, and debt crisis matters. Telephone: 1-800-532-5274. **Web site: http://www.patientadvocate.org**.

Patient Assistance Programs are offered by some pharmaceutical manufacturers to help pay for medications. To learn whether a specific drug might be available at reduced cost through such a program, talk with a physician or a medical social worker.

The State Children's Health Insurance Program

The State Children's Health Insurance Program (SCHIP) is a Federal-State partnership that offers low-cost or free health insurance coverage to uninsured children of low-wage, working parents. Callers will be referred to the SCHIP program in their state for further information about what the program covers, who is eligible, and the minimum qualifications. Telephone: 1-877-543-7669 (1-877-KIDS-NOW). Web site: **http://www.insurekidsnow.gov**.

Transportation

There are nonprofit organizations that arrange free or reduced cost air transportation for cancer patients going to or from cancer treatment centers. Financial need is not always a requirement. To find out about these programs, talk with a medical social worker. Ground transportation services may be offered or mileage reimbursed through the local ACS or your state or local Department of Social Services.

NORD's Medication Assistance Programs

Finally, the National Organization for Rare Disorders, Inc. (NORD) administers medication programs sponsored by humanitarian-minded pharmaceutical and biotechnology companies to help uninsured or under-insured individuals secure life-saving or life-sustaining drugs.[221] NORD programs ensure that certain vital drugs are available "to those families whose income is too high to qualify for Medicaid but too low to pay for their prescribed medications." The program has standards for fairness, equity, and unbiased eligibility. It currently covers some 14 programs for nine pharmaceutical companies. NORD also offers early access programs for investigational new drugs (IND) under the approved "Treatment INDs" programs of the Food and Drug Administration (FDA). In these programs, a

---

[221] Adapted from NORD: **http://www.rarediseases.org/cgi-bin/nord/progserv#patient?id=rPIzL9oD&mv_pc=30**.

limited number of individuals can receive investigational drugs that have yet to be approved by the FDA. These programs are generally designed for rare medical conditions. For more information, visit **www.rarediseases.org**.

Additional Resources

In addition to the references already listed in this chapter, you may need more information on health insurance, hospitals, or the healthcare system in general. The NIH has set up an excellent guidance Web site that addresses these and other issues. Topics include:[222]

- Health Insurance:
  http://www.nlm.nih.gov/medlineplus/healthinsurance.html
- Health Statistics:
  http://www.nlm.nih.gov/medlineplus/healthstatistics.html
- HMO and Managed Care:
  http://www.nlm.nih.gov/medlineplus/managedcare.html
- Hospice Care: **http://www.nlm.nih.gov/medlineplus/hospicecare.html**
- Medicaid: **http://www.nlm.nih.gov/medlineplus/medicaid.html**
- Medicare: **http://www.nlm.nih.gov/medlineplus/medicare.html**
- Nursing Homes and Long-term Care:
  http://www.nlm.nih.gov/medlineplus/nursinghomes.html
- Patient's Rights, Confidentiality, Informed Consent, Ombudsman Programs, Privacy and Patient Issues:
  http://www.nlm.nih.gov/medlineplus/patientissues.html
- Veteran's Health, Persian Gulf War, Gulf War Syndrome, Agent Orange:
  http://www.nlm.nih.gov/medlineplus/veteranshealth.html

Vocabulary Builder

Cervix: The lower, narrow end of the uterus that forms a canal between the uterus and vagina. [NIH]

Corticosteroids: Hormones that have antitumor activity in lymphomas and lymphoid leukemias; in addition, corticosteroids (steroids) may be used for hormone replacement and for the management of some of the complications

---

[222] You can access this information at:
http://www.nlm.nih.gov/medlineplus/healthsystem.html.

of cancer and its treatment. [NIH]

Erythrocytes: Cells that carry oxygen to all parts of the body. Also called red blood cells (RBCs). [NIH]

Immunosuppressive: Describes the ability to lower immune system responses. [NIH]

Inoperable: Not suitable to be operated upon. [EU]

Intermittent: Occurring at separated intervals; having periods of cessation of activity. [EU]

Lesion: An area of abnormal tissue change. [NIH]

Nausea: An unpleasant sensation, vaguely referred to the epigastrium and abdomen, and often culminating in vomiting. [EU]

Non-small cell lung cancer: A group of lung cancers that includes squamous cell carcinoma, adenocarcinoma, and large cell carcinoma. [NIH]

Prednisolone: A synthetic corticosteroid used in the treatment of blood cell cancers (leukemias) and lymph system cancers (lymphomas). [NIH]

Psychotherapy: A generic term for the treatment of mental illness or emotional disturbances primarily by verbal or nonverbal communication. [NIH]

Retreatment: The therapy of the same disease in a patient, with the same agent or procedure repeated after initial treatment, or with an additional or alternate measure or follow-up. It does not include therapy which requires more than one administration of a therapeutic agent or regimen. Retreatment is often used with reference to a different modality when the original one was inadequate, harmful, or unsuccessful. [NIH]

Topical: On the surface of the body. [NIH]

Vindesine: An anticancer drug that belongs to the family of plant drugs called vinca alkaloids. [NIH]

APPENDIX E. TALKING WITH YOUR CHILD ABOUT CANCER

Overview[223]

More children than ever are surviving childhood cancer. Over the last 30 years, survival into adulthood increased from 30 percent to 80 percent. There are new and better drugs and methods to help children deal with the side effects of treatment. And children who have had cancer now have a better quality of life throughout childhood and into adulthood; fewer long-term ill effects follow the treatment.

Yet, in spite of all this good news, cancer is still a serious disease. You are not alone in facing your fears; help is available. A treatment team - doctors, radiation therapists, rehabilitation specialists, dietitians, oncology nurses, and social workers, among others - can help you and your child deal with the disease. They will also help ensure that your child gets the best treatment available with as few ill effects as possible.

Your first question may be, "Should I tell my child about the cancer?" You may want to protect your child, but children usually know when something is wrong. Your child may not be feeling well, may be seeing the doctor often, and may have already had some tests. Your child may notice that you are afraid. No matter how hard you try to keep information about the illness and treatment from your child, others - such as family, friends, and clinic or hospital staff - may inadvertently say things that let your child know about the cancer. In addition, it will upset your child to find out that you were not telling the truth; your child depends on you for honest answers.

---

[223] Adapted from the NCI: **http://www.cancer.gov/CancerInformation/youngpeople**.

Why Should I Tell My Child?

Telling your child about his or her cancer is a personal matter, and family, cultural, or religious beliefs will come into play. It is important to be open and honest with your child because children who are not told about their illness often imagine things that are not true. For example, a child may think he or she has cancer as punishment for doing something wrong. Health professionals generally agree that telling children the truth about their illness leads to less stress and guilt. Children who know the truth are also more likely to cooperate with treatment. Finally, talking about cancer often helps to bring the family closer together and makes dealing with the cancer a little easier for everyone.

Parent's Questions

Parents have many questions about talking with their children about the diagnosis. Perhaps you have asked some of these yourself

When Should My Child Be Told?

Because you are probably the best judge of your child's personality and moods, you are the best person to decide when your child should be told. Keep in mind, though, that your child is likely to know early on that something is wrong, so you may want to tell your child soon after the diagnosis. In fact, most parents say it is easiest to tell them then. Waiting days or weeks may give your child time to imagine worse things than the truth and develop fears that may be hard to dispel later. Certainly, it would be easier for your child if he or she is told before treatment starts.

Who Should Tell My Child?

The answer to this question is personal. As a parent, you may feel that it is best for you to tell your child. Some parents, however, find it too painful to do so. Other family members or the treatment team - doctor, nurse, or social worker - may be able to help you. They may either tell your child for you or help you explain the illness.

Thinking about what you are going to say and how to say it will help you feel more relaxed. But how do you decide just what to say? Family and close friends, members of the treatment team, parents of other children who have cancer, members of support groups (you can find information about them at the end of this booklet), and clergy members can offer ideas.

Who Should Be There?

Your child needs love and support when hearing the diagnosis. Even if the doctor explains the illness, someone your child trusts and depends upon should be present. Having the support of other family members at this time can be very helpful.

What Should My Child Be Told?

How much information and the best way to relate this information depends on your child's age and what your child can understand. Being gentle, open, and honest is usually best.
The following sections describe what most children in various age groups are likely to understand. These guidelines are general; each child is different. Your child may fit into more than one or none of these categories.

Up to 2 Years Old

Children this young do not understand cancer. They understand what they can see and touch. Their biggest concern is what is happening to them right now. They worry most about being away from their parents.

After children are a year old, they think about how things feel and how to control things around them. Very young children are most afraid of medical tests. Many cry, run away, or squirm to try to control what is happening.

Because children begin to think about and understand what is going on around them at about 18 months, it is best to be honest. Be truthful about trips to the hospital and explain procedures that may hurt. You can tell your child that needle sticks will hurt a minute and that it is okay to cry. Being honest lets your child know that you understand and accept his or her feelings and helps your child trust you.

When you can, give your child choices. For example, if a medicine is taken by mouth, you might ask if your child would like it mixed in apple juice, grape juice, or applesauce.

2 to 7 Years Old

When children are between the ages of 2 and 7, they link events to one thing. For example, they usually tie illness to a specific event such as staying in bed or eating chicken soup. Children this age often think their illness is caused by a specific action. Therefore, getting better will "just happen" or will come if they follow a set of rules.

These approaches might help when talking with a child in this age group:

- Explain that treatment is needed so the hurting will go away or so the child can get better and play without getting so tired.

- Explain that the illness or treatment is not punishment for something the child has done, said, or thought.

- Be honest when you explain tests and treatments. Remind the child that all of these things are being done to get rid of the cancer and to help him or her get well.

- Use simple ways to explain the illness. For example, try talking about the cancer as a contest between "good" cells and "bad" cells. Having treatment will help the good cells to be stronger so that they can beat the bad cells.

7 to 12 Years Old

Children ages 7 to 12 are starting to understand links between things and events. For example, a child this age sees his or her illness as a set of symptoms, is less likely to believe that something he or she did caused the illness, understands that getting better comes from taking medicines and doing what the doctor says, and is able to cooperate with treatment.

You can give more details when explaining cancer, but you should still use situations your child may be used to. You might say that the body is made of up different types of cells, and these cells have different jobs to do. Like people, these cells must work together to get the job done. You might describe the cancer cells as "troublemakers" that get in the way of the work of the good cells. Treatment helps to get rid of the troublemakers so that other cells can work well together.

12 Years and Older

Children over 12 years old can often understand complicated relationships between events. They can think about things that have not happened to them. Teenagers tend to think of illness in terms of specific symptoms, such as tiredness, and in terms of limits or changes in their everyday activity. But because they also can understand the reason for their symptoms, you can explain cancer as a disease in which a few cells in the body go "haywire." These "haywire" cells grow more quickly than normal cells, invade other parts of the body, and get in the way of how the body usually works. The goal of treatment is to kill the "haywire" cells. The body can then work normally again, and the symptoms will go away.

Questions Children May Ask

Children are naturally curious about their disease and have many questions about cancer and cancer treatment. Your child will expect you to have answers to most questions. Children may begin to ask questions right after diagnosis or may wait until later. Here are some common questions and some ideas to help you answer them.

Why Me?

A child, like an adult, wonders "Why did I get cancer?" A child may feel that it is his or her fault, that somehow he or she caused the illness. Make it clear that not even the doctors know exactly what caused the cancer. Neither you, your child, nor his or her brothers or sisters did, said, or thought anything that caused the cancer. Stress also that cancer is not contagious, and your child did not "catch" it from someone else.

Will I Get Well?

Children often know about family members or friends who died of cancer. As a result, many children are afraid to ask if they will get well because they fear that the answer will be "no." Thus, you might tell your child that cancer is a serious disease, but that treatment - such as medicine, radiation, or an operation - has helped get rid of cancer in other children, and the doctors and nurses are trying their best to cure your child's cancer, too. Knowing that caring people - such as family, doctors, nurses, counselors, and others -

surround your child and your family may also help him or her feel more secure.

What Will Happen to Me?

When your child is first diagnosed with cancer, many new and scary things will happen. While at the doctor's office, hospital, or clinic, your child may see or play with other children with cancer who may not be feeling well, have lost their hair, or have had limbs removed because of cancer. Your child may wonder, "Will these things happen to me?" Yet, your child may be too afraid to ask questions. It is important to try to get your child to talk about these concerns. Explain ahead of time about the cancer, treatment, and possible side effects. Discuss what the doctor will do to help if side effects occur. You can also explain that there are many different types of cancer and that even when two children have the same cancer, what happens to one child will not always happen to the other.

Children should be told about any changes in their treatment schedule or in the type of treatment they receive. This information helps them prepare for visits to the doctor or hospital. You may want to help your child keep a calendar that shows the days for doctor visits, treatments, or tests. Do not tell younger children about upcoming treatments far ahead of time if it makes them nervous.

Why Do I Have to Take Medicine When I Feel Okay?

With cancer, your child may feel fine much of the time but need to take medicine often. Children do not understand why they have to take medicine when they feel well. You may want to remind your child of the reason for taking the medicine in the first place. For example, a child could be told: "Although you are feeling well, the bad cells are hiding. You must take the medicine for a while longer to find the bad cells and stop them from coming back."

Talking to Your Child with Late-Stage Cancer

During the past several years, health care professionals have become more aware of the needs of children who have late-stage cancer and of their families. For example, attending school half days or even for an hour a day - if possible - may make your child happier. Talking with your child about death and dying and giving your child as many choices as possible shows your child that you are being open and honest, and shows your support, love, and respect. Paying close attention to changes in your child's behavior may give you important clues as to what your child needs and whether he or she wants to talk about dying. Including all of your children in everyday activities - such as reading, doing homework, or watching a favorite television program or video together - can help keep the family close.

Vocabulary Builder

Fatigue: The state of weariness following a period of exertion, mental or physical, characterized by a decreased capacity for work and reduced efficiency to respond to stimuli. [NIH]

Lymphadenopathy: Disease or swelling of the lymph nodes. [NIH]

Oncology nurse: A nurse who specializes in treating and caring for people who have cancer. [NIH]

Palpitation: A subjective sensation of an unduly rapid or irregular heart beat. [EU]

Petechiae: Pinpoint, unraised, round red spots under the skin caused by bleeding. [NIH]

Physical Examination: Systematic and thorough inspection of the patient for physical signs of disease or abnormality. [NIH]

Platelet Count: A count of the number of platelets per unit volume in a sample of venous blood. [NIH]

Punishment: The application of an unpleasant stimulus or penalty for the purpose of eliminating or correcting undesirable behavior. [NIH]

Purpura: Purplish or brownish red discoloration, easily visible through the epidermis, caused by hemorrhage into the tissues. [NIH]

Shoulder Pain: Unilateral or bilateral pain of the shoulder. It is often caused by physical activities such as work or sports participation, but may also be pathologic in origin. [NIH]

ONLINE GLOSSARIES

The Internet provides access to a number of free-to-use medical dictionaries and glossaries. The National Library of Medicine has compiled the following list of online dictionaries:

- ADAM Medical Encyclopedia (A.D.A.M., Inc.), comprehensive medical reference: **http://www.nlm.nih.gov/medlineplus/encyclopedia.html**
- MedicineNet.com Medical Dictionary (MedicineNet, Inc.): **http://www.medterms.com/Script/Main/hp.asp**
- Merriam-Webster Medical Dictionary (Inteli-Health, Inc.): **http://www.intelihealth.com/IH/**
- Multilingual Glossary of Technical and Popular Medical Terms in Eight European Languages (European Commission) - Danish, Dutch, English, French, German, Italian, Portuguese, and Spanish: **http://allserv.rug.ac.be/~rvdstich/eugloss/welcome.html**
- On-line Medical Dictionary (CancerWEB): **http://www.graylab.ac.uk/omd/**
- Technology Glossary (National Library of Medicine) - Health Care Technology: **http://www.nlm.nih.gov/nichsr/ta101/ta10108.htm**
- Terms and Definitions (Office of Rare Diseases): **http://rarediseases.info.nih.gov/ord/glossary_a-e.html**

Beyond these, MEDLINEplus contains a very user-friendly encyclopedia covering every aspect of medicine (licensed from A.D.A.M., Inc.). The ADAM Medical Encyclopedia Web site address is **http://www.nlm.nih.gov/medlineplus/encyclopedia.html**. ADAM is also available on commercial Web sites such as drkoop.com (**http://www.drkoop.com/**) and Web MD (**http://my.webmd.com/adam/asset/adam_disease_articles/a_to_z/a**). Topics of interest can be researched by using keywords before continuing elsewhere, as these basic definitions and concepts will be useful in more advanced areas of research. You may choose to print various pages specifically relating to childhood acute lymphoblastic leukemia and keep them on file. The NIH, in particular, suggests that parents of children with childhood acute lymphoblastic leukemia visit the following Web sites in the ADAM Medical Encyclopedia:

- **Basic Guidelines for Childhood Acute Lymphoblastic Leukemia**

    Acute lymphocytic leukemia
    Web site:
    http://www.nlm.nih.gov/medlineplus/ency/article/000541.htm

- **Signs & Symptoms for Childhood Acute Lymphoblastic Leukemia**

    Anemia
    Web site:
    http://www.nlm.nih.gov/medlineplus/ency/article/000560.htm

    Ankle pain
    Web site:
    http://www.nlm.nih.gov/medlineplus/ency/article/003167.htm

    Bleeding gums
    Web site:
    http://www.nlm.nih.gov/medlineplus/ency/article/003062.htm

    Bleeding into the skin
    Web site:
    http://www.nlm.nih.gov/medlineplus/ency/article/003235.htm

    Bone pain or tenderness
    Web site:
    http://www.nlm.nih.gov/medlineplus/ency/article/003180.htm

    Bruising
    Web site:
    http://www.nlm.nih.gov/medlineplus/ency/article/003235.htm

    Ecchymoses
    Web site:
    http://www.nlm.nih.gov/medlineplus/ency/article/003235.htm

    Elbow pain
    Web site:
    http://www.nlm.nih.gov/medlineplus/ency/article/003172.htm

Enlarged liver
Web site:
http://www.nlm.nih.gov/medlineplus/ency/article/003275.htm

Fatigue
Web site:
http://www.nlm.nih.gov/medlineplus/ency/article/003088.htm

Fever
Web site:
http://www.nlm.nih.gov/medlineplus/ency/article/003090.htm

Foot pain
Web site:
http://www.nlm.nih.gov/medlineplus/ency/article/003183.htm

Gums, swollen
Web site:
http://www.nlm.nih.gov/medlineplus/ency/article/003066.htm

Hip pain
Web site:
http://www.nlm.nih.gov/medlineplus/ency/article/003179.htm

Joint pain
Web site:
http://www.nlm.nih.gov/medlineplus/ency/article/003261.htm

Knee pain
Web site:
http://www.nlm.nih.gov/medlineplus/ency/article/003187.htm

Leukemia
Web site:
http://www.nlm.nih.gov/medlineplus/ency/article/001299.htm

Menstrual periods, abnormal
Web site:
http://www.nlm.nih.gov/medlineplus/ency/article/003263.htm

Nosebleeds
Web site:
http://www.nlm.nih.gov/medlineplus/ency/article/003106.htm

Paleness
Web site:
http://www.nlm.nih.gov/medlineplus/ency/article/003244.htm

Palpitations
Web site:
http://www.nlm.nih.gov/medlineplus/ency/article/003081.htm

Petechiae
Web site:
http://www.nlm.nih.gov/medlineplus/ency/article/003235.htm

Pinpoint red spots
Web site:
http://www.nlm.nih.gov/medlineplus/ency/article/003235.htm

Purpura
Web site:
http://www.nlm.nih.gov/medlineplus/ency/article/003232.htm

Shortness of breath
Web site:
http://www.nlm.nih.gov/medlineplus/ency/article/003075.htm

Shoulder pain
Web site:
http://www.nlm.nih.gov/medlineplus/ency/article/003171.htm

Skin rash or lesion
Web site:
http://www.nlm.nih.gov/medlineplus/ency/article/003220.htm

Weight loss
Web site:
http://www.nlm.nih.gov/medlineplus/ency/article/003107.htm

Wrist pain
Web site:
http://www.nlm.nih.gov/medlineplus/ency/article/003175.htm

- **Diagnostics and Tests for Childhood Acute Lymphoblastic Leukemia**

    Blood cell differential
    Web site:
    http://www.nlm.nih.gov/medlineplus/ency/article/003657.htm

    Bone marrow aspiration
    Web site:
    http://www.nlm.nih.gov/medlineplus/ency/article/003658.htm

    CBC
    Web site:
    http://www.nlm.nih.gov/medlineplus/ency/article/003642.htm

    Cell surface antigen studies (B-cell, leukemia/lymphoma panel)
    Web site:
    http://www.nlm.nih.gov/medlineplus/ency/article/003518.htm

    Platelet count
    Web site:
    http://www.nlm.nih.gov/medlineplus/ency/article/003647.htm

    Platelets
    Web site:
    http://www.nlm.nih.gov/medlineplus/ency/article/003647.htm

    T(thymus derived) lymphocyte count
    Web site:
    http://www.nlm.nih.gov/medlineplus/ency/article/003516.htm

    WBC count
    Web site:
    http://www.nlm.nih.gov/medlineplus/ency/article/003643.htm

- **Nutrition for Childhood Acute Lymphoblastic Leukemia**

    Lymphadenopathy
    Web site:
    http://www.nlm.nih.gov/medlineplus/ency/article/001377.htm

- **Surgery and Procedures for Childhood Acute Lymphoblastic Leukemia**

    Bone marrow transplant
    Web site:
    http://www.nlm.nih.gov/medlineplus/ency/article/003009.htm

- **Background Topics for Childhood Acute Lymphoblastic Leukemia**

    Acute
    Web site:
    http://www.nlm.nih.gov/medlineplus/ency/article/002215.htm

    Aggravated by
    Web site:
    http://www.nlm.nih.gov/medlineplus/ency/article/002227.htm

    Bleeding
    Web site:
    http://www.nlm.nih.gov/medlineplus/ency/article/000045.htm

    Cancer - support group
    Web site:
    http://www.nlm.nih.gov/medlineplus/ency/article/002166.htm

    Chemotherapy
    Web site:
    http://www.nlm.nih.gov/medlineplus/ency/article/002324.htm

    Exercise
    Web site:
    http://www.nlm.nih.gov/medlineplus/ency/article/001941.htm

    Incidence
    Web site:
    http://www.nlm.nih.gov/medlineplus/ency/article/002387.htm

Leukemia - support group
Web site:
http://www.nlm.nih.gov/medlineplus/ency/article/002151.htm

Peripheral
Web site:
http://www.nlm.nih.gov/medlineplus/ency/article/002273.htm

Physical examination
Web site:
http://www.nlm.nih.gov/medlineplus/ency/article/002274.htm

Radiation therapy
Web site:
http://www.nlm.nih.gov/medlineplus/ency/article/001918.htm

Secondary infections
Web site:
http://www.nlm.nih.gov/medlineplus/ency/article/002300.htm

Toxins
Web site:
http://www.nlm.nih.gov/medlineplus/ency/article/002331.htm

Online Dictionary Directories

The following are additional online directories compiled by the National Library of Medicine, including a number of specialized medical dictionaries and glossaries:

- Medical Dictionaries: Medical & Biological (World Health Organization):
  http://www.who.int/hlt/virtuallibrary/English/diction.htm#Medical
- MEL-Michigan Electronic Library List of Online Health and Medical Dictionaries (Michigan Electronic Library):
  http://mel.lib.mi.us/health/health-dictionaries.html
- Patient Education: Glossaries (DMOZ Open Directory Project):
  http://dmoz.org/Health/Education/Patient_Education/Glossaries/
- Web of Online Dictionaries (Bucknell University):
  http://www.yourdictionary.com/diction5.html#medicine

CHILDHOOD ACUTE LYMPHOBLASTIC LEUKEMIA GLOSSARY

The following is a complete glossary of terms used in this sourcebook. The definitions are derived from official public sources including the National Institutes of Health [NIH] and the European Union [EU]. After this glossary, we list a number of additional hardbound and electronic glossaries and dictionaries that you may wish to consult.

506U78: An anticancer drug that belongs to the family of drugs called antimetabolites. [NIH]

Abdomen: The part of the body that contains the pancreas, stomach, intestines, liver, gallbladder, and other organs. [NIH]

Abscess: A localized collection of pus caused by suppuration buried in tissues, organs, or confined spaces. [EU]

Aclarubicin: An anthracycline antibiotic produced by Streptomyces galilaeus. It has potent antineoplastic activity, especially in the treatment of leukemias, with reduced cardiac toxicity in comparison to daunorubicin or doxorubicin. [NIH]

Adolescence: The period of life beginning with the appearance of secondary sex characteristics and terminating with the cessation of somatic growth. The years usually referred to as adolescence lie between 13 and 18 years of age. [NIH]

Alleles: Mutually exclusive forms of the same gene, occupying the same locus on homologous chromosomes, and governing the same biochemical and developmental process. [NIH]

Allogeneic: Taken from different individuals of the same species. [NIH]

Anemia: A condition in which the number of red blood cells is below normal. [NIH]

Anthracycline: A member of a family of anticancer drugs that are also antibiotics. [NIH]

Antibody: A type of protein made by certain white blood cells in response to a foreign substance (antigen). Each antibody can bind to only a specific antigen. The purpose of this binding is to help destroy the antigen. Antibodies can work in several ways, depending on the nature of the antigen. Some antibodies destroy antigens directly. Others make it easier for white blood cells to destroy the antigen. [NIH]

Anticonvulsants: Drugs that prevent, reduce, or stop convulsions or seizures. [NIH]

Antigens: Substances that cause the immune system to make a specific immune response. [NIH]

Antimetabolite: A chemical that is very similar to one required in a normal biochemical reaction in cells. Antimetabolites can stop or slow down the reaction. [NIH]

Apoptosis: A normal series of events in a cell that leads to its death. [NIH]

Aseptic: Free from infection or septic material; sterile. [EU]

Asparaginase: An anticancer drug that is an enzyme. [NIH]

Aspiration: Removal of fluid from a lump, often a cyst, with a needle and a syringe. [NIH]

Aspirin: A drug that reduces pain, fever, inflammation, and blood clotting. Aspirin belongs to the family of drugs called nonsteroidal anti-inflammatory agents. It is also being studied in cancer prevention. [NIH]

Assay: Determination of the amount of a particular constituent of a mixture, or of the biological or pharmacological potency of a drug. [EU]

Ataxia: Loss of muscle coordination. [NIH]

Autologous: Taken from an individual's own tissues, cells, or DNA. [NIH]

Bacteria: A large group of single-cell microorganisms. Some cause infections and disease in animals and humans. The singular of bacteria is bacterium. [NIH]

Bereavement: Refers to the whole process of grieving and mourning and is associated with a deep sense of loss and sadness. [NIH]

Biomarkers: Substances sometimes found in an increased amount in the blood, other body fluids, or tissues and that may suggest the presence of some types of cancer. Biomarkers include CA 125 (ovarian cancer), CA 15-3 (breast cancer), CEA (ovarian, lung, breast, pancreas, and GI tract cancers), and PSA (prostate cancer). Also called tumor markers. [NIH]

Biopsy: The removal of cells or tissues for examination under a microscope. When only a sample of tissue is removed, the procedure is called an incisional biopsy or core biopsy. When an entire tumor or lesion is removed, the procedure is called an excisional biopsy. When a sample of tissue or fluid is removed with a needle, the procedure is called a needle biopsy or fine-needle aspiration. [NIH]

Blasts: Immature blood cells. [NIH]

Blood transfusion: The administration of blood or blood products into a blood vessel. [NIH]

Carcinogen: Any substance that causes cancer. [NIH]

Carcinogenic: Producing carcinoma. [EU]

Cardiac: Having to do with the heart. [NIH]

Cardiomyopathy: A general diagnostic term designating primary myocardial disease, often of obscure or unknown etiology. [EU]

Carnitine: Constituent of striated muscle and liver. It is used therapeutically to stimulate gastric and pancreatic secretions and in the treatment of hyperlipoproteinemias. [NIH]

Catechol: A chemical originally isolated from a type of mimosa tree. Catechol is used as an astringent, an antiseptic, and in photography, electroplating, and making other chemicals. It can also be man-made. [NIH]

Cell: The individual unit that makes up all of the tissues of the body. All living things are made up of one or more cells. [NIH]

Cerebral: Of or pertaining of the cerebrum or the brain. [EU]

Cervical: Relating to the neck, or to the neck of any organ or structure. Cervical lymph nodes are located in the neck; cervical cancer refers to cancer of the uterine cervix, which is the lower, narrow end (the "neck") of the uterus. [NIH]

Cervix: The lower, narrow end of the uterus that forms a canal between the uterus and vagina. [NIH]

Charities: Social welfare organizations with programs designed to assist individuals in times of need. [NIH]

Chemotherapy: Treatment with anticancer drugs. [NIH]

Chromosomal: Pertaining to chromosomes. [EU]

Chromosome: Part of a cell that contains genetic information. Except for sperm and eggs, all human cells contain 46 chromosomes. [NIH]

Chronic: A disease or condition that persists or progresses over a long period of time. [NIH]

Cisplatin: An anticancer drug that belongs to the family of drugs called platinum compounds. [NIH]

CNS: Central nervous system. The brain and spinal cord. [NIH]

Corticosteroids: Hormones that have antitumor activity in lymphomas and lymphoid leukemias; in addition, corticosteroids (steroids) may be used for hormone replacement and for the management of some of the complications of cancer and its treatment. [NIH]

Cranial: Pertaining to the cranium, or to the anterior (in animals) or superior (in humans) end of the body. [EU]

CSF: Cerebrospinal fluid. The fluid flowing around the brain and spinal cord. CSF is produced in the ventricles of the brain. [NIH]

Curative: Tending to overcome disease and promote recovery. [EU]

Cyclic: Pertaining to or occurring in a cycle or cycles; the term is applied to chemical compounds that contain a ring of atoms in the nucleus. [EU]

Cyclophosphamide: An anticancer drug that belongs to the family of drugs called alkylating agents. [NIH]

Cyclosporine: A drug used to help reduce the risk of rejection of organ and bone marrow transplants by the body. It is also used in clinical trials to make cancer cells more sensitive to anticancer drugs. [NIH]

Cytarabine: An anticancer drug that belongs to the family of drugs called antimetabolites. [NIH]

Cytogenetics: A branch of genetics which deals with the cytological and molecular behavior of genes and chromosomes during cell division. [NIH]

Cytophotometry: A method for the study of certain organic compounds within cells, in situ, by measuring the light intensities of the selectively stained areas of cytoplasm. The compounds studied and their locations in the cells are made to fluoresce and are observed under a microscope. [NIH]

Cytosine: A pyrimidine base that is a fundamental unit of nucleic acids. [NIH]

Daunorubicin: An anticancer drug that belongs to the family of drugs called antitumor antibiotics. [NIH]

Decitabine: An anticancer drug that belongs to the family of drugs called antimetabolites. [NIH]

Dermatology: A medical specialty concerned with the skin, its structure, functions, diseases, and treatment. [NIH]

Dexamethasone: A synthetic steroid (similar to steroid hormones produced naturally in the adrenal gland). Dexamethasone is used to treat leukemia and lymphoma and may be used to treat some of the problems caused by other cancers and their treatment. [NIH]

Dexrazoxane: A drug used to protect the heart from the toxic effects of anthracycline drugs such as doxorubicin. It belongs to the family of drugs called chemoprotective agents. [NIH]

Disposition: A tendency either physical or mental toward certain diseases. [EU]

Docetaxel: An anticancer drug that belongs to the family of drugs called mitotic inhibitors. [NIH]

Doxorubicin: An anticancer drug that belongs to the family of drugs called antitumor antibiotics. It is an anthracycline. [NIH]

Eagles: Members of the Falconiformes order of birds, family Accipitridae. They are characterized by their powerful talons, which carry long, curved, pointed claws and by their opposable hindtoe. [NIH]

Encephalopathy: A disorder of the brain that can be caused by disease, injury, drugs, or chemicals. [NIH]

Endogenous: Produced inside an organism or cell. The opposite is external (exogenous) production. [NIH]

Enzyme: A protein that speeds up chemical reactions in the body. [NIH]

Erwinia: A genus of gram-negative, facultatively anaerobic, rod-shaped bacteria whose organisms are associated with plants as pathogens, saprophytes, or as constituents of the epiphytic flora. [NIH]

Erythrocytes: Cells that carry oxygen to all parts of the body. Also called red blood cells (RBCs). [NIH]

Erythroleukemia: Cancer of the blood-forming tissues in which large numbers of immature, abnormal red blood cells are found in the blood and bone marrow. [NIH]

Etoposide: An anticancer drug that is a podophyllotoxin derivative and belongs to the family of drugs called mitotic inhibitors. [NIH]

Exogenous: Developed or originating outside the organism, as exogenous disease. [EU]

Fatigue: The state of weariness following a period of exertion, mental or physical, characterized by a decreased capacity for work and reduced efficiency to respond to stimuli. [NIH]

Filgrastim: A colony-stimulating factor that stimulates the production of neutrophils (a type of white blood cell). It is a cytokine that belongs to the family of drugs called hematopoietic (blood-forming) agents. Also called granulocyte colony-stimulating factor (G-CSF). [NIH]

Filtration: The passage of a liquid through a filter, accomplished by gravity, pressure, or vacuum (suction). [EU]

Fludarabine: An anticancer drug that belongs to the family of drugs called antimetabolites. [NIH]

Fluorescence: The property of emitting radiation while being irradiated. The radiation emitted is usually of longer wavelength than that incident or absorbed, e.g., a substance can be irradiated with invisible radiation and emit visible light. X-ray fluorescence is used in diagnosis. [NIH]

Gemcitabine: An anticancer drug that belongs to the family of drugs called antimetabolites. [NIH]

Genotype: The genetic constitution of the individual; the characterization of the genes. [NIH]

Glucocorticoid: A compound that belongs to the family of compounds called corticosteroids (steroids). Glucocorticoids affect metabolism and have anti-inflammatory and immunosuppressive effects. They may be naturally produced (hormones) or synthetic (drugs). [NIH]

Glycoprotein: A protein that has sugar molecules attached to it. [NIH]

Graft: Healthy skin, bone, or other tissue taken from one part of the body and used to replace diseased or injured tissue removed from another part of the body. [NIH]

Granulocyte: A type of white blood cell that fights bacterial infection. Neutrophils, eosinophils, and basophils are granulocytes. [NIH]

Haploidy: The number of chromosomes in the gametes, which is half the number normally found in somatic cells. Symbol: N. [NIH]

Hematologist: A doctor who specializes in treating diseases of the blood. [NIH]

Hematology: A subspecialty of internal medicine concerned with morphology, physiology, and pathology of the blood and blood-forming tissues. [NIH]

Hematopoiesis: The forming of new blood cells. [NIH]

Hepatic: Refers to the liver. [NIH]

Herbicide: A chemical that kills plants. [NIH]

Histiocytosis: General term for the abnormal appearance of histiocytes in the blood. Based on the pathological features of the cells involved rather than on clinical findings, the histiocytic diseases are subdivided into three groups: histiocytosis, langerhans cell; histiocytosis, non-langerhans cell; and histiocytic disorders, malignant. [NIH]

Humoral: Of, relating to, proceeding from, or involving a bodily humour - now often used of endocrine factors as opposed to neural or somatic. [EU]

Hunger: The desire for food generated by a sensation arising from the lack of food in the stomach. [NIH]

Hybridization: The genetic process of crossbreeding to produce a hybrid. Hybrid nucleic acids can be formed by nucleic acid hybridization of DNA and RNA molecules. Protein hybridization allows for hybrid proteins to be formed from polypeptide chains. [NIH]

Hydrocortisone: A drug used to relieve the symptoms of certain hormone shortages and to suppress an immune response. [NIH]

Hypoglycemia: Abnormally low blood sugar [NIH]

Idarubicin: An anticancer drug that belongs to the family of drugs called antitumor antibiotics. Also called 4-demethoxydaunorubicin. [NIH]

Ifosfamide: An anticancer drug that belongs to the family of drugs called alkylating agents. [NIH]

Immunity: The condition of being immune; the protection against infectious disease conferred either by the immune response generated by immunization or previous infection or by other nonimmunologic factors (innate i.). [EU]

Immunization: The induction of immunity. [EU]

Immunocompromised: Having a weakened immune system caused by certain diseases or treatments. [NIH]

Immunoglobulin: A protein that acts as an antibody. [NIH]

Immunosuppressive: Describes the ability to lower immune system responses. [NIH]

Immunotherapy: Treatment to stimulate or restore the ability of the immune system to fight infection and disease. Also used to lessen side effects that may be caused by some cancer treatments. Also called biological therapy or biological response modifier (BRM) therapy. [NIH]

Induction: The act or process of inducing or causing to occur, especially the production of a specific morphogenetic effect in the developing embryo through the influence of evocators or organizers, or the production of anaesthesia or unconsciousness by use of appropriate agents. [EU]

Infusion: A method of putting fluids, including drugs, into the bloodstream. Also called intravenous infusion. [NIH]

Inoperable: Not suitable to be operated upon. [EU]

Interferon: A biological response modifier (a substance that can improve the body's natural response to disease). Interferons interfere with the division of cancer cells and can slow tumor growth. There are several types of interferons, including interferon-alpha, -beta, and -gamma. These substances are normally produced by the body. They are also made in the laboratory for use in treating cancer and other diseases. [NIH]

Intermittent: Occurring at separated intervals; having periods of cessation of activity. [EU]

Interphase: The interval between two successive cell divisions during which the chromosomes are not individually distinguishable and DNA replication occurs. [NIH]

Intramuscular: IM. Within or into muscle. [NIH]

Intrathecal: Describes the fluid-filled space between the thin layers of tissue that cover the brain and spinal cord. Drugs can be injected into the fluid or a sample of the fluid can be removed for testing. [NIH]

Intravenous: IV. Into a vein. [NIH]

Invasive: 1. having the quality of invasiveness. 2. involving puncture or incision of the skin or insertion of an instrument or foreign material into the body; said of diagnostic techniques. [EU]

Lesion: An area of abnormal tissue change. [NIH]

Leucovorin: A drug used to protect normal cells from high doses of the anticancer drug methotrexate. It is also used to increase the antitumor effects of fluorouracil and tegafur-uracil, an oral treatment alternative to intravenous fluorouracil. [NIH]

Leukaemia: An acute or chronic disease of unknown cause in man and other warm-blooded animals that involves the blood-forming organs, is characterized by an abnormal increase in the number of leucocytes in the tissues of the body with or without a corresponding increase of those in the circulating blood, and is classified according of the type leucocyte most prominently involved. [EU]

Leukemia: Cancer of blood-forming tissue. [NIH]

Leukocytosis: A transient increase in the number of leukocytes in a body fluid. [NIH]

LH: A small glycoprotein hormone secreted by the anterior pituitary. LH plays an important role in controlling ovulation and in controlling secretion of hormones by the ovaries and testes. [NIH]

Lymphadenopathy: Disease or swelling of the lymph nodes. [NIH]

Lymphocyte: A white blood cell. Lymphocytes have a number of roles in the immune system, including the production of antibodies and other substances that fight infection and diseases. [NIH]

Lymphocytic: Referring to lymphocytes, a type of white blood cell. [NIH]

Lymphoid: Referring to lymphocytes, a type of white blood cell. Also refers to tissue in which lymphocytes develop. [NIH]

Lymphoma: Cancer that arises in cells of the lymphatic system. [NIH]

Malignancy: A cancerous tumor that can invade and destroy nearby tissue and spread to other parts of the body. [NIH]

Mammography: The use of x-rays to create a picture of the breast. [NIH]

Membrane: A very thin layer of tissue that covers a surface. [NIH]

Mercaptopurine: An anticancer drug that belongs to the family of drugs called antimetabolites. [NIH]

Metabolite: Any substance produced by metabolism or by a metabolic process. [EU]

Methotrexate: An anticancer drug that belongs to the family of drugs called antimetabolites. [NIH]

Molecule: A chemical made up of two or more atoms. The atoms in a molecule can be the same (an oxygen molecule has two oxygen atoms) or different (a water molecule has two hydrogen atoms and one oxygen atom).

Biological molecules, such as proteins and DNA, can be made up of many thousands of atoms. [NIH]

Morphology: The science of the form and structure of organisms (plants, animals, and other forms of life). [NIH]

Mutagenic: Inducing genetic mutation. [EU]

Myelogenous: Produced by, or originating in, the bone marrow. [NIH]

Myelosuppression: A condition in which bone marrow activity is decreased, resulting in fewer red blood cells, white blood cells, and platelets. Myelosuppression is a side effect of some cancer treatments. [NIH]

Nausea: An unpleasant sensation, vaguely referred to the epigastrium and abdomen, and often culminating in vomiting. [EU]

Necrosis: Refers to the death of living tissues. [NIH]

Neuroendocrine: Having to do with the interactions between the nervous system and the endocrine system. Describes certain cells that release hormones into the blood in response to stimulation of the nervous system. [NIH]

Neurosurgeon: A doctor who specializes in surgery on the brain, spine, and other parts of the nervous system. [NIH]

Neurotoxicity: The tendency of some treatments to cause damage to the nervous system. [NIH]

Non-small cell lung cancer: A group of lung cancers that includes squamous cell carcinoma, adenocarcinoma, and large cell carcinoma. [NIH]

Occult: Obscure; concealed from observation, difficult to understand. [EU]

Oncogene: A gene that normally directs cell growth. If altered, an oncogene can promote or allow the uncontrolled growth of cancer. Alterations can be inherited or caused by an environmental exposure to carcinogens. [NIH]

Oncologist: A doctor who specializes in treating cancer. Some oncologists specialize in a particular type of cancer treatment. For example, a radiation oncologist specializes in treating cancer with radiation. [NIH]

Oncology: The study of cancer. [NIH]

Oncology nurse: A nurse who specializes in treating and caring for people who have cancer. [NIH]

Osteonecrosis: Death of a bone or part of a bone, either atraumatic or posttraumatic. [NIH]

Osteosarcoma: A cancer of the bone that affects primarily children and adolescents. Also called osteogenic sarcoma. [NIH]

Palliative: 1. affording relief, but not cure. 2. an alleviating medicine. [EU]

Palpitation: A subjective sensation of an unduly rapid or irregular heart beat. [EU]

Paradoxical: Occurring at variance with the normal rule. [EU]

Paralysis: Loss of ability to move all or part of the body. [NIH]

Pathologist: A doctor who identifies diseases by studying cells and tissues under a microscope. [NIH]

Pediatrics: A medical specialty concerned with maintaining health and providing medical care to children from birth to adolescence. [NIH]

Pegaspargase: A modified form of asparaginase, an anticancer drug that belongs to the family of drugs derived from enzymes. [NIH]

Pelvis: The lower part of the abdomen, located between the hip bones. [NIH]

Petechiae: Pinpoint, unraised, round red spots under the skin caused by bleeding. [NIH]

Pharmacodynamics: The study of the biochemical and physiological effects of drugs and the mechanisms of their actions, including the correlation of actions and effects of drugs with their chemical structure; also, such effects on the actions of a particular drug or drugs. [EU]

Pharmacokinetics: The activity of drugs in the body over a period of time, including the processes by which drugs are absorbed, distributed in the body, localized in the tissues, and excreted. [NIH]

Phenobarbital: A sedative/anticonvulsant barbiturate that has been used to treat diarrhea and to increase the antitumor effect of other therapies. [NIH]

Phenotype: The outward appearance of the individual. It is the product of interactions between genes and between the genotype and the environment. This includes the killer phenotype, characteristic of yeasts. [NIH]

Physical Examination: Systematic and thorough inspection of the patient for physical signs of disease or abnormality. [NIH]

Plasma: The clear, yellowish, fluid part of the blood that carries the blood cells. The proteins that form blood clots are in plasma. [NIH]

Platelet Count: A count of the number of platelets per unit volume in a sample of venous blood. [NIH]

Platelets: A type of blood cell that helps prevent bleeding by causing blood clots to form. Also called thrombocytes. [NIH]

Ploidy: The number of sets of chromosomes in a cell or an organism. For example, haploid means one set and diploid means two sets. [NIH]

Polyethylene: A vinyl polymer made from ethylene. It can be branched or linear. Branched or low-density polyethylene is tough and pliable but not to the same degree as linear polyethylene. Linear or high-density polyethylene has a greater hardness and tensile strength. Polyethylene is used in a variety of products, including implants and prostheses. [NIH]

Postnatal: Occurring after birth, with reference to the newborn. [EU]

Preclinical: Before a disease becomes clinically recognizable. [EU]

Precursor: Something that precedes. In biological processes, a substance from which another, usually more active or mature substance is formed. In clinical medicine, a sign or symptom that heralds another. [EU]

Prednisolone: A synthetic corticosteroid used in the treatment of blood cell cancers (leukemias) and lymph system cancers (lymphomas). [NIH]

Prednisone: Belongs to the family of drugs called steroids and is used to treat several types of cancer and other disorders. Prednisone also inhibits the body's immune response. [NIH]

Prenatal: Existing or occurring before birth, with reference to the fetus. [EU]

Prevalence: The total number of cases of a given disease in a specified population at a designated time. It is differentiated from incidence, which refers to the number of new cases in the population at a given time. [NIH]

Prophylaxis: An attempt to prevent disease. [NIH]

Prostate: A gland in males that surrounds the neck of the bladder and the urethra. It secretes a substance that liquifies coagulated semen. It is situated in the pelvic cavity behind the lower part of the pubic symphysis, above the deep layer of the triangular ligament, and rests upon the rectum. [NIH]

Proteins: Polymers of amino acids linked by peptide bonds. The specific sequence of amino acids determines the shape and function of the protein. [NIH]

Proteoglycan: A molecule that contains both protein and glycosaminoglycans, which are a type of polysaccharide. Proteoglycans are found in cartilage and other connective tissues. [NIH]

Pseudomonas: A genus of gram-negative, aerobic, rod-shaped bacteria widely distributed in nature. Some species are pathogenic for humans, animals, and plants. [NIH]

Psychotherapy: A generic term for the treatment of mental illness or emotional disturbances primarily by verbal or nonverbal communication. [NIH]

Pulse: The rhythmical expansion and contraction of an artery produced by waves of pressure caused by the ejection of blood from the left ventricle of the heart as it contracts. [NIH]

Purpura: Purplish or brownish red discoloration, easily visible through the epidermis, caused by hemorrhage into the tissues. [NIH]

Randomized: Describes an experiment or clinical trial in which animal or human subjects are assigned by chance to separate groups that compare different treatments. [NIH]

Receptor: A molecule inside or on the surface of a cell that binds to a specific substance and causes a specific physiologic effect in the cell. [NIH]

Recombinant: 1. a cell or an individual with a new combination of genes not found together in either parent; usually applied to linked genes. [EU]

Recurrence: The return of cancer, at the same site as the original (primary) tumor or in another location, after the tumor had disappeared. [NIH]

Refractory: Not readily yielding to treatment. [EU]

Regimen: A treatment plan that specifies the dosage, the schedule, and the duration of treatment. [NIH]

Remission: A decrease in or disappearance of signs and symptoms of cancer. In partial remission, some, but not all, signs and symptoms of cancer have disappeared. In complete remission, all signs and symptoms of cancer have disappeared, although there still may be cancer in the body. [NIH]

Retreatment: The therapy of the same disease in a patient, with the same agent or procedure repeated after initial treatment, or with an additional or alternate measure or follow-up. It does not include therapy which requires more than one administration of a therapeutic agent or regimen. Retreatment is often used with reference to a different modality when the original one was inadequate, harmful, or unsuccessful. [NIH]

Retrospective: Looking back at events that have already taken place. [NIH]

Screening: Checking for disease when there are no symptoms. [NIH]

Seizures: Convulsions; sudden, involuntary movements of the muscles. [NIH]

Serum: The clear liquid part of the blood that remains after blood cells and clotting proteins have been removed. [NIH]

Shoulder Pain: Unilateral or bilateral pain of the shoulder. It is often caused by physical activities such as work or sports participation, but may also be pathologic in origin. [NIH]

Sinusitis: Inflammation of a sinus. The condition may be purulent or nonpurulent, acute or chronic. Depending on the site of involvement it is known as ethmoid, frontal, maxillary, or sphenoid sinusitis. [EU]

Solvent: 1. dissolving; effecting a solution. 2. a liquid that dissolves or that is capable of dissolving; the component of a solution that is present in greater amount. [EU]

Somatic: 1. pertaining to or characteristic of the soma or body. 2. pertaining to the body wall in contrast to the viscera. [EU]

Somnolence: Sleepiness; also unnatural drowsiness. [EU]

Spleen: An organ that is part of the lymphatic system. The spleen produces lymphocytes, filters the blood, stores blood cells, and destroys old blood cells. It is located on the left side of the abdomen near the stomach. [NIH]

Staging: Performing exams and tests to learn the extent of the cancer within the body, especially whether the disease has spread from the original site to other parts of the body. [NIH]

Steroids: Drugs used to relieve swelling and inflammation. [NIH]

STI571: A drug that is being studied for its ability to inhibit the growth of certain cancers. It interferes with a portion of the protein produced by the bcr/abl oncogene. [NIH]

Strabismus: Deviation of the eye which the patient cannot overcome. The visual axes assume a position relative to each other different from that required by the physiological conditions. The various forms of strabismus are spoken of as tropias, their direction being indicated by the appropriate prefix, as cyclo tropia, esotropia, exotropia, hypertropia, and hypotropia. Called also cast, heterotropia, manifest deviation, and squint. [EU]

Subacute: Somewhat acute; between acute and chronic. [EU]

Systemic: Affecting the entire body. [NIH]

Telangiectasia: The permanent enlargement of blood vessels, causing redness in the skin or mucous membranes. [NIH]

Teniposide: An anticancer drug that is a podophyllotoxin derivative and belongs to the family of drugs called mitotic inhibitors. [NIH]

Testicular: Pertaining to a testis. [EU]

Thymus: An organ that is part of the lymphatic system, in which T lymphocytes grow and multiply. The thymus is in the chest behind the breastbone. [NIH]

Tonsils: Small masses of lymphoid tissue on either side of the throat. [NIH]

Topical: On the surface of the body. [NIH]

Toxicity: The quality of being poisonous, especially the degree of virulence of a toxic microbe or of a poison. [EU]

Transplantation: The replacement of an organ with one from another person. [NIH]

Trimetrexate: A nonclassical folic acid inhibitor through its inhibition of the enzyme dihydrofolate reductase. It is being tested for efficacy as an antineoplastic agent and as an antiparasitic agent against Pneumocystis carinii pneumonia in AIDS patients. Myelosuppression is its dose-limiting toxic effect. [NIH]

Trisomy: The possession of a third chromosome of any one type in an otherwise diploid cell. [NIH]

Vaccination: Treatment with a vaccine. [NIH]

Vaccine: A substance or group of substances meant to cause the immune system to respond to a tumor or to microorganisms, such as bacteria or viruses. [NIH]

Varicella: Chicken pox. [EU]

Vincristine: An anticancer drug that belongs to the family of plant drugs called vinca alkaloids. [NIH]

Vindesine: An anticancer drug that belongs to the family of plant drugs called vinca alkaloids. [NIH]

Viral: Pertaining to, caused by, or of the nature of virus. [EU]

General Dictionaries and Glossaries

While the above glossary is essentially complete, the dictionaries listed here cover virtually all aspects of medicine, from basic words and phrases to more advanced terms (sorted alphabetically by title; hyperlinks provide rankings, information and reviews at Amazon.com):

- **The Cancer Dictionary** by Roberta Altman, Michael J., Md Sarg; Paperback - 368 pages, 2nd Revised edition (November 1999), Checkmark Books; ISBN: 0816039542;
  http://www.amazon.com/exec/obidos/ASIN/0816039542/icongroupinterna

- **Dictionary of Medical Acronymns & Abbreviations** by Stanley Jablonski (Editor), Paperback, 4th edition (2001), Lippincott Williams & Wilkins Publishers, ISBN: 1560534605,
  http://www.amazon.com/exec/obidos/ASIN/1560534605/icongroupinterna

- **Dictionary of Medical Terms : For the Nonmedical Person (Dictionary of Medical Terms for the Nonmedical Person, Ed 4)** by Mikel A. Rothenberg, M.D, et al, Paperback - 544 pages, 4th edition (2000), Barrons Educational Series, ISBN: 0764112015,
  http://www.amazon.com/exec/obidos/ASIN/0764112015/icongroupinterna

- **A Dictionary of the History of Medicine** by A. Sebastian, CD-Rom edition (2001), CRC Press-Parthenon Publishers, ISBN: 185070368X,
  http://www.amazon.com/exec/obidos/ASIN/185070368X/icongroupinterna

- **Dorland's Illustrated Medical Dictionary (Standard Version)** by Dorland, et al, Hardcover - 2088 pages, 29th edition (2000), W B Saunders Co, ISBN: 0721662544,
  http://www.amazon.com/exec/obidos/ASIN/0721662544/icongroupinterna

- **Dorland's Electronic Medical Dictionary** by Dorland, et al, Software, 29th Book & CD-Rom edition (2000), Harcourt Health Sciences, ISBN: 0721694934,
  http://www.amazon.com/exec/obidos/ASIN/0721694934/icongroupinterna

- **Dorland's Pocket Medical Dictionary (Dorland's Pocket Medical Dictionary, 26th Ed)** Hardcover - 912 pages, 26th edition (2001), W B Saunders Co, ISBN: 0721682812,
  http://www.amazon.com/exec/obidos/ASIN/0721682812/icongroupinterna/103-4193558-7304618

- **Melloni's Illustrated Medical Dictionary (Melloni's Illustrated Medical Dictionary, 4th Ed)** by Melloni, Hardcover, 4th edition (2001), CRC Press-Parthenon Publishers, ISBN: 85070094X,
  http://www.amazon.com/exec/obidos/ASIN/85070094X/icongroupinterna

- **Stedman's Electronic Medical Dictionary Version 5.0 (CD-ROM for Windows and Macintosh, Individual)** by Stedmans, CD-ROM edition (2000), Lippincott Williams & Wilkins Publishers, ISBN: 0781726328,
  http://www.amazon.com/exec/obidos/ASIN/0781726328/icongroupinterna

- **Stedman's Medical Dictionary** by Thomas Lathrop Stedman, Hardcover - 2098 pages, 27th edition (2000), Lippincott, Williams & Wilkins, ISBN: 068340007X,
  http://www.amazon.com/exec/obidos/ASIN/068340007X/icongroupinterna

- **Stedman's Oncology Words** by Beverly J. Wolpert (Editor), Stedmans; Paperback - 502 pages, 3rd edition (June 15, 2000), Lippincott, Williams & Wilkins; ISBN: 0781726549;
  http://www.amazon.com/exec/obidos/ASIN/0781726549/icongroupinterna

- **Tabers Cyclopedic Medical Dictionary (Thumb Index)** by Donald Venes (Editor), et al, Hardcover - 2439 pages, 19th edition (2001), F A Davis Co, ISBN: 0803606540,
  http://www.amazon.com/exec/obidos/ASIN/0803606540/icongroupinterna

INDEX

A
Abdomen 12, 27, 261, 287, 288, 291
Adolescence 25, 49, 144, 279, 288
Alleles 92
Allogeneic 14, 113, 165, 181, 181, 182, 228, 235
Anemia 12
Anthracycline 126, 127, 137, 166, 174, 230, 279, 282
Antibody 183, 195, 196, 279, 285
Anticonvulsants 171
Antigens 125, 152, 154, 195, 279
Antimetabolite 156, 157, 159, 172, 173, 174
Apoptosis 98, 102, 109, 155
Aseptic 167, 177
Asparaginase 95, 106, 119, 165, 167, 168, 173, 175, 196, 228, 230, 233, 288
Aspiration 26, 275, 280
Assay 94
Ataxia 146
Autologous 14, 121, 227, 228

B
Bacteria 12, 26, 87, 127, 129, 280, 283, 289, 292
Bereavement 36
Biopsy 12, 26, 183, 280
Blasts 11, 100, 160, 168

C
Carcinogen 122
Cardiac 95, 112, 137, 279
Cardiomyopathy 95
Carnitine 95
Catechol 99
Cerebral 170
Cervical 34, 48, 281
Chromosomal 97, 105, 109, 151, 156, 162
Chromosome ... 65, 67, 99, 112, 117, 149, 155, 156, 157, 158, 160, 165, 178, 180, 197, 291
Chronic... 12, 27, 65, 67, 69, 87, 133, 140, 191, 197, 251, 286, 290, 291
Cisplatin 96
Corticosteroids 127, 260, 281, 283
Cranial 121, 146, 163, 169, 170, 171, 172, 176, 183, 235
Curative 36, 94, 147, 180
Cyclophosphamide 174, 179, 227, 228, 229, 231
Cyclosporine 64
Cytarabine 163, 168
Cytogenetics 122, 124
Cytophotometry 132
Cytosine 133, 229, 231

D
Daunorubicin 112, 137, 279
Decitabine 72
Dexamethasone.. 165, 167, 168, 172, 176
Dexrazoxane 95, 179
Disposition 99
Docetaxel 63
Doxorubicin ... 95, 126, 137, 235, 279, 282

E
Encephalopathy 101
Endogenous 102
Enzyme 87, 117, 126, 167, 171, 176, 225, 280, 291
Erythrocytes 236
Erythroleukemia 140
Etoposide 99, 228, 233
Exogenous 102, 127, 283

F
Filgrastim 64
Filtration 134
Fludarabine 65
Fluorescence 115, 127, 283

G
Gemcitabine 66
Genotype 101, 120, 288
Glucocorticoid 108
Glycoprotein 107, 109, 128, 286
Graft 62
Granulocyte 86, 133, 283

H
Haploidy 115
Hematology 140, 141, 142
Hepatic 122
Histiocytosis 110
Humoral 125
Hybridization 109, 112, 115, 124
Hydrocortisone 168
Hypoglycemia 107

I
Idarubicin 179
Immunity 26, 125, 285
Immunization 128, 285
Immunoglobulin 152, 153, 159
Immunosuppressive 127, 236, 283
Immunotherapy 229
Infusion 128, 169, 178, 285
Inoperable 225
Interferon 121, 128, 285
Intermittent 231

Intramuscular 167
Intrathecal 14, 16, 95, 146, 160, 163, 165, 168, 169, 170, 171, 172, 176, 182
Intravenous ... 87, 128, 166, 172, 173, 174, 175, 178, 285, 286
Invasive 209

L
Lesion 26, 274, 280
Leucovorin 59, 169, 172, 175, 178
Leukocytosis 154
Lymphocyte 229, 275
Lymphocytic ... 11, 20, 56, 60, 63, 67, 141, 148, 161, 172, 173, 174, 272
Lymphoid 4, 27, 55, 172, 260, 281, 291
Lymphoma 20, 21, 22, 23, 58, 59, 60, 61, 68, 69, 146, 152, 153, 162, 179, 191, 195, 275, 282

M
Malignancy 93, 95, 97, 141
Mammography 34
Membrane 100
Mercaptopurine .. 115, 117, 166, 173, 174, 176
Metabolite 100
Millimeter 170, 196
Molecular .. 96, 97, 99, 110, 122, 126, 148, 158, 161, 184, 187, 189, 282
Molecule 96, 118, 128, 129, 196, 286, 289, 290
Morphology 48, 134, 140, 152, 153, 284
Mutagenic 100
Myelogenous 65, 66, 67, 69, 132, 134, 141
Myelosuppression 165

N
Nausea 224
Necrosis 102, 104, 167, 177, 228
Neuroendocrine 170
Neurotoxicity 168, 169, 170, 172
Non-small cell lung cancer 225

O
Occult 183
Oncologist 49, 287
Oncology 18, 46, 144, 151, 263
Oncology nurse 263
Osteonecrosis 175
Osteosarcoma 58, 59

P
Palliative 36
Paradoxical 101
Paralysis 170
Pegaspargase 167
Pelvis 12
Pharmacokinetics 115
Phenobarbital 171

Phenotype 99, 101, 102, 129, 153, 154, 288
Plasma 100, 129, 288
Platelets 11, 12, 196, 269, 287, 288
Ploidy 101
Polyethylene 167, 196, 288
Postnatal 92, 145
Preclinical 210
Precursor ... 104, 121, 147, 148, 151, 152, 153, 154, 155, 156, 157, 158, 162, 172, 174, 174, 179
Prednisolone 228
Prednisone 123, 160, 165, 167, 169, 172, 176, 177, 229, 230, 233, 236
Prenatal 92, 145, 147
Prevalence 121
Prophylaxis ... 14, 124, 134, 163, 169, 170, 171, 172
Prostate 126, 191, 219, 225, 280
Proteins .. 97, 99, 127, 128, 129, 197, 211, 284, 287, 288, 290
Psychotherapy 219
Pulse 132
Punishment 264, 266

R
Randomized 95, 106, 111, 112, 167, 173, 174, 174, 176
Receptor 108, 133, 147
Recombinant 103, 231
Recurrence 107, 180, 181, 232
Refractory 55, 59, 63, 66, 72, 102
Regimen 58, 59, 61, 62, 67, 95, 114, 163, 166, 169, 172, 173, 174, 175, 176, 178, 179, 261, 290
Retreatment 234
Retrospective 181, 236

S
Screening 76, 78, 79, 94
Seizures 170, 171, 195, 280
Serum 167
Sinusitis 27, 290
Solvent 108
Somatic 25, 97, 127, 279, 284
Somnolence 170
Spleen 12, 27, 163, 290
Staging 13
Steroids 67, 127, 129, 175, 260, 281, 283, 289
Strabismus 130, 291
Subacute 170
Systemic 14, 15, 16, 99, 146, 152, 153, 163, 168, 169, 170, 172, 182, 232

T
Telangiectasia 146, 190
Teniposide 99

Testicular....147, 151, 161, 176, 177, 182, 183, 236
Thymus 12, 27, 145, 275, 291
Tonsils..12
Toxicity....... 95, 117, 137, 164, 166, 167, 170, 171, 174, 176, 279
Trimetrexate 59
Trisomy 161

V
Vaccination.. 125
Vaccine 70, 130, 292
Vincristine ..165, 167, 175, 176, 177, 227, 228, 229, 230, 236
Vindesine 230
Viral 125